# Interstitial Lung Disease

# Interstitial Lung Disease

HAROLD R. COLLARD, MD
Division of Pulmonary and Critical Care Medicine
Department of Medicine
University of California San Francisco
San Francisco, CA, United States

LUCA RICHELDI, MD, PhD
Division of Pulmonary Medicine
Agostino Gemelli University Hospital
Catholic University of the Sacred Heart
Rome, Italy

ELSEVIER

# ELSEVIER

1600 John F. Kennedy Blvd.
Ste 1800
Philadelphia, PA 19103-2899

*Content Strategist:* Patrick Manley
*Content Development Specialist:* Meredith Clinton
*Design Direction:* Renee Duenow

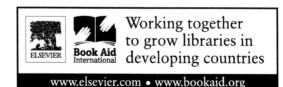

Working together
to grow libraries in
developing countries

www.elsevier.com • www.bookaid.org

# Contributors

**Danielle Antin-Ozerkis, MD**
Associate Professor of Medicine
Director, Yale Interstitial Lung Disease Program
Pulmonary and Critical Care Medicine Section
Department of Internal Medicine
Yale University School of Medicine
New Haven, CT, United States

**Jürgen Behr, MD**
Department of Internal Medicine V
University of Munich
Asklepios Kliniken München-Gauting Comprehensive
    Pneumology Center
Member, German Center for Lung Research
Munich, Germany

**Stefania Cerri, MD, PhD**
Center for Rare Lung Disease
University Hospital of Modena
Modena, Italy

**Sonye K. Danoff, MD, PhD**
Department of Medicine
Pulmonary and Critical Care Medicine
Johns Hopkins University School of Medicine
Baltimore, MD, United States

**Janine Evans, MD**
Associate Professor of Medicine
Rheumatology Section
Department of Internal Medicine
Yale University School of Medicine
New Haven, CT, United States

**Charlene D. Fell, MD, MSc, FRCPC**
Division of Respirology
Department of Medicine
University of Calgary
Calgary, AB, Canada

**Christine Kim Garcia, MD, PhD**
McDermott Center for Human Growth and
    Development
Department of Internal Medicine, Division of
    Pulmonary and Critical Care
University of Texas Southwestern Medical Center
Dallas, TX, United States

**Robert J. Homer, MD, PhD**
Professor of Pathology and Medicine (Pulmonary)
Yale University School of Medicine
New Haven, CT, United States

**Kirk D. Jones, MD**
Professor
Department of Pathology
University of California, San Francisco, School of
    Medicine
San Francisco, CA, United States

**Dong Soon Kim, MD, PhD**
Emeritus Professor
University of Ulsan
Seoul, South Korea

**Kathleen Oare Lindell, PhD, RN**
Research Assistant Professor of Medicine
Clinical Nurse Specialist
Dorothy P. & Richard P. Simmons Center for
    Interstitial Lung Disease
Pulmonary, Allergy and Critical Care Medicine
The University of Pittsburgh
Pittsburgh, PA, United States

**Fabrizio Luppi, MD, PhD**
Center for Rare Lung Disease
University Hospital of Modena
Modena, Italy

**Richard A. Matthay, MD**
Boehringer Ingelheim Emeritus Professor of Medicine
    and Senior Research Scientist
Pulmonary and Critical Care Medicine Section
Department of Internal Medicine
Yale University School of Medicine
New Haven, CT, United States

**Amy L. Olson, MD, MSPH**
Assistant Professor
Department of Medicine
Division of Pulmonary, Critical Care and Sleep
    Medicine
National Jewish Health
Denver, CO, United States;
Department of Medicine
Division of Pulmonary Sciences and Critical Care
    Medicine
University of Colorado, Denver
Aurora, CO, United States

**Luca Paoletti, MD**
Assistant Professor
Division of Pulmonary and Critical Care Medicine
Medical University of South Carolina
Charleston, SC, United States

**Silvia Puglisi, MD**
Regional Referral Centre for Rare Lung Diseases
University of Catania
University-Hospital Policlinico–Vittorio Emanuele
Catania, Italy

**Luca Richeldi, MD, PhD**
Division of Pulmonary Medicine
Agostino Gemelli University Hospital
Catholic University of the Sacred Heart
Rome, Italy

**Ami Rubinowitz, MD**
Associate Professor of Diagnostic Radiology
Chief of Thoracic Imaging
Department of Diagnostic Radiology and Biomedical
    Imaging
Yale University School of Medicine
New Haven, CT, United States

**Jay H. Ryu, MD**
Division of Pulmonary and Critical Care Medicine
Mayo Clinic
Rochester, MN, United States

**Giacomo Sgalla, MD**
National Institute for Health Research
Respiratory Biomedical Research Unit
University Hospital Southampton
Southampton, United Kingdom

**Aditi Shah, MD**
Division of Respirology, Critical Care, and Sleep
    Medicine
Department of Medicine
University of Saskatchewan
Saskatoon, SK, Canada

**Leann L. Silhan, MD**
Department of Medicine
Pulmonary and Critical Care Medicine
Johns Hopkins University School of Medicine
Baltimore, MD, United States

**Paolo Spagnolo, MD, PhD**
Respiratory Disease Unit
Department of Cardiac, Thoracic, and Vascular
    Sciences
University of Padua
Padua, Italy

**Jeffrey J. Swigris, DO, MS**
Associate Professor
Department of Medicine
Division of Pulmonary, Critical Care and Sleep
    Medicine
National Jewish Health
Denver, CO, United States;
Department of Medicine
Division of Pulmonary Sciences and Critical Care
    Medicine
University of Colorado, Denver
Aurora, CO, United States

**Anatoly Urisman, MD, PhD**
Assistant Professor
Department of Pathology
University of California, San Francisco, School of
    Medicine
San Francisco, CA, United States

**Carlo Vancheri, MD, PhD**
Regional Referral Centre for Rare Lung Diseases
University of Catania
University-Hospital Policlinico–Vittorio Emanuele
Catania, Italy

**Robert Vassallo, MD**
Division of Pulmonary and Critical Care Medicine
Departments of Medicine, Physiology and Biomedical
    Engineering
Mayo Clinic
Rochester, MN, United States

**Timothy P.M. Whelan, MD**
Professor of Medicine
Division of Pulmonary and Critical Care Medicine
Medical University of South Carolina
Charleston, SC, United States

**Zulma X. Yunt, MD**
Assistant Professor
Department of Medicine
Division of Pulmonary, Critical Care and Sleep
    Medicine
National Jewish Health
Denver, CO, United States;
Department of Medicine
Division of Pulmonary Sciences and Critical Care
    Medicine
University of Colorado, Denver
Aurora, CO, United States

# Preface

The interstitial lung diseases (ILDs) are a large and heterogeneous group of disease entities that differ significantly with respect to presentation, cause, prevention, therapy, and prognosis. Many of them have no clear etiology. However, in recent years considerable progress has been made in our understanding of these entities. In *Interstitial Lung Disease*, we discuss the most important of the ILDs and update the reader about their management.

Arriving at the correct diagnosis often requires correlation with clinical, radiologic, and pathologic findings. The diagnostic strategy that should be employed when faced with a patient with ILD is described. Given the important role of high-resolution computed tomography (HRCT) in the diagnosis of ILD, we introduce pulmonologists and clinicians to the imaging appearances of ILDs by providing a pattern approach to the evaluation of HRCT. In addition, a focused discussion of the HRCT findings in the common ILDs is presented.

Idiopathic pulmonary fibrosis (IPF) is the most common of the idiopathic interstitial pneumonias. Over the past decade, our thinking about IPF has been reshaped and guidelines have been revised using an evidence-based approach. A number of epidemiologic studies have identified potential risk factors for IPF. We summarize the approach to diagnosing IPF and review its epidemiology. With improved understanding of IPF, we now recognize that there may also be distinct phenotypes among this group of patients. Furthermore, we describe how the identification and management of comorbidities may improve the overall quality of life and well-being of these patients. It has become clear that the clinical course of individual patients with IPF is variable and that the sudden deterioration of a patient's respiratory condition during a relatively stable course is possible. This deterioration can result from well-known causes such as infection, pulmonary embolism, congestive heart failure, pneumothorax, or drugs. However, in many cases the etiology is not certain despite rigorous searches. The current state of our understanding of this important manifestation of IPF is discussed. Also, the mechanisms of action of current and potential IPF therapies are reviewed, with particular reference to current disease understanding and to highlight areas of IPF disease biology that afford attractive targets for the development of the new treatments. The general management of a patient with IPF is described, especially the management of important comorbidities (e.g., pulmonary hypertension and gastroesophageal reflux) and symptoms (e.g., dyspnea, exercise limitation, fatigue, anxiety, mood disturbance, sleep disorders) that dramatically affect IPF patients' lives. Furthermore, the increasingly important role of lung transplantation in the treatment of patients with ILD is discussed, especially the evidence suggesting that patients with pulmonary fibrosis undergoing lung transplantation have a favorable long-term survival compared with other disease indications.

Finally, several chapters review important individual ILD entities, including inherited fibrotic lung diseases, nonspecific interstitial pneumonia, ILD associated with connective tissue diseases, chronic hypersensitivity pneumonitis, and smoking-related ILDs.

**Harold R. Collard, MD**
*Division of Pulmonary and Critical Care Medicine*
*Department of Medicine*
*University of California San Francisco*
*San Francisco, CA, USA*

**Luca Richeldi, MD, PhD**
*Division of Pulmonary Medicine*
*Agostino Gemelli University Hospital*
*Catholic University of the Sacred Heart*
*Rome, Italy*

# Contents

# CHAPTER 1

# Genetic Interstitial Lung Disease

CHRISTINE KIM GARCIA

**KEY POINTS**

- The interstitial lung diseases (ILDs), or diffuse parenchymal lung diseases, are a heterogeneous collection of more than 100 different pulmonary disorders that affect the tissue and spaces surrounding the alveoli.
- Many of the genes involve pathways that lead to altered surfactant metabolism, increased ER stress signaling, and telomere shortening.
- Genetics provides a molecular framework for explaining phenotypes and, sometimes, provides information that directly affects patient care.

The interstitial lung diseases (ILDs) include a wide variety of relatively uncommon disorders. Technologic advances in sequencing and genotyping have led to an explosion of genetic discoveries, shedding new light on the underlying pathogenesis of ILD. New monogenic syndromes have been described, often with clinically diverse and extreme phenotypes, based on the discovery of single gene mutations. In addition, many apparently disparate clinical presentations have been linked together through the discovery of mutations in the same gene or mutations in multiple genes sharing a common pathway. These genetic discoveries have only further increased the number of discrete ILDs. The genetic etiology provides a molecular framework for the disease and provides patients and their treating physicians with an explanation of phenotypes that are often seen across multiple organs. As more cohorts of patients are described with these rare syndromes, more information will be gleaned about the natural history of disease and best practices for surveillance and treatment. The goal of this chapter is to summarize (1) genetic syndromes involving multiple organs, in which ILD is one of many different phenotypes, and (2) genetic disorders in which ILD is the dominant phenotype.

As a rule, manifestations of ILD even within a single gene syndrome are generally characterized by a spectrum of clinical presentations, a wide range in age of onset, and incomplete penetrance. Thus, a high level of suspicion is needed for many of these disorders. Detecting a pattern of inheritance in large, extended kindreds across multiple generations separated by time and space strongly supports a genetic

mechanism of disease. A detailed family history also provides important information about personal and family member phenotypes, providing important clues that may suggest a certain genetic diagnosis. For example, a personal or family history of bone marrow failure, early graying, or liver disease in a patient with adult-onset pulmonary fibrosis suggests a short telomere syndrome. Younger and more severely affected individuals in later generations may reflect genetic anticipation, which can also be seen in short telomere syndromes. Some diseases show a predisposition for affecting a certain gender, for example, affected males and asymptomatic carrier females suggest an X-linked disorder.

All ILDs arise from the infiltration of inflammatory and fibrotic mediators into the lung parenchyma. Very few cells normally reside within the interstitium, which is the delicate space between the alveolar epithelial cells and the capillary vascular endothelial cells. The filling of the interstitial space with inflammatory cells, activated fibroblasts, and extracellular matrix causes irreversible architectural distortion and impairs gas exchange. Most ILDs share similar clinical signs and symptoms, including respiratory distress and cough. Pulmonary restriction and a decreased diffusion capacity are frequently found, as well as radiographic evidence of parenchymal abnormalities. However, the radiographic and histopathologic features of ILDs vary widely. Historically, the type of infiltrating cells, the pattern of infiltration (nodular, reticular, alveolar), the nature of extracellular protein deposits (collagen, elastin, periodic acid–Schiff [PAS]-positive), the location of abnormalities (peripheral, alveolar, peribronchio-lar), the pattern of the fibrotic response (fibroblastic foci, temporal/spatial homogeneity, or heterogeneity), and the form of lung destruction (cysts, bronchiectasis, honeycombing) have been used to describe different clinical forms of ILD. Now that genetic underpinnings of some monogenic ILDs are being established, classification by genetic etiology may ultimately supplant historical classification schemes. This will occur most readily for those disorders in which the genetic classification predicts specific treatments (e.g., sirolimus for tuberous sclerosis complex [TSC]–lymphangioleiomyomatosis [LAM]). A genetic classification of ILD is also advisable for those diseases in which the genetic information provides information relevant to patient care. For example, regular screening may lead to earlier interventions to remove premalignant renal cancers in patients with Birt-Hogg-Dubé syndrome (BHDS). Similarly, knowledge of a monogenic short telomere syndrome provides prognostic information regarding the rate of ILD progression and the nature of specific post–lung transplant complications.

In this chapter, I focus primarily on disorders caused by rare mutations and include selected common variants that significantly increase susceptibility to ILD. The nomenclature of diseases follows the genetic classification system adopted by the Online Mendelian Inheritance in Man (http://www.omim.org). Other pulmonary genetic diseases are not covered. I refer to other excellent resources for reviews of alpha-1-antitrypsin deficiency, cystic fibrosis and *CFTR*-related disorders, primary ciliary dyskinesia, pulmonary capillary or veno-occlusive disease, pulmonary malformation syndromes, and disorders that primarily affect the thoracic cage.

## GENETIC DISORDERS AFFECTING MULTIPLE ORGANS, INCLUDING THE LUNG

Table 1.1 lists the defined genetic disorders that are associated with ILDs, with the lung being only one of the many different affected organs. In this broad category that encompasses many different disorders, ILD may be a more severe or life-threatening manifestation of disease or one of the more common features associated with the disease.

### Lymphangioleiomyomatosis and Tuberous Sclerosis Complex

Pulmonary LAM is a rare disease that almost exclusively affects women. It is caused by proliferating smooth muscle–like cells, which can involve small airways, the pulmonary vasculature, and intrathoracic and extrathoracic lymphatic structures. The hallmark feature of the disease is the radiographically apparent numerous, round, thin-walled cysts, generally between 2 and 60 mm in diameter, which are found throughout the lung. Extraparenchymal lung abnormalities include pneumothorax and chylous pleural effusions. Eighty percent of patients develop a pneumothorax at some time during the course of their disease. Pleural effusions are characterized by elevated triglyceride levels and an abundance of chylomicrons. Obstructive and mixed obstructive-restrictive ventilator defects are observed. Renal angiomyolipomas occur in ~30% of sporadic LAM patients and in >90% of TSC-LAM patients.[1]

LAM can occur either in patients with sporadic (non-inherited) disease or in 1–3% of patients with TSC, an autosomal dominant multisystem disorder characterized by hamartomas in multiple organ systems, including the brain, skin, heart, kidneys, and lungs. The ILD manifestation of TSC patients is indistinguishable from sporadic LAM.[2] TSC patients who develop LAM are often women over 30 years of age who have little or no mental retardation. Extrapulmonary features include facial angiofibromas (or adenoma sebaceum), hypomelanotic macules (which are most easily visualized with a Wood light), rough, yellow thickening of skin over the lumbosacral area (shagreen patch), ungual or periungual fibromas, renal angiomyolipomas, renal cysts, subependymal giant cell astrocytomas, brain cysts, hamartomas, cardiac rhabdomyomas, dental pits, epilepsy, learning difficulties, and mental retardation.

TSC is characterized by autosomal dominant inheritance. However, about two-thirds of patients have de novo mutations. There are two genes associated with this syndrome. Mutations in *TSC2* occur more frequently, accounting for 75–80% of all cases.[3] Mutations in *TSC1* are less common.[3] There are no mutational hot spots within these two genes. In general, *TSC2* mutations are associated with more severe disease, more frequent and severe epilepsy, mental retardation, and cortical tubers. Inactivation of both alleles of *TSC1* or *TSC2* is needed for the development of tumors. Loss of heterozygosity is frequently found in renal angiomyolipomas and supports Knudson's two-hit model tumor suppressor pathogenesis.[4]

Most sporadic LAM results from two somatic mutations in the *TSC2* gene, although rare cases are caused by germline *TSC1* mutations.[5-7] In contrast with TSC patients in whom germline mutations are present in tumor and normal tissue, the mutations in LAM patients are generally not present in normal tissues. This suggests that two mutations arise in a precursor cell of origin and that the mutation-carrying smooth muscle–like cells spread to various organs (lungs, kidneys).

**TABLE 1.1**
**Genetic Interstitial Lung Disease (ILD): Disorders Affecting Multiple Organs, Including the Lung**

| Disease | Inheritance | Gene | Pathogenesis | Pulmonary Involvement | ILD Presentation |
|---|---|---|---|---|---|
| LAM/tuberous sclerosis | Sporadic, AD | *TSC1, TSC2* | mTOR activation | ~100% | Multiple cysts |
| Birt-Hogg-Dubé syndrome | AD | *FLCN* | Loss of folliculin | ~90% | Multiple cysts |
| Dyskeratosis congenita | XLR, AD, AR | *DKC1, TERC, TERT, NOP10, NHP2, TINF2, WRAP53, RTEL1, ACD, CTC1, PARN* | Telomere shortening | Second most serious complication | Inflammatory infiltrates and interstitial fibrosis |
| RIDDLE syndrome | AR | *RNF168* | DSB repair defect | 50% | Pulmonary fibrosis |
| Hermansky-Pudlak syndrome | AR | *HPS1, AP3B1, HPS3, HPS4, HPS5, HPS6, DTNBP1, BLOC1S3, BLOC1S6* | Cytoplasmic organelle defect | Described for those with HPS1, HPS2, and HPS4 | Fibrosis, foamy type II pneumocytes |
| NKX2-1 related disorders | AD | *NPX2-1* | Transcription factor defect | ~50% | Respiratory distress, NEHI, pulmonary fibrosis |
| Neurofibromatosis | AD | *NF1* | Loss of tumor suppressor | ~10% | Pulmonary fibrosis, bullae |
| Poikiloderma with tendon contractures and pulmonary fibrosis | AD | *FAM111B* | Unknown | >50% | UIP |
| ILD, nephrotic syndrome, and epidermolysis bullosa | AR | *ITGA3* | Integrin defect | 100% | Abnormal alveolarization |
| STING-associated vasculopathy | AD | *TMEM173* | Increased interferon | >50% | Alveolitis with fibrosis |
| Autoimmune disease with facial dysmorphism | AR | *ITCH* | E3 ubiquitin ligase defect | ~90% | NSIP |
| Autoimmune interstitial lung, joint, and kidney disease | AD | *COPA* | ER stress | ~100% | Lymphocytic infiltration |
| GATA2 deficiency | Sporadic, AD | *GATA2* | Transcription factor defect | ~60% | PAP |
| CVID syndromes | Sporadic, AR, AD | *ICOS, CD19, CD20, CD21, CD81, TNFRSF13B, TNFRSF13C, LRBA, IL21, NFKB1, NFKB2, IKZF1* | Variable antibody deficiencies | 55–90% | Bronchiectasis, GLILD, organizing pneumonia |
| Agammaglobulinemia | X-linked, AR, AD | *BTK, IGHM, IGLL1, CD79A, CD79B, BLNK, TCF3* | B cell defect | ~25% | Bronchiectasis |

*Continued*

**TABLE 1.1**
**Genetic Interstitial Lung Disease (ILD): Disorders Affecting Multiple Organs, Including the Lung—cont'd**

| Disease | Inheritance | Gene | Pathogenesis | Pulmonary Involvement | ILD Presentation |
|---|---|---|---|---|---|
| Hyper IgE syndrome | Sporadic, AD | STAT3 | STAT3 defect, Lack of Th17 cells | ~70% | Bronchiectasis, pneumatoceles |
| Activated PI3K-δ syndrome | AD | PIK3CD | Activation of PI3K | ~75% | Lymphoid aggregates |
| CTLA4 deficiency | AD | CTLA4 | Activated T cells | ~75% | GLILD |
| X-linked reticulate pigmentary | X-linked | POLA1 | Increased type 1 interferons | ~100% | Bronchiectasis |
| Gaucher disease, type I | AR | GBA | Deficiency of acid β-glucosidase | ~65% | Gaucher cell infiltration |
| Niemann-Pick disease, types A, B, C1, and C2 | AR | SMPD1, NPC1, NPC2 | Deficiency of acid sphingomyelinase; defective intracellular lipid movement | Various | GGO and septal thickening |
| Lysinuric protein intolerance | AR | SLC7A7 | Defect of cationic amino acid transport | | PAP, septal thickening |

*AD*, autosomal dominant; *AR*, autosomal recessive; *DSB*, double-stranded DNA break; *GGO*, ground-glass opacities; *GLILD*, granulomatous lymphocytic interstitial lung disease; *mTOR*, mammalian target of rapamycin; *NEHI*, neuroendocrine cell hyperplasia of infancy; *NSIP*, nonspecific interstitial pneumonia; *PAP*, pulmonary alveolar proteinosis; *UIP*, usual interstitial pneumonia; *XLR*, X-linked recessive.

The proteins encoded by these two genes regulate the mammalian target of rapamycin (mTOR) pathway.[8] Inhibition of the mTOR complex corrects the specific molecular defects underlying TSC. mTOR inhibitors cause shrinkage of renal or retroperitoneal angiomyolipomas and subependymal giant cell astrocytomas in TSC patients.[9–11] In addition, sirolimus stabilizes lung function, reduces respiratory symptoms, and improves the quality of life of LAM patients.[12]

**Birt-Hogg-Dubé Syndrome**

This disorder, which is also known as Hornstein-Knickenberg syndrome,[13] is characterized by the autosomal dominant inheritance of multiple benign skin tumors, which are usually characterized as fibrofolliculomas. Approximately 90% of affected individuals have evidence of lung cysts,[14] and up to 34% develop kidney tumors.[15] The disease is caused by loss-of-function mutations in the folliculin (*FLCN*) gene.[16] Two different studies, one using whole-genome linkage analysis and the other a candidate gene approach, independently found that kindreds presenting solely with familial spontaneous pneumothorax and/or lung cysts have mutations in *FLCN*

and represent a *forme fruste* of BHDS.[17,18] Nearly all mutations, including the common mutation hot spot that introduces a frameshift mutation (c.1285insC and c.1285delC), predict a truncated protein product.[15] The pulmonary cysts are generally bilateral, are usually located in a subpleural distribution in the mid- and lower-lung zones, and are of varying sizes, ranging from round, oval, lentiform, to multiseptated shapes.[19,20] Because the skin findings typically appear in the fourth decade and the renal malignancy can be a late finding (mean age of 48 years), a spontaneous pneumothorax in the second or third decade of life is often the presenting manifestation.[15,18] The molecular mechanism of lung cyst formation is incompletely understood.

Genetic testing is indicated for all individuals with suspected BHDS because the presence of a mutation prompts screening for renal cancer for which surgical resection may be curative. As was described in a past case,[21] the phenotype of familial spontaneous pneumothorax may be the presenting feature for the index case that then leads to the identification of an occult renal malignancy in a family member with a *FLCN* mutation. All first-degree relatives have a 50% chance of having the same germline *FLCN* mutation.

## Dyskeratosis Congenita

Dyskeratosis congenita (DC) is a rare multisystem disorder characterized by the classic triad of a lacy reticular pigmentation on the upper chest and neck, nail dystrophy, and oral leukoplakia. The prevalence is approximately 1 in 1,000,000, with death occurring at a median age of 16 years.[22] Patients are usually healthy at birth and then develop different organ dysfunction, including bone marrow failure, pulmonary fibrosis, and eye, tooth, gastrointestinal, endocrine, skeletal, urologic, and immunologic abnormalities. Significant developmental delay is found for the more severe clinical variants of DC. There is a wide variation in the severity and spectrum of clinical findings, which is only partly explained by locus heterogeneity. The mode of inheritance varies by gene mutation. Most patients in a large international registry are male with X-linked recessive inheritance.[23] Kindreds with autosomal recessive and autosomal dominant patterns of inheritance are less common. For affected male patients, the classic skin and nail findings are present in ~90%. The abnormal skin findings have been described as poikiloderma vascularis atrophicans or a latticework hypo- and hyperpigmentation defect found especially on the neck, upper chest, and proximal limbs.[23,24] Bone marrow failure is very common (>85%) and is the leading cause of death.

After bone marrow failure, pulmonary fibrosis is the most serious and life-threatening complication of DC. In most cases it presents either after hematopoietic cell transplantation[25,26] or as a later manifestation of disease in those over the age of 30 years.[27-29] Patients with pulmonary disease have rales, digital clubbing, a restrictive pulmonary defect, a reduced diffusion capacity, and diffuse interstitial markings on high-resolution computed tomography (HRCT) imaging of the chest. Lung histopathology generally features a mixture of cellular inflammatory infiltrates and interstitial fibrosis.[30,31] Clinical survival of DC patients after the development of ILD is poor as pulmonary disease is generally rapidly progressive. Death is usually 12–40 months after the onset of clinical symptoms.[28]

Mutations in 11 different genes have been described in DC patients. Regardless of the pattern of genetic inheritance or the individual genetic mutation, all DC patients exhibit short telomere lengths for their age.[32] Telomeres are specialized structures essential for maintenance of integrity of chromosomal ends composed of nucleotide repeats $(TTAGGG)_n$ and telomere-specific accessory proteins. Positional cloning first led to the identification of mutations in the *DKC1* gene in those with the X-linked recessive form of the disease.[33] Dyskerin is a nucleolar protein that copurifies with the catalytically active RNA and protein component of telomerase.[34] Mutations in both genes encoding telomerase (hTR, encoded by *TERC* gene and *TERT*) have been found in patients with autosomal dominant DC[35,36]; biallelic mutations in *TERT* have been found in patients with autosomal recessive DC.[37,38] Germline mutations in *TINF2*, a component of the shelterin complex that protects the telomeric ends of chromosomes, mostly occur de novo and are found in patients with autosomal dominant DC.[39,40] Mutations in the gene *ACD*, encoding another member of the shelterin complex, TPP1, have been found in two kindreds with DC.[41,42] Compound heterozygous mutations in *CTC1* were first described in patients with Coats plus and in the phenotypically similar disorder cranioretinal microangiopathy with calcifications and cysts and then were later described in patients with autosomal recessive DC.[43,44] CTC1 is part of the trimeric telomere capping complex that cooperates with the shelterin complex to protect telomeres. Homozygous mutations in *NOLA2* and *NOLA3* account for less than 1% of DC mutations; these genes encode NHP2 and NOP10, respectively, which maintain the stability and proper trafficking of a complex of H/ACA small nucleolar RNAs, including the telomerase RNA, hTR.[45-47] Mutations in *WRAP53* have been described linked to DC; this gene encodes TCAB1 that binds telomerase and directs its localization to nuclear Cajal bodies, an important step in telomere maintenance.[48] Whole exome sequencing has led to the identification of heterozygous or compound heterozygous mutations in *RTEL1*.[49-51] This gene encodes a DNA helicase that is crucial for telomere maintenance and DNA repair. Homozygous or compound heterozygous mutations in *PARN* have most recently been linked to autosomal recessive DC.[52-54] The PARN protein belongs to a family of conserved exoribonucleases that shorten the poly(A) tail of messenger RNA through deadenylation. One of the RNA species that is modified by PARN is hTR or the RNA component of telomerase.[54] Thus, mutations in *PARN* lead to defective hTR and telomerase biogenesis and telomere disease.

Genetic anticipation has been seen in DC kindreds with *TERC* and *TERT* mutations. Inheritance of progressively shorter telomere lengths in each subsequent generation of mutation carriers provides a molecular explanation for the observation of an earlier age of onset in more severely affected individuals with each successive generation.[36,55] Siblings who do not inherit the mutated gene can inherit short telomere lengths from the affected parent.[56] Thus, DC patients have to inherit both short telomere lengths and a deleterious telomerase mutation to demonstrate anticipation.

## RIDDLE Syndrome

Patients with this very rare autosomal recessive disorder have a syndrome of increased sensitivity to radiation, immunodeficiency, learning difficulties, dysmorphic features, short stature, and pulmonary fibrosis in later years.[57,58] The syndrome is caused by homozygous or compound heterozygous mutations in the *RNF168* gene, an E3 ubiquitin ligase critical for double-stranded DNA break (DSB) repair. It promotes ubiquitination of H2A and H2AX, which, in turn, mediates accumulation of 53BP1 and BRACA1 at DSBs to promote DNA repair.[59,60] It also has a role in TRF2-mediated protection of telomeres.[61]

## Hermansky-Pudlak Syndrome

Hermansky-Pudlak syndrome (HPS) is an autosomal recessive disease first described in 1959.[62] It is characterized by oculocutaneous albinism, a bleeding diathesis resulting from platelet storage pool deficiency, and in some cases, pulmonary fibrosis.[63] It is now known that HPS is caused by defects of multiple cytoplasmic organelles, including melanosomes, platelet-dense granules, and lysosomes leading to diverse clinical features. Other clinical features of the disease include granulomatous colitis, neutropenia, immunodeficiency, cutaneous malignancies, cardiomyopathy, and renal failure. Currently the diagnosis is confirmed by the absence of dense bodies on whole-mount electron microscopy of platelets.[64] Mutations in nine different genes cause this disease. Each of these genes functions in trafficking of vesicular cargo proteins to cytoplasmic organelles or in organelle biogenesis and maturation.[65–70] HPS is the most common single gene disorder in Puerto Rico with an estimated frequency of about 1 in 1800 and a carrier frequency of 1 in 21.[71] Mutations in *HPS1* and *HPS3* are found in 75% and 25% of Puerto Rican patients, respectively.

ILD generally causes symptoms in the 30s and, when it occurs, is generally fatal within a decade. Patients have progressive restrictive disease with a highly variable course.[63,72] Pulmonary fibrosis has been described most frequently in patients with *HPS1* mutations, and more rarely in patients with *HPS2* or *HPS4* mutations.[72–77] In this regard, molecular subtyping is important to assess the risk of developing pulmonary fibrosis. In one of the largest studies, the mean age of onset was 35 years with a range of 15–53 years.[72] The variability of pulmonary findings was generally not attributable to prior environmental exposures. Over 80% of patients had abnormalities on CT scans, which were generally predictive of the degree of physiologic impairment and mortality. Most patients demonstrate

a peripheral distribution of HRCT reticulations with a trend toward increasing involvement of the central portions of the lungs with progressive severity as a result of peribronchovascular thickening and bronchiectasis.[73] Surgical lung biopsies demonstrate lung remodeling, numerous chronic inflammatory cells, and distinctive clusters of clear vacuolated type II pneumocytes with florid foamy swelling and degeneration ("giant lamellar body degeneration").[78,79] Despite an early positive study,[76] a follow-up clinical trial showed no benefit of pirfenidone for the treatment of Hermansky-Pudlak pulmonary fibrosis.[80]

Pathogenesis of pulmonary fibrosis is incompletely understood. Studies of a mouse model of disease that is homozygous for both *HPS1* and *HPS2* mutations demonstrate additive effects of the genetic defects toward the development of spontaneous pulmonary fibrosis.[81] Subpleural reticulations begin at 3 months and extensive fibrosis is seen by 9 months.[82] The histology of the mouse lung replicates the human phenotype with "giant lamellar body degeneration" of the type II cells and demonstrates decreased phospholipid and surfactant protein (SP)-B and C secretion.[81,83] The underlying molecular mechanism of murine HPS-associated pulmonary fibrosis seems related to endoplasmic reticulum (ER) stress and chronic alveolar epithelial type II cell injury.[82]

### NKX2-1–Related Disorders

These disorders include benign hereditary chorea, neonatal respiratory distress, and congenital hypothyroidism; it is also known as brain-lung-thyroid syndrome. Childhood-onset chorea is the hallmark clinical feature of this disorder. Pulmonary disease is the second most common presentation, with nearly half of the patients having some type of pulmonary manifestation.[84] These include neonatal respiratory distress with or without pulmonary hypertension, neuroendocrine cell hyperplasia, ILD in children between the ages of 4 months to 7 years, and pulmonary fibrosis in older individuals.[85–87] Defective surfactant homeostasis and recurrent respiratory infections have been found to be a prominent feature in some subjects.[86,88] Mutations include missense, nonsense, and deletions of the *NKX2-1* gene.

## Neurofibromatosis

Neurofibromatosis (NF1) is an autosomal dominant disorder that affects all ethnic groups. Type I, von Recklinghausen disease or classic NF1, is characterized by multiple (>6) café au lait spots, axillary and inguinal freckling, multiple cutaneous neurofibromas, and iris Lisch nodules. Pulmonary manifestations are less common. The incidence of ILD in NF1 has been estimated at 6–12%.[89–91] It is characterized by lower lobe–predominant diffuse interstitial fibrosis and honeycombing. Thin-walled bullae are present in almost all patients with ILD or may be seen in isolation; they are large, asymmetric, and typically involve the upper lobes.[91] Histologic evidence of an alveolitis and interstitial fibrosis has been found in patients with normal chest X-rays or those with only apical bullae.[90] Although there is near complete penetrance of the disease after childhood, the ILD is not observed until adulthood, typically in patients older than 40 years of age.[90] The disease is often progressive and may lead to pulmonary hypertension and right-sided heart failure.[92] The pathogenesis of NF-associated ILD is unknown.

## Poikiloderma, With Tendon Contractures, Myopathy, and Pulmonary Fibrosis

This rare disorder usually affects individuals from early childhood; presenting features include thin hair, telangiectasias and pigmentary abnormalities on sun-exposed areas, and tendon contractures frequently involving the ankles and feet.[93] There is incomplete penetrance of pulmonary fibrosis; >50% of cases have lung involvement. When it is present, the pulmonary fibrosis generally develops during the second decade of life, is progressive, and can lead to death. The histopathology for at least one case was consistent with usual interstitial pneumonia.[93] Different missense mutations in the FAM111B gene have been found in unrelated cases of different ancestry.[94] The function of this gene is unclear.

## Interstitial Lung Disease, Nephrotic Syndrome, and Epidermolysis Bullosa

Infants with this congenital autosomal recessive disorder present with disease in multiple organs. The pulmonary and renal features cause significant morbidity and mortality, although dermatologic features are common (epidermolysis bullosa, thin hair, dystrophic nails, onycholysis). The lung involvement is characterized radiographically by diffuse ground-glass opacity and interlobular septal thickening. Histology demonstrates abnormal alveolarization with poorly septated ("simplified") alveolar spaces.[95,96] All mutations are homozygous deletion/frameshift or missense mutations in ITGA3, which encode an integrin alpha chain belonging to a family of cell surface adhesion proteins. One of the missense mutations prevents proper post-translational modification of the integrin alpha chain with defective cell surface expression.

## Stimulator of Interferon Genes–Associated Vasculopathy, Infantile-Onset

Patients with this autosomal dominant disorder have an autoimmune vasculopathy that causes severe skin lesions affecting the face, ears, nose, and digits, resulting in ulceration and necrosis beginning in infancy. Over 85% have an ILD apparent on HRCT chest imaging. Lung biopsy samples demonstrate a scattered mix of lymphocytic inflammatory infiltrate, follicular hyperplasia and B-cell germinal centers, interstitial fibrosis, and emphysematous changes.[97,98] Patients can have livedo reticularis, Raynaud phenomenon, myositis, joint involvement, immune complex deposition, hypergammaglobulinemia, leukopenia, and autoantibodies (antinuclear, antiphospholipid, anticardiolipin). All cases are caused by heterozygous, missense, gain-of-function mutations in the TMEM173 gene, which encodes the STING (stimulator of interferon genes).[97,98] Mutations lead to activation of STAT1.[97]

## Autoimmune Disease With Facial Dysmorphism

This autosomal recessive disease has been described only in children with features of failure to thrive, developmental delay, dysmorphic features, autoantibodies, and inflammatory cell infiltration of the lungs, liver, and gut. Chronic lung disease was found in 9 of 10 children. Three had a chronic oxygen requirement and died of respiratory failure. Surgical lung biopsy from one case showed a cellular, nonspecific interstitial pneumonitis (NSIP). All affected children in one large Amish kindred were homozygous for a frameshift mutation in the ITCH gene that is predicted to cause a truncation of an E3 ubiquitin ligase.[99] Of note, mice with a small genomic inversion that disrupts the Itch and agouti genes develop a similar spectrum of immunologic disease of the spleen, lymph nodes, stomach, and skin, as well as chronic pulmonary interstitial inflammation and alveolar proteinosis.[100,101]

## Autoimmune Interstitial Lung, Joint, and Kidney Disease

This rare syndrome was recently elucidating by whole exome sequencing of patients from five unrelated families with autoimmune interstitial lung, joint, and kidney disease.[102] All patients had high-titer autoantibodies, ILD, and inflammatory arthritis. The average age at presentation was 3.5 years, with a range of 6 months to 22 years. Some patients presented with pulmonary hemorrhage that required immunosuppression. Lung biopsies showed lymphocytic interstitial infiltration with lung-infiltrating CD4+ T cells and CD20+ B cells within germinal centers. All mutations affect the same functional domain of the COPA protein, impair intracellular ER-Golgi transport, and lead to ER stress and upregulation of cytokines.

## GATA2 Deficiency

Haploinsufficiency of the hematopoietic transcription factor GATA2 leads to a wide spectrum of diseases including primary immunodeficiency syndromes such as dendritic cell, monocyte, B lymphocyte, and NK lymphocyte deficiency (DCML) and monocytopenia and mycobacterial infection syndrome (MONOMAC); primary lymphedema with myelodysplasia (Emberger syndrome); and susceptibility to myelodysplastic syndrome and acute myeloid leukemia. Besides immunodeficiency (with predisposition especially to severe viral, disseminated nontuberculous mycobacterial, and invasive fungal infections), pulmonary disease, vascular/lymphatic dysfunction, and hearing loss are common.[103–107] Most individuals have some manifestation of pulmonary disease; 79% have a diffusion defect, 63% with abnormal pulmonary function tests, 18% with biopsy-proved pulmonary alveolar proteinosis (PAP), and 9% with pulmonary arterial hypertension.[107] All lack anti–GM-CSF antibodies and are resistant to subcutaneous or inhaled granulocyte-macrophage colony–stimulating factor (GM-CSF) therapy. Chest CT findings include reticulonodular opacities, "crazy paving," and paraseptal emphysema. Median age at first presentation is 20 years, but is highly variable (5 months to 78 years). Most mutations are predicted to cause a loss of function of the mutated allele, leading to haploinsufficiency and autosomal dominant inheritance.[106,108] Hematopoietic stem cell transplantation is indicated for severe disease.

## Immunodeficiency Syndromes

*Common variable immunodeficiency (CVID) syndromes* are all associated with an increased susceptibility to recurrent infections, especially sinopulmonary infections. There is a high variability of clinical features. Respiratory complications are frequently responsible for patient morbidity and mortality and include acute infections, sequelae of infections (bronchiectasis), noninfectious immune-mediated infiltrates such as granulomatous lymphocytic interstitial lung disease (GLILD) and lymphoma, and progressive respiratory failure.[109,110] When severe, bronchiectasis is generally associated with obstructive lung disease; GLILD is typically associated with restrictive physiology and decreased diffusion capacity.[111] Lung disease is frequently found in patients with CVID, as >90% have radiographic abnormalities apparent on chest CT.[112]

This genetically heterogeneous group of diseases includes those with variable antibody and B-cell, T-cell, and NK-cell deficiencies, as well as defective responses to vaccination. Mutations in multiple genes, including *ICOS*,[113] *TNFRSF13B* (encoding the transmembrane activator and CAML interactor TACI),[114,115] *TNFRSF13C* (encoding the B-cell activating factor),[116] *CD19*,[117] *CD20*,[118] *CD81*,[119] *CD21*,[120] *LRBA*,[121,122] *IL21*,[123] *NFKB1*,[124] *NFKB2*,[125] and *IKZF1* (encoding the hematopoietic zinc finger transcription factor),[126,127] lead to sporadic, autosomal recessive, and autosomal dominant patterns of disease.

*X-linked agammaglobulinemia (XLA)* is an immunodeficiency disorder that occurs almost exclusively in males from a failure of B-cell maturation. Although there is a high prevalence of pneumonia in XLA, there is a lower prevalence of chronic lung disease with 47% and 25% demonstrating abnormal pulmonary function studies and bronchiectasis, respectively.[109] Although the degree of immune dysregulation may be lower,[109] the rate of progression of lung function decline is greater for those with XLA.[128] Between 85% and 90% of cases are caused by mutations in *BTK*, the gene encoding Bruton tyrosine kinase and a key regulator in B-cell development.[129] The remaining cases include a genetically heterogeneous group of patients with mutations in *IGHM* (encoding the mu heavy-chain),[130] *IGLL1* (encoding immunoglobulin lambda-like-1),[130,131] *CD79A*,[132] *BLNK*,[133] *CD79B*,[134] and *TCF3*.[135]

*Autosomal dominant hyper-IgE syndrome* is an immune deficiency disorder characterized by the triad of recurrent staphylococcal skin abscesses, pneumonias, and elevations of IgE (usually >2000 IU/mL). Survival is typically into adulthood, but death is usually secondary to infections. Diagnosis requires a high level of suspicion due to variability of phenotypic features. A clinical scoring system has been developed that combines immunologic (elevated IgE, eosinophilia >700/μL, decreased T-helper [Th]17 cells, recurrent infections) and nonimmune features (retained primary teeth, scoliosis, joint hyperextensibility, bone fractures following minimal trauma, a typical facial appearance, and vascular abnormalities). Pneumatoceles and bronchiectasis, which result from aberrant healing of the pneumonias, are seen in ~70% of patients and lead to significant mortality.[136,137] Patients have heterozygous missense, splice site, or small deletions in the *STAT3* gene.[138] Most mutations cluster in the DNA-binding domain of this transcription factor, which regulates responses to many different cytokines. Patients' purified native T cells are unable to differentiate in vitro into IL-17–producing Th17 cells, which play a critical role in the clearance of fungal and extracellular bacterial infections of the lung and skin.[139] Most patients represent sporadic cases, but autosomal dominant transmission has been seen in some kindreds.

*Activated PI3K-delta syndrome* is a monogenic autosomal dominant disease that leads to overactivation of the PI3K signaling pathway and lymphoproliferation. This autosomal dominant disease is characterized by recurrent sinopulmonary infections, reduced IgG2, increased serum IgM, and impaired vaccine responses. In one series, 75% of patients had CT evidence of bronchiectasis or mosaic attenuation.[140] The lymphoid aggregates within the lung and can lead to the compression of nearby bronchi.[110] Heterozygous missense mutations in *PIK3CD* result in increased phosphorylation of AKT, consistent with a gain of function.[140,141]

*CTLA4 deficiency* syndrome is an autosomal dominant immunodeficiency characterized by T-cell immune dysregulation. Pulmonary manifestations mirror CVID with recurrent respiratory infections and GLILD. Lymphocytic infiltration is found for other organs, including the bone marrow, kidney, brain, liver, spleen, and lymph nodes. Heterozygous loss-of-function mutations in *CTLA4* have been recently described.[142,143]

*X-linked reticulate pigmentary disorder* is a rare immunodeficiency disorder with features of recurrent infections and systemic sterile inflammation. Affected patients typically develop recurrent pneumonias in the first few months of life. By childhood, affected males develop diffuse skin hyperpigmentation with a distinctive reticulate pattern, bronchiectasis, hypohidrosis, corneal scarring, enterocolitis, and recurrent urethral strictures.[144-146] A recurrent intronic mutation has been found that disrupts the expression of the catalytic subunit of DNA polymerase-alpha (*POLA1*) and leads to increased production of type I interferons.[147]

### Inborn Errors of Metabolism

*Gaucher disease* is an autosomal recessive lysosomal storage disease characterized by the accumulation of the glycolipid glucosylceramide due to the deficiency of the enzyme acid-beta glucosidase. Diagnosis relies on the demonstration of deficient enzyme activity in cells or the identification of two disease-causing mutations in the *GBA* gene. Patients can display a large variety of symptoms, ranging from patients who are completely asymptomatic to those who present with perinatal lethality. The usual clinical findings include hepatosplenomegaly, anemia, thrombocytopenia,

and bone manifestations including osteopenia, lytic lesions, bone crisis, and skeletal deformities. Infiltration of Gaucher cells into the alveoli, interstitium, and pulmonary capillaries can lead to lung involvement. Over 65% of patients with type I disease have pulmonary function abnormalities, but only a fraction (<5%) have diffuse lower lobe linear infiltrates, restrictive physiologic impairment, and a reduced diffusion capacity consistent with ILD.[148,149] Enzyme replacement therapy can reduce organ volumes and improve the hematologic parameters and bone pain but is usually poorly effective in treating the lung manifestations of this disease.[150] Other therapeutic treatments, such as substrate reduction therapy as well as others, are in development.[151]

*Niemann–Pick disease* types A and B are caused by an inherited deficiency of acid sphingomyelinase activity. Type C is caused by defective movement of lipids, including cholesterol, from endosomes and lysosomes. Patients demonstrate a range of ages and can have diverse symptoms affecting the lung, liver, spleen, bone marrow, skeleton, brain, muscle, mental ability, and movement. The pulmonary manifestations include ILD and recurrent lung infections. In some patients the ILD is predominantly in the bases with thickened interlobular septa, interlobular lines, and ground-glass opacities.[153]

*Lysinuric protein intolerance* is an autosomal recessive disease caused by an inherited defect of cationic amino acid transport. There is excess urinary clearance of these amino acids and deficient intestinal absorption, which leads to depleted body pools. Most patients present in infancy with failure to thrive, growth retardation, protein aversion, muscular hypotonia, hepatosplenomegaly, and osteoporosis. In one study, all patients who developed a fatal respiratory insufficiency, usually PAP, were children less than 15 years of age.[154] Most adult patients have evidence of an ILD on CT scans with interlobular and intralobular septal thickening and subpleural cysts, but only a few are symptomatic.[154]

### GENETIC DISEASES IN WHICH INTERSTITIAL LUNG DISEASE IS THE DOMINANT PHENOTYPE

Table 1.2 lists the genetic disorders in which an ILD is the dominant clinical feature. Included in this group are the surfactant disorders. Pulmonary surfactant is a mixture of phospholipids and associated proteins that covers the alveolar surface at the gas-alveolus interface, where it functions to reduce surface tension and prevent atelectasis. A group of genetic disorders

**TABLE 1.2**
**Genetic Interstitial Lung Disease (ILD): Disorders in Which ILD Is the Dominant Phenotype**

| Disease | Inheritance | Gene | Pathogenesis | Presentation |
|---|---|---|---|---|
| Surfactant metabolism dysfunction 1 | AR | SFTPB | Absent SP-B | Neonatal respiratory failure |
| Surfactant metabolism dysfunction 2 | AD | SFTPC | Lack of SP-C and ER stress | Neonatal respiratory distress, NSIP, UIP |
| Surfactant metabolism dysfunction 3 | AR | ABCA3 | Phospholipid transport defect | Neonatal respiratory distress, PAP |
| Surfactant metabolism dysfunction 4 | AR | CSF2RA CSF2RB | GM-CSF signaling defect | PAP |
| Interstitial lung and liver disease | AR | MARS | Methionine tRNA ligase defect | PAP |
| Pulmonary fibrosis, telomere related, type 1 | AD | TERT | Short telomere length | Pulmonary fibrosis |
| Pulmonary fibrosis, telomere related, type 2 | AD | TERC | Short telomere length | Pulmonary fibrosis |
| Pulmonary fibrosis, telomere related, type 3 | AD | RTEL1 | Short telomere length | Pulmonary fibrosis |
| Pulmonary fibrosis, telomere related, type 4 | AD | PARN | Short telomere length | Pulmonary fibrosis |
| Pulmonary fibrosis, telomere related | Various | DKC1, TINF2, NAF1 | Short telomere length | Pulmonary fibrosis |
| Pulmonary fibrosis and adenocarcinoma | AD | SFTPA1, SFTPA2 | ER stress | Pulmonary fibrosis, adenocarcinoma, respiratory distress in infancy |
| Pulmonary fibrosis susceptibility | Sporadic | MUC5B | ER stress? | UIP, ILAs |
| Pulmonary fibrosis susceptibility | Sporadic | TERT, TERC, OBFC1 | Short telomere length | UIP |
| Pulmonary alveolar microlithiasis | AR | SLC34A2 | Phosphate transport defect | Microliths |

*ER*, endoplasmic reticulum; *GM-CSF*, granulocyte-macrophage colony-stimulating factor; *ILA*, interstitial lung abnormalities; *NSIP*, nonspecific interstitial pneumonia; *PAP*, pulmonary alveolar proteinosis; *SP*, surfactant protein; *UIP*, usual interstitial pneumonia.

involving the production, processing, and clearance of surfactant has been recognized as an important cause of neonatal and pediatric respiratory illness. This group, collectively referred to as surfactant dysfunction disorders,[155] encompasses a variety of mutations involving the genes that encode SP-B (*SFTPB*), SP-C (*SFTPC*), the ATP-binding cassette transporter A3 (*ABCA3*), and the receptor for granulocyte-macrophage colony–stimulating factor (*CSF2RA* and *CSF2RB*). ABCA3 deficiency is the most prevalent for the surfactant disorders that present in the neonatal period with severe respiratory distress. Mutations in *SFTPB*, *SFTPC*, and *NKX2-1* are more rare. Of all the

surfactant dysfunction disorders, patients with mutations in *SFTPC* display the broadest range in age of onset, with affected neonates to older adults.

### Surfactant Metabolism Dysfunction, Type 1: *SFTPB* Mutations

SP-B deficiency is inherited in an autosomal recessive manner, and the majority of affected patients develop respiratory failure in the neonatal period with rapid progression of disease and death at 3–6 months.[156-161] A few mutations that seem to confer a milder phenotype have been found. Children with these mutations have partial expression of the

SP-B protein, survive longer, and go on to develop a chronic ILD.[162,163]

## Surfactant Metabolism Dysfunction, Type 2: SFTPC Mutations

Autosomal dominant lung disease due to mutations in the gene encoding SP-C, *SFTPC*, was first described in 2001 by Nogee and colleagues.[164] The index case was a full-term infant who developed respiratory symptoms at 6 weeks of age. An open lung biopsy revealed histologic features of NSIP. The child's mother had been diagnosed with desquamative interstitial pneumonitis at 1 year of age, and the child's maternal grandfather had died from lifelong respiratory illness of unknown cause. Both the mother and her infant had a heterozygous mutation at the splice donor site in intron 4 (c.460+1G>A), which resulted in skipping of exon 4 and deletion of 37 amino acids.[164] In the next year, a large five-generation kindred was described with 14 affected family members.[165] The age at diagnosis for the affected individuals ranged from 4 months to 57 years and included four adults with surgical lung biopsy evidence of usual interstitial pneumonitis and three children with NSIP. Genomic sequencing revealed a rare heterozygous missense SP-C mutation (L188Q) in all analyzed individuals. Human type II alveolar epithelial cells from one of the patients and mouse lung epithelial cells producing the mutant SP-C protein showed abnormal lamellar bodies. Since these two studies, over 30 different mutations in *SFTPC* have been identified in children and adults. A missense mutation (c.218T>C) that changes a conserved isoleucine at position 73 to a threonine is one of the more common and accounts for 25–35% of abnormal alleles.[155,166-171] There is incomplete penetrance of the ILD phenotype and phenotypic heterogeneity. The disease ranges from severe respiratory distress in infants to IPF in older adults. Mutations of *SFTPC* are rare in individuals without a family history of pulmonary fibrosis.[171-173] At present, the disease phenotype is thought to be caused by aberrant protein-folding, which elicits the unfolded protein response, ER stress, and apoptosis of alveolar epithelial cells.[155,174-178]

## Surfactant Metabolism Dysfunction, Type 3: ABCA3 Mutations

There is a significant amount of phenotypic overlap between patients with *SFTPB* mutations and those with defects in *ABCA3*. Like SP-B deficiency, the disease is inherited in an autosomal recessive manner. Since the first mutation was discovered in 2004, more than 200 different mutations have been found. Mutations in *ABCA3* are the most common inherited defects in surfactant metabolism presenting either with severe neonatal disease or as diffuse lung disease in infancy or childhood.[155,174,179,180] *ABCA3* is an ATP-binding cassette transporter that localizes to the limiting membrane of lamellar bodies where it functions in translocating phospholipids, primarily phosphatidylcholine, into these organelles for assembly and storage of surfactant in type II AECs.[181,182] The functional consequences of the *ABCA3* mutations include decreased expression of the protein, abnormal localization of the protein to the lamellar membrane, production of surfactant that is deficient in phosphatidylcholine, and increased alveolar surface tension.[183-185]

## Surfactant Metabolism Dysfunction, Types 4 and 5: CSF2RA and CSF3RB Mutations

Protein alveolar proteinosis (PAP) is a rare form of lung disease characterized by intraalveolar accumulation of surfactant, which results in respiratory insufficiency. Histopathology specimens from affected patients demonstrate distal airspaces filled with foamy alveolar macrophages and a granular, eosinophilic material that stains positively with PAS reagent. In general, the underlying lung architecture is normal unless infection is present.[186] When the accumulated surfactant is removed, as is done with whole-lung lavage, the gas exchange properties of the lung improve.[186] Approximately 90% of PAP cases are acquired and are referred to as primary PAP.[187-189] Circulating autoantibodies to GM-CSF can be found in over 92% of patients with primary PAP.[190-193] These antibodies block GM-CSF signaling in vivo, reduce alveolar macrophage surfactant catabolism, and impair surfactant clearance.[186,193-196] Secondary PAP occurs in several different clinical settings, such as in association with hematologic malignancies, immunosuppression, inhalation of inorganic dusts, and certain infections.

The GM-CSF receptor is composed of an α- and a β-chain, encoded by the *CSF2RA* and *CSF2RB* genes, respectively.[197] Mutations in both *CSF2RA* and *CSF2RB* have been identified in children with PAP.[198,199] In 2011, a case of adult-onset hereditary PAP was reported in Japan.[200] Here, a 36-year-old woman with PAP had elevated circulating levels of GM-CSF, no measurable anti-GM-CSF antibodies, and reduced expression of the GM-CSF receptor β-chain. Genetic sequencing revealed a homozygous, single-base deletion at nucleotide 631 in exon 6 of *CSF2RB*. Both of the patient's parents were heterozygous for the mutation. Hereditary PAP follows an autosomal recessive pattern. Mice with deletion of the gene encoding GM-CSF or its receptor demonstrate a phenotype very similar to adults with primary PAP.[186,201-204]

## Interstitial Lung and Liver Disease

A specific and severe type of PAP has been described affecting infants and children on Réunion Island.[205] Since 1970, 34 children have been diagnosed and treated, giving rise to an incidence of disease of 1 in at least 10,000 newborns. The lung disease progresses to lung fibrosis despite regular whole-lung lavage. It has recently been found that patients have biallelic mutations in *MARS*, the gene encoding methionine tRNA ligase.[205] Compound heterozygous mutations in the same gene have been found in one patient with multiorgan disease, predominated by liver failure.[206] The increased prevalence of disease on Réunion Island and in nearby Tunisia and France is due to founder mutations. A potential benefit of high-dose methionine supplementation has not yet been studied in these patients.

## Pulmonary Fibrosis, Telomere Related, Type 1

Heterozygous mutations in the gene encoding the protein component (*TERT*) of telomerase have been found in ~15% of patients with autosomal dominant familial pulmonary fibrosis.[207,208] The frequency of *TERT* mutations in patients with sporadic adult-onset ILD is less common.[208,209] Telomerase is a multimeric ribonucleoprotein enzyme that catalyzes the addition of a repetitive DNA sequence to the ends of chromosomes known as telomeres. Each of the mutations is rare and associated with decreased in vitro activity of telomerase and short leukocyte telomere lengths. *TERT* mutations are the most common genetic mutations found in adult patients with ILD.[210] In addition, adult-onset pulmonary fibrosis is the most common manifestation of *TERT* mutations.[211] Other clinical manifestations of *TERT* mutations include DC (see earlier discussion), aplastic anemia and other forms of bone marrow failure,[212] liver disease including liver cirrhosis,[213,214] early graying of hair,[215] and an increased risk for myelodysplastic syndrome and acute myeloid leukemia.[216,217] Altogether, disparate clinical presentations and diseases linked together by defects in telomere-related genes and characterized by short telomere lengths are known as monogenic short telomere syndromes or telomeropathies.

The penetrance of pulmonary fibrosis in *TERT* mutation carriers is age and gender dependent.[210] The penetrance of pulmonary fibrosis for men aged 40–49, 50–59, and >60 years is 14%, 38%, and 60%, respectively. Women show the same age-dependent increase in penetrance. Microscopic honeycombing and fibroblastic foci are commonly found in surgical lung biopsies.[210,218] While approximately half of patients carry a diagnosis of idiopathic pulmonary fibrosis (IPF), others have diagnoses of another idiopathic interstitial pneumonia, unclassifiable lung fibrosis, chronic hypersensitivity pneumonitis, pleuroparenchymal fibroelastosis, idiopathic fibrosis with autoimmune features, or, rarely, a connective tissue disease–associated ILD.[218] Many *TERT* mutation carriers with pulmonary fibrosis report past cigarette smoking or an exposure to a fibrogenic environmental insult, suggesting that injurious environmental exposures in conjunction with the underlying inherited genetic predisposition lead to the lung disease. Disease progression is inexorable, with a mean transplant-free survival of <3 years after diagnosis. *TERT* mutation patients undergoing lung transplant generally have a higher risk of cytopenias and other extrapulmonary complications.[219–221]

Genetic anticipation is seen for *TERT* mutation patients, with an earlier age of diagnosis of lung fibrosis in subsequent generations.[218] Similar to DC, progressively shorter telomere lengths are found in subsequent generations of *TERT* mutation carriers, and these shorter telomere lengths explain genetic anticipation seen in kindreds.[36,210,218]

## Pulmonary Fibrosis, Telomere Related, Type 2

Heterozygous mutations in the gene encoding the RNA component (*TERC*) of telomerase have been found in ~3% of patients with autosomal dominant familial pulmonary fibrosis.[207,208] Each of the mutations is rare and associated with decreased in vitro activity of telomerase and short leukocyte telomere lengths. A wide range of progressive adult-onset pulmonary fibrosis subtypes are seen in patients with *TERC* mutations.[218] Patients with *TERC* mutations are generally diagnosed with ILD at an earlier age (51 years) than *TERT* mutation carriers (58 years). In addition, they have a higher incidence of hematologic comorbidities, especially leukopenia, thrombocytopenia, aplastic anemia, or myelodysplastic syndrome.

## Pulmonary Fibrosis, Telomere Related, Type 3

Autosomal dominant pulmonary fibrosis with incomplete penetrance has been linked to rare mutations in *RTEL1*.[222–224] *RTEL1* surpassed the threshold for genomewide significance when comparing the number of observed versus expected novel damaging or conserved missense mutations in familial pulmonary fibrosis cases and controls.[223] Across independent studies, *RTEL1* mutations are rare and associated with short leukocyte telomere lengths. This gene encodes the regulator of telomere elongation helicase 1 and has a known role in telomere maintenance. Mutations in *RTEL1* were previously shown to cause Hoyeraal-Hreidarsson syndrome, a severe variant of DC (see earlier discussion), in which affected children generally have very short telomere lengths and biallelic mutations. In contrast, those affected with adult-onset pulmonary fibrosis are heterozygous for rare missense or loss-of-function *RTEL1* mutations. Similar to patients with *TERT* mutations, ~50% of heterozygous *RTEL1* mutation carriers have hematologic manifestations such as anemia or macrocytosis.[218] A wide range of progressive adult-onset pulmonary fibrosis subtypes are seen in patients with *RTEL1* mutations. Genetic anticipation is also seen in *RTEL1* kindreds.

### Pulmonary Fibrosis, Telomere Related, Type 4

Exome sequencing has linked autosomal dominant pulmonary fibrosis with incomplete penetrance to mutations in *PARN*, the gene encoding a polyadenylate-specific ribonuclease.[223] *PARN* surpassed the threshold for genomewide significance when comparing the number of observed versus expected novel damaging mutations in cases and controls.[223] Most mutations are predicted to cause protein loss of function (splice site, nonsense, and frameshift). One large kindred was identified by linking together two smaller and previously unknowingly related kindreds with familial pulmonary fibrosis and an identical splice-site *PARN* mutation. The kinship of the two families was confirmed by demonstrating that the two probands share ~6% of their overall genome, including the genomic segment on which the *PARN* mutation is located. As a further test for the relevance of the *PARN* mutations, the cosegregation of the mutations with pulmonary fibrosis was compared across extended kindreds. The overall backward LOD score across all informative *PARN* kindreds was 3.6, reflecting an odds ratio of 1:4096 in favor of linkage.

Other clinical manifestations of *PARN* mutations include DC (see earlier discussion), in which biallelic mutations in the gene are frequently found.[52-54] Patient cells show deficiencies in trimming of small nucleolar RNAs, including abnormally adenylated hTR.[54] In general, leukocyte telomere lengths of *PARN* mutation patients are shorter than in controls, but longer than in subjects with *TERT*, *TERC*, or *RTEL1* mutations.[223] Patients with *PARN* mutations are generally diagnosed with ILD at an older age (64 years) than *TERT* mutation carriers (58 years).[218] However, once pulmonary fibrosis is diagnosed, the respiratory disease progresses and patients have a mean transplant-free survival of 5.7 years from diagnosis.

### Pulmonary Fibrosis, Other Telomere Related

Genes found to be mutated in DC patients are candidate genes for patients with adult-onset pulmonary fibrosis and short telomere lengths. Similar to the other short telomere syndromes mentioned earlier, many individuals have clinical features that overlap with DC, including bone marrow abnormalities and skin changes. A missense mutation in the *DKC1*, encoding dyskerin, has been reported in a kindred with two affected older males with interstitial fibrosis, hyperpigmented skin changes, dyskeratotic nails, and macrocytic anemia.[225] Blood leukocyte telomere lengths were short. The expression of hTR in a lymphoblastoid cell line derived from the proband was lower than that of controls, even though expression of *DKC1* was not reduced. Female mutation carriers were unaffected.

*TINF2* encodes one of the shelterin complex proteins that functions to protect the telomeric ends of chromosomes. Exome sequencing revealed a complex spice acceptor site and missense mutation on the same *TINF2* allele, with predominant expression of the missense mutation in lung-derived DNA from a female patient with pulmonary fibrosis and infertility.[226] Heterozygous loss of function mutations in *NAF1* have most recently been linked to pulmonary fibrosis-emphysema, short telomere lengths, bone marrow failure, and liver disease.[226a] *NAF1* has been shown to be essential for the biogenesis of telomerase RNA.

### Pulmonary Fibrosis and Adenocarcinoma, Related to Surfactant A Mutations

Novel missense mutations in the gene encoding SP-A2 (*SFTPA2*) were discovered by genomewide linkage followed by sequencing candidate genes within the linked region.[227] Affected individuals have evidence of pulmonary fibrosis and/or lung adenocarcinoma with features of bronchoalveolar cell carcinoma. A second study reported three additional rare *SFTPA2* mutations in patients with adult-onset pulmonary fibrosis and a personal or family history of adenocarcinoma.[228] A third study has recently described the cosegregation of ILD and lung adenocarcinoma in an extended kindred with a germline mutation in *SFTPA1* that is predicted to change a conserved tryptophan at position 211 (Trp211Arg).[229] While most of the affected individuals in the *SFTPA1* kindred were affected with an ILD after age 30 (range 31–69 years at diagnosis), one was diagnosed at 7 months of age and died of respiratory failure 2 months later.[229] Thus, a wide range of age at the time of diagnosis is observed, from respiratory insufficiency in infancy to lung fibrosis and adenocarcinoma in adulthood. All known mutations in the surfactant A genes affect highly conserved residues in the carbohydrate recognition domain of the proteins. Two of the mutations are predicted to alter the same glycine at amino acid position 231 (Gly231Val, Gly231Arg).

Cells expressing mutant proteins fail to secrete mature protein into the culture media.[227,229] In addition, expression of these mutant proteins led to fewer intracellular oligomers, greater protein instability, and increased markers of ER stress.[230] Family members with these heterozygous mutations secrete comparable amounts of total SP-A into the alveolar space, as compared with control family members, suggesting that the pathogenic mechanism may be related to ER stress of the resident epithelial alveolar cells.[230]

## Susceptibility to Pulmonary Fibrosis, Common Variants

Using a genomewide screen, a common variant located 3 kb upstream of the *MUC5B* transcription start site (rs35705950) was found to be present at a higher frequency in IPF patients. This variant is found in ~9% of controls (an overall allele frequency of 0.10) and 38% of patients with IPF. The odds ratio for IPF disease among subjects who are heterozygous or homozygous for the minor allele of this single nucleotide polymorphism (SNP) was 9.0 (CI 6.2–13.1) and 21.8 (5.1–93.5), respectively.[231] The variant allele was associated with upregulation of *MUC5B* expression (up to 37.4 times as high when compared with those homozygous for the wild-type allele) in lung tissue of unaffected subjects.[231]

A genomewide association study (GWAS) was performed comparing the frequency of common SNPs in patients with fibrotic idiopathic interstitial pneumonia (n = 1616) with controls (n = 4683). A replication analysis included 876 cases and 1890 controls. A *MUC5B* promoter variant (rs868903) was again found to be significantly associated with fibrotic lung disease, with a metaanalysis $P$ value of $9.2 \times 10^{-26}$.[232] A broad region on 11p15, including the *MUC5B*, *MUC2*, and *TOLLIP* genes, was found to demonstrate genomewide significance. After adjusting for the *MUC5B* promoter SNP found in the earlier study (rs35705950),[231] most of the variants in this broad region were no longer significantly associated, suggesting that the associations seen for the other SNPs may be due to linkage disequilibrium. The *MUC5B* promoter (rs35705950) has been found in the Framingham Heart Study[233] to be associated with interstitial lung abnormalities, thus linking it to an early manifestation of IPF. Mucins undergo a complex maturation process in airway cells, with glycosylation and disulfide multimerization, before secretion. As genetic perturbations leading to increased mucin production cause elevated ER stress signaling,[234–236] it is interesting to speculate that the *MUC5B* promoter variant may lead to increased susceptibility to lung fibrosis through its effects on increased mucin expression and ER stress.

The GWAS study confirmed the association of IPF with variants in the *TERT*[237] and *TERC* genes, with metaanalysis $p$ values of $1.7 \times 10^{-19}$ and $4.5 \times 10^{-8}$, respectively.[232] Overall, common variants in three telomere length–related genes (*TERT*, *TERC*, and *OBFC1*)[238–240] were found to be associated with lung fibrosis in this study. The GWAS study also found seven new loci that reached genomewide statistical significance.[232] These loci are located near genes involved with host defense, cell-cell adhesion, and DNA repair.

## Pulmonary Alveolar Microlithiasis

Pulmonary alveolar microlithiasis (PAM) is a rare disorder characterized by laminated calcium phosphate concretions within the alveoli. PAM is inherited in an autosomal recessive manner and is particularly prevalent in Turkey, Italy, the United States, and Japan.[241] The chest radiographs of patients with PAM show diffuse, bilateral, micronodular opacities, which obscure the heart border, mediastinum, and diaphragmatic surfaces. Despite the "sandstormlike" appearance, the clinical presentation of PAM is variable.[242–245] Early in the disease course, patients are often asymptomatic, but over time develop cough, dyspnea, and a restrictive defect with reduced diffusion. In 2006, Corut et al. reported the discovery of several mutations in the gene encoding the type IIb sodium-phosphate cotransporter protein (*SCL34A2*) in individuals with PAM.[246] The group used linkage analysis of a large consanguineous family in which six members were affected by PAM, and ultimately identified six homozygous mutations in *SCL34A2* that predict loss of protein function. A separate group in Japan used genomewide SNP mapping to identify candidate genes in six patients with PAM, and they independently identified *SCL34A2* as a gene of interest.[247] Two patients had homozygous frameshift mutations and four had splice-site mutations of the gene. None of the mutations was identified in normal controls. Since these initial discoveries, additional missense and frameshift mutations, as well as intragenetic deletions, have been identified.[248–250] The gene is expressed in high levels in the lung, predominantly in type II epithelial cells.[251–253] Epithelial deletion of the mouse *Npt2b* gene in the lung leads to a progressive pulmonary process characterized by diffuse alveolar microliths, restrictive physiology, and alveolar phospholipidosis.[254] Microliths are readily dissolved by whole-lung EDTA lavage. A low-phosphate diet prevents microlith formation in young mice and decreases the burden of pulmonary calcium deposits in older mice. The effectiveness of such a diet has not yet been studied in human patients.

**TABLE 1.3**
**Genetic Interstitial Lung Disease: Pathogenesis**

| Pathway | Surfactant Metabolism | ER Stress | Telomere Shortening |
|---|---|---|---|
| Rare variants | *NKX2.1* | *SFTPC* | *TERT, TERC* |
| | *ABCA3* | *SFTPA1, SFTPA2* | *RTEL1* |
| | *SFTPB* | *HPS1, HPS2, HPS4* | *PARN* |
| | *SFTPC* | *COPA* | *DKC1, TINF2* |
| | *SFTPA1, SFTPA2* | | Other DC genes |
| | *CSF2RA, SFT2RB* | | |
| Common variants | | *MUC5B?* | *TERT, TERC* |
| | | | *OBFC1* |

*DC*, dyskeratosis congenita; *ER*, endoplasmic reticulum.

## CONCLUSION

Discoveries of the genetic underpinnings of ILD have demonstrated a few consistent themes. Many of the genes involve common pathways that lead to altered surfactant metabolism, increased ER stress signaling, and telomere shortening (Table 1.3). Mutations, or pathologic ultrarare variants, have been found in genes involved with the metabolism of pulmonary surfactant. Given the central role surfactant has for reducing surface tension of the lung, opsonizing respiratory pathogens, and regulating inflammatory responses in the alveolar space, it is not surprising that patients with mutations in these genes have a wide range of ILD presentations.

Another common pathway, increased ER stress signaling, has been elucidated by genetic variants linked to various ILD subtypes.[255,256] Production of misfolded (missense) surfactant proteins in type 2 alveolar epithelial cells leads to increased ER stress. Mutations in the *HPS* and *COPA* genes alter intracellular protein transport and also upregulate ER stress pathways and lead to lung fibrosis. As the common variant located in the *MUC5B* promoter increases gene expression, this SNP may lead to increased susceptibility to lung fibrosis through its effects on increased mucin expression and increased ER stress. Finally, many different rare and common variants linked to genetic ILD share a common pathway of telomere shortening. Pulmonary fibrosis has been estimated to be the most common manifestation of the monogenic short telomere syndromes, and SNPs in three telomere-related genes reach genomewide significance in a large GWAS study. The link between telomere attrition and lung fibrosis is further strengthened by the finding that telomere length predicts transplant-free survival in patients with sporadic (noninherited) IPF across independent cohorts.[257,258] Thus, the study of rare human patients and families has led to the identification of genes relevant to the molecular pathogenesis of more common manifestations of ILD. How this knowledge leads to effective treatments across the spectrum of genetic ILD will be the next grand opportunity to improve patient care.

## REFERENCES

1. Avila NA, Dwyer AJ, Rabel A, Moss J. Sporadic lymphangioleiomyomatosis and tuberous sclerosis complex with lymphangioleiomyomatosis: comparison of CT features. *Radiology.* 2007;242(1):277–285.
2. Lenoir S, Grenier P, Brauner MW, et al. Pulmonary lymphangiomyomatosis and tuberous sclerosis: comparison of radiographic and thin-section CT findings. *Radiology.* 1990;175(2):329–334.
3. Curatolo P, Bombardieri R, Jozwiak S. Tuberous sclerosis. *Lancet.* 2008;372(9639):657–668.
4. Henske EP, Wessner LL, Golden J, et al. Loss of tuberin in both subependymal giant cell astrocytomas and angiomyolipomas supports a two-hit model for the pathogenesis of tuberous sclerosis tumors. *Am J Pathol.* 1997;151(6):1639–1647.
5. Carsillo T, Astrinidis A, Henske EP. Mutations in the tuberous sclerosis complex gene TSC2 are a cause of sporadic pulmonary lymphangioleiomyomatosis. *Proc Natl Acad Sci USA.* 2000;97(11):6085–6090.
6. Sato T, Seyama K, Fujii H, et al. Mutation analysis of the TSC1 and TSC2 genes in Japanese patients with pulmonary lymphangioleiomyomatosis. *J Hum Genet.* 2002;47(1):20–28.
7. Smolarek TA, Wessner LL, McCormack FX, Mylet JC, Menon AG, Henske EP. Evidence that lymphangiomyomatosis is caused by TSC2 mutations: chromosome 16p13 loss of heterozygosity in angiomyolipomas and lymph nodes from women with lymphangiomyomatosis. *Am J Hum Genet.* 1998;62(4):810–815.
8. Henske EP, McCormack FX. Lymphangioleiomyomatosis – a wolf in sheep's clothing. *J Clin Invest.* 2012;122(11):3807–3816.

9. Bissler JJ, McCormack FX, Young LR, et al. Sirolimus for angiomyolipoma in tuberous sclerosis complex or lymphangioleiomyomatosis. *N Engl J Med.* 2008;358(2):140–151.

10. Morton JM, McLean C, Booth SS, Snell GI, Whitford HM. Regression of pulmonary lymphangioleiomyomatosis (PLAM)-associated retroperitoneal angiomyolipoma post-lung transplantation with rapamycin treatment. *J Heart Lung Transplant.* 2008;27(4):462–465.

11. Krueger DA, Care MM, Holland K, et al. Everolimus for subependymal giant-cell astrocytomas in tuberous sclerosis. *N Engl J Med.* 2010;363(19):1801–1811.

12. McCormack FX, Inoue Y, Moss J, et al. Efficacy and safety of sirolimus in lymphangioleiomyomatosis. *N Engl J Med.* 2011;364(17):1595–1606.

13. Hornstein OP, Knickenberg M. Perifollicular fibromatosis cutis with polyps of the colon–a cutaneointestinal syndrome sui generis. *Arch Dermatol Res.* 1975;253(2):161–175.

14. Toro JR, Pautler SE, Stewart L, et al. Lung cysts, spontaneous pneumothorax, and genetic associations in 89 families with Birt-Hogg-Dube syndrome. *Am J Respir Crit Care Med.* 2007;175(10):1044–1053.

15. Toro JR, Wei MH, Glenn GM, et al. BHD mutations, clinical and molecular genetic investigations of Birt-Hogg-Dube syndrome: a new series of 50 families and a review of published reports. *J Med Genet.* 2008;45(6):321–331.

16. Nickerson ML, Warren MB, Toro JR, et al. Mutations in a novel gene lead to kidney tumors, lung wall defects, and benign tumors of the hair follicle in patients with the Birt-Hogg-Dube syndrome. *Cancer Cell.* 2002;2(2):157–164.

17. Painter JN, Tapanainen H, Somer M, Tukiainen P, Aittomaki KA. 4-bp deletion in the Birt-Hogg-Dube gene (FLCN) causes dominantly inherited spontaneous pneumothorax. *Am J Hum Genet.* 2005;76(3):522–527.

18. Graham RB, Nolasco M, Peterlin B, Garcia CK. Nonsense mutations in folliculin presenting as isolated familial spontaneous pneumothorax in adults. *Am J Respir Crit Care Med.* 2005;172(1):39–44.

19. Agarwal PP, Gross BH, Holloway BJ, Seely J, Stark P, Kazerooni EA. Thoracic CT findings in Birt-Hogg-Dube syndrome. *AJR Am J Roentgenol.* 2011;196(2):349–352.

20. Tobino K, Gunji Y, Kurihara M, et al. Characteristics of pulmonary cysts in Birt-Hogg-Dube syndrome: thin-section CT findings of the chest in 12 patients. *Eur J Radiol.* 2011;77(3):403–409.

21. Devine MS, Garcia CK. Genetic interstitial lung disease. *Clin Chest Med.* 2012;33(1):95–110.

22. Drachtman RA, Alter BP. Dyskeratosis congenita. *Dermatol Clin.* 1995;13(1):33–39.

23. Dokal I. Dyskeratosis congenita in all its forms. *Br J Haematol.* 2000;110(4):768–779.

24. Zinsser F. Atrophia Cutis Reticularis cum Pigmentations, Dystrophia Unguium et Leukoplakis oris (Poikioodermia atrophicans vascularis Jacobi). *Ikonogr Dermatol.* 1910;5:219–223.

25. de la Fuente J, Dokal I. Dyskeratosis congenita: advances in the understanding of the telomerase defect and the role of stem cell transplantation. *Pediatr Transplant.* 2007;11(6):584–594.

26. Giri N, Lee R, Faro A, et al. Lung transplantation for pulmonary fibrosis in dyskeratosis congenita: Case Report and systematic literature review. *BMC Blood Disord.* 2011;11:3.

27. Imokawa S, Sato A, Toyoshima M, et al. Dyskeratosis congenita showing usual interstitial pneumonia. *Intern Med.* 1994;33(4):226–230.

28. Verra F, Kouzan S, Saiag P, Bignon J, de Cremoux H. Bronchoalveolar disease in dyskeratosis congenita. *Eur Respir J.* 1992;5(4):497–499.

29. Parry EM, Alder JK, Qi X, Chen JJ, Armanios M. Syndrome complex of bone marrow failure and pulmonary fibrosis predicts germline defects in telomerase. *Blood.* 2011;117(21):5607–5611.

30. Yabe M, Yabe H, Hattori K, et al. Fatal interstitial pulmonary disease in a patient with dyskeratosis congenita after allogeneic bone marrow transplantation. *Bone Marrow Transplant.* 1997;19(4):389–392.

31. Rocha V, Devergie A, Socie G, et al. Unusual complications after bone marrow transplantation for dyskeratosis congenita. *Br J Haematol.* 1998;103(1):243–248.

32. Alter BP, Baerlocher GM, Savage SA, et al. Very short telomere length by flow FISH identifies patients with Dyskeratosis Congenita. *Blood.* 2007;110(5):1439–1447.

33. Heiss NS, Knight SW, Vulliamy TJ, et al. X-linked dyskeratosis congenita is caused by mutations in a highly conserved gene with putative nucleolar functions. *Nat Genet.* 1998;19(1):32–38.

34. Cohen SB, Graham ME, Lovrecz GO, Bache N, Robinson PJ, Reddel RR. Protein composition of catalytically active human telomerase from immortal cells. *Science.* 2007;315(5820):1850–1853.

35. Vulliamy T, Marrone A, Goldman F, et al. The RNA component of telomerase is mutated in autosomal dominant dyskeratosis congenita. *Nature.* 2001;413(6854):432–435.

36. Armanios M, Chen JL, Chang YP, et al. Haploinsufficiency of telomerase reverse transcriptase leads to anticipation in autosomal dominant dyskeratosis congenita. *Proc Natl Acad Sci USA.* 2005;102(44):15960–15964.

37. Du HY, Pumbo E, Manley P, et al. Complex inheritance pattern of dyskeratosis congenita in two families with 2 different mutations in the telomerase reverse transcriptase gene. *Blood.* 2008;111(3):1128–1130.

38. Aspesi A, Vallero S, Rocci A, et al. Compound heterozygosity for two new TERT mutations in a patient with aplastic anemia. *Pediatr Blood Cancer.* 2010;55(3):550–553.

39. Savage SA, Giri N, Baerlocher GM, Orr N, Lansdorp PM, Alter BP. TINF2, a component of the shelterin telomere protection complex, is mutated in dyskeratosis congenita. *Am J Hum Genet.* 2008;82(2):501–509.

40. Walne AJ, Vulliamy T, Beswick R, Kirwan M, Dokal I. TINF2 mutations result in very short telomeres: analysis of a large cohort of patients with dyskeratosis congenita and related bone marrow failure syndromes. *Blood.* 2008;112(9):3594–3600.

41. Guo Y, Kartawinata M, Li J, et al. Inherited bone marrow failure associated with germline mutation of ACD, the gene encoding telomere protein TPP1. *Blood.* 2014;124(18):2767–2774.

42. Kocak H, Ballew BJ, Bisht K, et al. Hoyeraal-Hreidarsson syndrome caused by a germline mutation in the TEL patch of the telomere protein TPP1. *Genes Dev.* 2014;28(19):2090–2102.

43. Keller RB, Gagne KE, Usmani GN, et al. CTC1 Mutations in a patient with dyskeratosis congenita. *Pediatr Blood Cancer.* 2012;59(2):311–314.

44. Walne AJ, Bhagat T, Kirwan M, et al. Mutations in the telomere capping complex in bone marrow failure and related syndromes. *Haematologica.* 2013;98(3):334–338.

45. Walne AJ, Vulliamy T, Marrone A, et al. Genetic heterogeneity in autosomal recessive dyskeratosis congenita with one subtype due to mutations in the telomerase-associated protein NOP10. *Hum Mol Genet.* 2007;16(13):1619–1629.

46. Trahan C, Martel C, Dragon F. Effects of dyskeratosis congenita mutations in dyskerin, NHP2 and NOP10 on assembly of H/ACA pre-RNPs. *Hum Mol Genet.* 2010;19(5):825–836.

47. Vulliamy T, Beswick R, Kirwan M, et al. Mutations in the telomerase component NHP2 cause the premature ageing syndrome dyskeratosis congenita. *Proc Natl Acad Sci USA.* 2008;105(23):8073–8078.

48. Zhong F, Savage SA, Shkreli M, et al. Disruption of telomerase trafficking by TCAB1 mutation causes dyskeratosis congenita. *Genes Dev.* 2011;25(1):11–16.

49. Walne AJ, Vulliamy T, Kirwan M, Plagnol V, Dokal I. Constitutional mutations in RTEL1 cause severe dyskeratosis congenita. *Am J Hum Genet.* 2013;92(3):448–453.

50. Le Guen T, Jullien L, Touzot F, et al. Human RTEL1 deficiency causes Hoyeraal-Hreidarsson syndrome with short telomeres and genome instability. *Hum Mol Genet.* 2013;22(16):3239–3249.

51. Ballew BJ, Yeager M, Jacobs K, et al. Germline mutations of regulator of telomere elongation helicase 1, RTEL1, in Dyskeratosis congenita. *Hum Genet.* 2013;132(4):473–480.

52. Tummala H, Walne A, Collopy L, et al. Poly(A)-specific ribonuclease deficiency impacts telomere biology and causes dyskeratosis congenita. *J Clin Invest.* 2015;125(5):2151–2160.

53. Dhanraj S, Gunja SM, Deveau AP, et al. Bone marrow failure and developmental delay caused by mutations in poly(A)-specific ribonuclease (PARN). *J Med Genet.* 2015;52(11):738–748.

54. Moon DH, Segal M, Boyraz B, et al. Poly(A)-specific ribonuclease (PARN) mediates 3′-end maturation of the telomerase RNA component. *Nat Genet.* 2015;47(12):1482–1488.

55. Vulliamy T, Marrone A, Szydlo R, Walne A, Mason PJ, Dokal I. Disease anticipation is associated with progressive telomere shortening in families with dyskeratosis congenita due to mutations in TERC. *Nat Genet.* 2004;36(5):447–449.

56. Goldman F, Bouarich R, Kulkarni S, et al. The effect of TERC haploinsufficiency on the inheritance of telomere length. *Proc Natl Acad Sci USA.* 2005;102(47):17119–17124.

57. Devgan SS, Sanal O, Doil C, et al. Homozygous deficiency of ubiquitin-ligase ring-finger protein RNF168 mimics the radiosensitivity syndrome of ataxia-telangiectasia. *Cell Death Differ.* 2011;18(9):1500–1506.

58. Stewart GS, Stankovic T, Byrd PJ, et al. RIDDLE immunodeficiency syndrome is linked to defects in 53BP1-mediated DNA damage signaling. *Proc Natl Acad Sci USA.* 2007;104(43):16910–16915.

59. Doil C, Mailand N, Bekker-Jensen S, et al. RNF168 binds and amplifies ubiquitin conjugates on damaged chromosomes to allow accumulation of repair proteins. *Cell.* 2009;136(3):435–446.

60. Stewart GS, Panier S, Townsend K, et al. The RIDDLE syndrome protein mediates a ubiquitin-dependent signaling cascade at sites of DNA damage. *Cell.* 2009;136(3):420–434.

61. Okamoto K, Bartocci C, Ouzounov I, Diedrich JK, Yates 3rd JR, Denchi EL. A two-step mechanism for TRF2-mediated chromosome-end protection. *Nature.* 2013;494(7438):502–505.

62. Hermansky F, Pudlak P. Albinism associated with hemorrhagic diathesis and unusual pigmented reticular cells in the bone marrow: report of two cases with histochemical studies. *Blood.* 1959;14(2):162–169.

63. Gahl WA, Brantly M, Kaiser-Kupfer MI, et al. Genetic defects and clinical characteristics of patients with a form of oculocutaneous albinism (Hermansky-Pudlak syndrome). *N Engl J Med.* 1998;338(18):1258–1264.

64. Witkop CJ, Krumwiede M, Sedano H, White JG. Reliability of absent platelet dense bodies as a diagnostic criterion for Hermansky-Pudlak syndrome. *Am J Hematol.* 1987;26(4):305–311.

65. Dell'Angelica EC, Shotelersuk V, Aguilar RC, Gahl WA, Bonifacino JS. Altered trafficking of lysosomal proteins in Hermansky-Pudlak syndrome due to mutations in the beta 3A subunit of the AP-3 adaptor. *Mol Cell.* 1999;3(1):11–21.

66. Morgan NV, Pasha S, Johnson CA, et al. A germline mutation in BLOC1S3/reduced pigmentation causes a novel variant of Hermansky-Pudlak syndrome (HPS8). *Am J Hum Genet.* 2006;78(1):160–166.

67. Martina JA, Moriyama K, Bonifacino JS. BLOC-3, a protein complex containing the Hermansky-Pudlak syndrome gene products HPS1 and HPS4. *J Biol Chem.* 2003;278(31):29376–29384.

68. Suzuki T, Li W, Zhang Q, et al. The gene mutated in cocoa mice, carrying a defect of organelle biogenesis, is a homologue of the human Hermansky-Pudlak syndrome-3 gene. *Genomics.* 2001;78(1–2):30–37.

69. Zhang Q, Zhao B, Li W, et al. Ru2 and Ru encode mouse orthologs of the genes mutated in human Hermansky-Pudlak syndrome types 5 and 6. *Nat Genet*. 2003;33(2):145–153.

70. Li W, Zhang Q, Oiso N, et al. Hermansky-Pudlak syndrome type 7 (HPS-7) results from mutant dysbindin, a member of the biogenesis of lysosome-related organelles complex 1 (BLOC-1). *Nat Genet*. 2003;35(1): 84–89.

71. Wildenberg SC, Oetting WS, Almodovar C, Krumwiede M, White JG, King RA. A gene causing Hermansky-Pudlak syndrome in a Puerto Rican population maps to chromosome 10q2. *Am J Hum Genet*. 1995;57(4):755–765.

72. Brantly M, Avila NA, Shotelersuk V, Lucero C, Huizing M, Gahl WA. Pulmonary function and high-resolution CT findings in patients with an inherited form of pulmonary fibrosis, Hermansky-Pudlak syndrome, due to mutations in HPS-1. *Chest*. 2000;117(1):129–136.

73. Avila NA, Brantly M, Premkumar A, Huizing M, Dwyer A, Gahl WA. Hermansky-Pudlak syndrome: radiography and CT of the chest compared with pulmonary function tests and genetic studies. *AJR Am J Roentgenol*. 2002;179(4):887–892.

74. Anderson PD, Huizing M, Claassen DA, White J, Gahl WA. Hermansky-Pudlak syndrome type 4 (HPS-4): clinical and molecular characteristics. *Hum Genet*. 2003;113(1):10–17.

75. Bachli EB, Brack T, Eppler E, et al. Hermansky-Pudlak syndrome type 4 in a patient from Sri Lanka with pulmonary fibrosis. *Am J Med Genet A*. 2004;127A(2):201–207.

76. Gahl WA, Brantly M, Troendle J, et al. Effect of pirfenidone on the pulmonary fibrosis of Hermansky-Pudlak syndrome. *Mol Genet Metab*. 2002;76(3):234–242.

77. Gochuico BR, Huizing M, Golas GA, et al. Interstitial lung disease and pulmonary fibrosis in Hermansky-Pudlak syndrome type 2, an adaptor protein-3 complex disease. *Mol Med*. 2012;18:56–64.

78. Nakatani Y, Nakamura N, Sano J, et al. Interstitial pneumonia in Hermansky-Pudlak syndrome: significance of florid foamy swelling/degeneration (giant lamellar body degeneration) of type-2 pneumocytes. *Virchows Arch*. 2000;437(3):304–313.

79. Pierson DM, Ionescu D, Qing G, et al. Pulmonary fibrosis in hermansky-pudlak syndrome. a case report and review. *Respiration*. 2006;73(3):382–395.

80. O'Brien K, Troendle J, Gochuico BR, et al. Pirfenidone for the treatment of Hermansky-Pudlak syndrome pulmonary fibrosis. *Mol Genet Metab*. 2011;103(2):128–134.

81. Lyerla TA, Rusiniak ME, Borchers M, et al. Aberrant lung structure, composition, and function in a murine model of Hermansky-Pudlak syndrome. *Am J Physiol Lung Cell Mol Physiol*. 2003;285(3):L643–L653.

82. Mahavadi P, Korfei M, Henneke I, et al. Epithelial stress and apoptosis underlie Hermansky-Pudlak syndrome-associated interstitial pneumonia. *Am J Respir Crit Care Med*. 2010;182(2):207–219.

83. Guttentag SH, Akhtar A, Tao JQ, et al. Defective surfactant secretion in a mouse model of Hermansky-Pudlak syndrome. *Am J Respir Cell Mol Biol*. 2005;33(1):14–21.

84. Gras D, Jonard L, Roze E, et al. Benign hereditary chorea: phenotype, prognosis, therapeutic outcome and long term follow-up in a large series with new mutations in the TITF1/NKX-1 gene. *J Neurol Neurosurg Psychiatry*. 2012;83(10):956–962.

85. Young LR, Deutsch GH, Bokulic RE, Brody AS, Nogee LM. A mutation in TTF1/NKX2.1 is associated with familial neuroendocrine cell hyperplasia of infancy. *Chest*. 2013;144(4):1199–1206.

86. Hamvas A, Deterding RR, Wert SE, et al. Heterogeneous pulmonary phenotypes associated with mutations in the thyroid transcription factor gene NKX2-1. *Chest*. 2013;144(3):794–804.

87. Carre A, Szinnai G, Castanet M, et al. Five new TTF1/NKX2.1 mutations in brain-lung-thyroid syndrome: rescue by PAX8 synergism in one case. *Hum Mol Genet*. 2009;18(12):2266–2276.

88. Peca D, Petrini S, Tzialla C, et al. Altered surfactant homeostasis and recurrent respiratory failure secondary to TTF-1 nuclear targeting defect. *Respir Res*. 2011;12:115.

89. Burkhalter JL, Morano JU, McCay MB. Diffuse interstitial lung disease in neurofibromatosis. *South Med J*. 1986;79(8):944–946.

90. Massaro D, Katz S. Fibrosing alveolitis: its occurrence, roentgenographic, and pathologic features in von Recklinghausen's neurofibromatosis. *Am Rev Respir Dis*. 1966;93(6):934–942.

91. Webb WR, Goodman PC. Fibrosing alveolitis in patients with neurofibromatosis. *Radiology*. 1977;122(2):289–293.

92. Porterfield JK, Pyeritz RE, Traill TA. Pulmonary hypertension and interstitial fibrosis in von Recklinghausen neurofibromatosis. *Am J Med Genet*. 1986;25(3):531–535.

93. Khumalo NP, Pillay K, Beighton P, et al. Poikiloderma, tendon contracture and pulmonary fibrosis: a new autosomal dominant syndrome? *Br J Dermatol*. 2006;155(5):1057–1061.

94. Mercier S, Kury S, Shaboodien G, et al. Mutations in FAM111B cause hereditary fibrosing poikiloderma with tendon contracture, myopathy, and pulmonary fibrosis. *Am J Hum Genet*. 2013;93(6):1100–1107.

95. Has C, Sparta G, Kiritsi D, et al. Integrin alpha3 mutations with kidney, lung, and skin disease. *N Engl J Med*. 2012;366(16):1508–1514.

96. Yalcin EG, He Y, Orhan D, Pazzagli C, Emiralioglu N, Has C. Crucial role of posttranslational modifications of integrin alpha3 in interstitial lung disease and nephrotic syndrome. *Hum Mol Genet*. 2015;24(13):3679–3688.

97. Liu Y, Jesus AA, Marrero B, et al. Activated STING in a vascular and pulmonary syndrome. *N Engl J Med*. 2014;371(6):507–518.

98. Jeremiah N, Neven B, Gentili M, et al. Inherited STING-activating mutation underlies a familial inflammatory syndrome with lupus-like manifestations. *J Clin Invest*. 2014;124(12):5516–5520.

99. Lohr NJ, Molleston JP, Strauss KA, et al. Human ITCH E3 ubiquitin ligase deficiency causes syndromic multisystem autoimmune disease. *Am J Hum Genet.* 2010;86(3):447–453.

100. Hustad CM, Perry WL, Siracusa LD, et al. Molecular genetic characterization of six recessive viable alleles of the mouse agouti locus. *Genetics.* 1995;140(1):255–265.

101. Perry WL, Hustad CM, Swing DA, O'Sullivan TN, Jenkins NA, Copeland NG. The itchy locus encodes a novel ubiquitin protein ligase that is disrupted in a18H mice. *Nat Genet.* 1998;18(2):143–146.

102. Watkin LB, Jessen B, Wiszniewski W, et al. COPA mutations impair ER-Golgi transport and cause hereditary autoimmune-mediated lung disease and arthritis. *Nat Genet.* 2015;47(6):654–660.

103. Ostergaard P, Simpson MA, Connell FC, et al. Mutations in GATA2 cause primary lymphedema associated with a predisposition to acute myeloid leukemia (Emberger syndrome). *Nat Genet.* 2011;43(10):929–931.

104. Hahn CN, Chong CE, Carmichael CL, et al. Heritable GATA2 mutations associated with familial myelodysplastic syndrome and acute myeloid leukemia. *Nat Genet.* 2011;43(10):1012–1017.

105. Dickinson RE, Griffin H, Bigley V, et al. Exome sequencing identifies GATA-2 mutation as the cause of dendritic cell, monocyte, B and NK lymphoid deficiency. *Blood.* 2011;118(10):2656–2658.

106. Hsu AP, Sampaio EP, Khan J, et al. Mutations in GATA2 are associated with the autosomal dominant and sporadic monocytopenia and mycobacterial infection (Mono-MAC) syndrome. *Blood.* 2011;118(10):2653–2655.

107. Spinner MA, Sanchez LA, Hsu AP, et al. GATA2 deficiency: a protean disorder of hematopoiesis, lymphatics, and immunity. *Blood.* 2014;123(6):809–821.

108. Hsu AP, Johnson KD, Falcone EL, et al. GATA2 haploinsufficiency caused by mutations in a conserved intronic element leads to MonoMAC syndrome. *Blood.* 2013;121(19):3830–3837. S3831–S3837.

109. Aghamohammadi A, Allahverdi A, Abolhassani H, et al. Comparison of pulmonary diseases in common variable immunodeficiency and X-linked agammaglobulinaemia. *Respirology.* 2010;15(2):289–295.

110. Verma N, Grimbacher B, Hurst JR. Lung disease in primary antibody deficiency. *Lancet Respir Med.* 2015;3(8):651–660.

111. Maarschalk-Ellerbroek LJ, de Jong PA, van Montfrans JM, et al. CT screening for pulmonary pathology in common variable immunodeficiency disorders and the correlation with clinical and immunological parameters. *J Clin Immunol.* 2014;34(6):642–654.

112. Gregersen S, Aalokken TM, Mynarek G, et al. High resolution computed tomography and pulmonary function in common variable immunodeficiency. *Respir Med.* 2009;103(6):873–880.

113. Grimbacher B, Hutloff A, Schlesier M, et al. Homozygous loss of ICOS is associated with adult-onset common variable immunodeficiency. *Nat Immunol.* 2003;4(3):261–268.

114. Salzer U, Chapel HM, Webster AD, et al. Mutations in TNFRSF13B encoding TACI are associated with common variable immunodeficiency in humans. *Nat Genet.* 2005;37(8):820–828.

115. Castigli E, Wilson SA, Garibyan L, et al. TACI is mutant in common variable immunodeficiency and IgA deficiency. *Nat Genet.* 2005;37(8):829–834.

116. Warnatz K, Salzer U, Rizzi M, et al. B-cell activating factor receptor deficiency is associated with an adult-onset antibody deficiency syndrome in humans. *Proc Natl Acad Sci USA.* 2009;106(33):13945–13950.

117. van Zelm MC, Reisli I, van der Burg M, et al. An antibody-deficiency syndrome due to mutations in the CD19 gene. *N Engl J Med.* 2006;354(18):1901–1912.

118. Kuijpers TW, Bende RJ, Baars PA, et al. CD20 deficiency in humans results in impaired T cell-independent antibody responses. *J Clin Invest.* 2010;120(1):214–222.

119. van Zelm MC, Smet J, Adams B, et al. CD81 gene defect in humans disrupts CD19 complex formation and leads to antibody deficiency. *J Clin Invest.* 2010;120(4):1265–1274.

120. Thiel J, Kimmig L, Salzer U, et al. Genetic CD21 deficiency is associated with hypogammaglobulinemia. *J Allergy Clin Immunol.* 2012;129(3):801–810.e806.

121. Lopez-Herrera G, Tampella G, Pan-Hammarstrom Q, et al. Deleterious mutations in LRBA are associated with a syndrome of immune deficiency and autoimmunity. *Am J Hum Genet.* 2012;90(6):986–1001.

122. Alangari A, Alsultan A, Adly N, et al. LPS-responsive beige-like anchor (LRBA) gene mutation in a family with inflammatory bowel disease and combined immunodeficiency. *J Allergy Clin Immunol.* 2012;130(2):481–488.e482.

123. Salzer E, Kansu A, Sic H, et al. Early-onset inflammatory bowel disease and common variable immunodeficiency-like disease caused by IL-21 deficiency. *J Allergy Clin Immunol.* 2014;133(6):1651–1659.e1612.

124. Fliegauf M, Bryant VL, Frede N, et al. Haploinsufficiency of the NF-kappaB1 Subunit p50 in common variable immunodeficiency. *Am J Hum Genet.* 2015;97(3):389–403.

125. Chen K, Coonrod EM, Kumanovics A, et al. Germline mutations in NFKB2 implicate the noncanonical NF-kappaB pathway in the pathogenesis of common variable immunodeficiency. *Am J Hum Genet.* 2013;93(5):812–824.

126. Goldman FD, Gurel Z, Al-Zubeidi D, et al. Congenital pancytopenia and absence of B lymphocytes in a neonate with a mutation in the Ikaros gene. *Pediatr Blood Cancer.* 2012;58(4):591–597.

127. Kuehn HS, Boisson B, Cunningham-Rundles C, et al. Loss of B cells in patients with heterozygous mutations in IKAROS. *N Engl J Med.* 2016;374(11):1032–1043.

128. Chen Y, Stirling RG, Paul E, Hore-Lacy F, Thompson BR, Douglass JA. Longitudinal decline in lung function in patients with primary immunoglobulin deficiencies. *J Allergy Clin Immunol.* 2011;127(6):1414–1417.

129. Vetrie D, Vorechovsky I, Sideras P, et al. The gene involved in X-linked agammaglobulinaemia is a member of the src family of protein-tyrosine kinases. *Nature.* 1993;361(6409):226–233.

130. Yel L, Minegishi Y, Coustan-Smith E, et al. Mutations in the mu heavy-chain gene in patients with agammaglobulinemia. *N Engl J Med.* 1996;335(20):1486–1493.

131. Minegishi Y, Coustan-Smith E, Wang YH, Cooper MD, Campana D, Conley ME. Mutations in the human lambda5/14.1 gene result in B cell deficiency and agammaglobulinemia. *J Exp Med.* 1998;187(1):71–77.

132. Minegishi Y, Coustan-Smith E, Rapalus L, Ersoy F, Campana D, Conley ME. Mutations in Igalpha (CD79a) result in a complete block in B-cell development. *J Clin Invest.* 1999;104(8):1115–1121.

133. Minegishi Y, Rohrer J, Coustan-Smith E, et al. An essential role for BLNK in human B cell development. *Science.* 1999;286(5446):1954–1957.

134. Dobbs AK, Yang T, Farmer D, Kager L, Parolini O, Conley ME. Cutting edge: a hypomorphic mutation in Igbeta (CD79b) in a patient with immunodeficiency and a leaky defect in B cell development. *J Immunol.* 2007;179(4):2055–2059.

135. Boisson B, Wang YD, Bosompem A, et al. A recurrent dominant negative E47 mutation causes agammaglobulinemia and BCR(-) B cells. *J Clin Invest.* 2013;123(11):4781–4785.

136. Freeman AF, Holland SM. Clinical manifestations, etiology, and pathogenesis of the hyper-IgE syndromes. *Pediatr Res.* 2009;65(5 Pt 2):32R–37R.

137. Freeman AF, Kleiner DE, Nadiminti H, et al. Causes of death in hyper-IgE syndrome. *J Allergy Clin Immunol.* 2007;119(5):1234–1240.

138. Minegishi Y, Saito M, Tsuchiya S, et al. Dominant-negative mutations in the DNA-binding domain of STAT3 cause hyper-IgE syndrome. *Nature.* 2007;448(7157):1058–1062.

139. Milner JD, Brenchley JM, Laurence A, et al. Impaired T(H)17 cell differentiation in subjects with autosomal dominant hyper-IgE syndrome. *Nature.* 2008;452(7188):773–776.

140. Angulo I, Vadas O, Garcon F, et al. Phosphoinositide 3-kinase delta gene mutation predisposes to respiratory infection and airway damage. *Science.* 2013;342(6160):866–871.

141. Lucas CL, Kuehn HS, Zhao F, et al. Dominant-activating germline mutations in the gene encoding the PI(3)K catalytic subunit p110delta result in T cell senescence and human immunodeficiency. *Nat Immunol.* 2014;15(1):88–97.

142. Kuehn HS, Ouyang W, Lo B, et al. Immune dysregulation in human subjects with heterozygous germline mutations in CTLA4. *Science.* 2014;345(6204):1623–1627.

143. Schubert D, Bode C, Kenefeck R, et al. Autosomal dominant immune dysregulation syndrome in humans with CTLA4 mutations. *Nature Med.* 2014;20(12):1410–1416.

144. Partington MW, Prentice RS. X-linked cutaneous amyloidosis: further clinical and pathological observations. *Am J Med Genet.* 1989;32(1):115–119.

145. Ades LC, Rogers M, Sillence DO. An X-linked reticulate pigmentary disorder with systemic manifestations: report of a second family. *Pediatr Dermatol.* 1993;10(4):344–351.

146. Anderson RC, Zinn AR, Kim J, Carder KR. X-linked reticulate pigmentary disorder with systemic manifestations: report of a third family and literature review. *Pediatr Dermatol.* 2005;22(2):122–126.

147. Starokadomskyy P, Gemelli T, Rios JJ, et al. DNA polymerase-alpha regulates the activation of type I interferons through cytosolic RNA: DNA synthesis. *Nat Immunol.* 2016;17(5):495–504.

148. Kerem E, Elstein D, Abrahamov A, et al. Pulmonary function abnormalities in type I Gaucher disease. *Eur Respir J.* 1996;9(2):340–345.

149. Miller A, Brown LK, Pastores GM, Desnick RJ. Pulmonary involvement in type 1 Gaucher disease: functional and exercise findings in patients with and without clinical interstitial lung disease. *Clin Genet.* 2003;63(5):368–376.

150. Goitein O, Elstein D, Abrahamov A, et al. Lung involvement and enzyme replacement therapy in Gaucher's disease. *QJM.* 2001;94(8):407–415.

151. Jmoudiak M, Futerman AH. Gaucher disease: pathological mechanisms and modern management. *Br J Haematol.* 2005;129(2):178–188.

152. McGovern MM, Wasserstein MP, Giugliani R, et al. A prospective, cross-sectional survey study of the natural history of Niemann-Pick disease type B. *Pediatrics.* 2008;122(2):e341–e349.

153. Mendelson DS, Wasserstein MP, Desnick RJ, et al. Type B Niemann-Pick disease: findings at chest radiography, thin-section CT, and pulmonary function testing. *Radiology.* 2006;238(1):339–345.

154. Parto K, Svedstrom E, Majurin ML, Harkonen R, Simell O. Pulmonary manifestations in lysinuric protein intolerance. *Chest.* 1993;104(4):1176–1182.

155. Nogee LM. Genetic basis of children's interstitial lung disease. *Pediatr Allergy Immunol Pulmonol.* 2010;23(1).

156. Nogee LM, de Mello DE, Dehner LP, Colten HR. Brief report: deficiency of pulmonary surfactant protein B in congenital alveolar proteinosis. *N Engl J Med.* 1993;328(6):406–410.

157. Nogee LM, Garnier G, Dietz HC, et al. A mutation in the surfactant protein B gene responsible for fatal neonatal respiratory disease in multiple kindreds. *J Clin Invest.* 1994;93(4):1860–1863.

158. Andersen C, Ramsay JA, Nogee LM, et al. Recurrent familial neonatal deaths: hereditary surfactant protein B deficiency. *Am J Perinatol.* 2000;17(4):219–224.

159. Cole FS, Hamvas A, Rubinstein P, et al. Population-based estimates of surfactant protein B deficiency. *Pediatrics.* 2000;105(3 Pt 1):538–541.

160. Somaschini M, Wert S, Mangili G, Colombo A, Nogee L. Hereditary surfactant protein B deficiency resulting from a novel mutation. *Intensive Care Med.* 2000;26(1):97–100.

161. Wegner DJ, Hertzberg T, Heins HB, et al. A major deletion in the surfactant protein-B gene causing lethal respiratory distress. *Acta Paediatr.* 2007;96(4): 516–520.

162. Dunbar 3rd AE, Wert SE, Ikegami M, et al. Prolonged survival in hereditary surfactant protein B (SP-B) deficiency associated with a novel splicing mutation. *Pediatr Res.* 2000;48(3):275–282.

163. Ballard PL, Nogee LM, Beers MF, et al. Partial deficiency of surfactant protein B in an infant with chronic lung disease. *Pediatrics.* 1995;96(6):1046–1052.

164. Nogee LM, Dunbar 3rd AE, Wert SE, Askin F, Hamvas A, Whitsett JA. A mutation in the surfactant protein C gene associated with familial interstitial lung disease. *N Engl J Med.* 2001;344(8):573–579.

165. Thomas AQ, Lane K, Phillips 3rd J, et al. Heterozygosity for a surfactant protein C gene mutation associated with usual interstitial pneumonitis and cellular nonspecific interstitial pneumonitis in one kindred. *Am J Respir Crit Care Med.* 2002;165(9): 1322–1328.

166. Abou Taam R, Jaubert F, Emond S, et al. Familial interstitial disease with I73T mutation: a mid- and long-term study. *Pediatr Pulmonol.* 2009;44(2):167–175.

167. Brasch F, Griese M, Tredano M, et al. Interstitial lung disease in a baby with a de novo mutation in the SFTPC gene. *Eur Respir J.* 2004;24(1):30–39.

168. Bullard JE, Nogee LM. Heterozygosity for ABCA3 mutations modifies the severity of lung disease associated with a surfactant protein C gene (SFTPC) mutation. *Pediatr Res.* 2007;62(2):176–179.

169. Cameron HS, Somaschini M, Carrera P, et al. A common mutation in the surfactant protein C gene associated with lung disease. *J Pediatr.* 2005;146(3):370–375.

170. Soraisham AS, Tierney AJ, Amin HJ. Neonatal respiratory failure associated with mutation in the surfactant protein C gene. *J Perinatol.* 2006;26(1):67–70.

171. van Moorsel CH, van Oosterhout MF, Barlo NP, et al. Surfactant protein C mutations are the basis of a significant portion of adult familial pulmonary fibrosis in a dutch cohort. *Am J Respir Crit Care Med.* 2010;182(11):1419–1425.

172. Lawson WE, Grant SW, Ambrosini V, et al. Genetic mutations in surfactant protein C are a rare cause of sporadic cases of IPF. *Thorax.* 2004;59(11):977–980.

173. Markart P, Ruppert C, Wygrecka M, et al. Surfactant protein C mutations in sporadic forms of idiopathic interstitial pneumonias. *Eur Respir J.* 2007;29(1): 134–137.

174. Wert SE, Whitsett JA, Nogee LM. Genetic disorders of surfactant dysfunction. *Pediatr Dev Pathol.* 2009;12(4): 253–274.

175. Mulugeta S, Maguire JA, Newitt JL, Russo SJ, Kotorashvili A, Beers MF. Misfolded BRICHOS SP-C mutant proteins induce apoptosis via caspase-4- and cytochrome c-related mechanisms. *Am J Physiol Lung Cell Mol Physiol.* 2007;293(3):L720–L729.

176. Stevens PA, Pettenazzo A, Brasch F, et al. Nonspecific interstitial pneumonia, alveolar proteinosis, and abnormal proprotein trafficking resulting from a spontaneous mutation in the surfactant protein C gene. *Pediatr Res.* 2005;57(1):89–98.

177. Woischnik M, Sparr C, Kern S, et al. A non-BRICHOS surfactant protein c mutation disrupts epithelial cell function and intercellular signaling. *BMC Cell Biol.* 2010;11:88.

178. Bridges JP, Xu Y, Na CL, Wong HR, Weaver TE. Adaptation and increased susceptibility to infection associated with constitutive expression of misfolded SP-C. *J Cell Biol.* 2006;172(3):395–407.

179. Garmany TH, Wambach JA, Heins HB, et al. Population and disease-based prevalence of the common mutations associated with surfactant deficiency. *Pediatr Res.* 2008;63(6):645–649.

180. Somaschini M, Nogee LM, Sassi I, et al. Unexplained neonatal respiratory distress due to congenital surfactant deficiency. *J Pediatr.* 2007;150(6):649–653. 653.e641.

181. Weaver TE. Synthesis, processing and secretion of surfactant proteins B and C. *Biochim Biophys Acta.* 1998;1408(2–3):173–179.

182. Serrano AG, Perez-Gil J. Protein-lipid interactions and surface activity in the pulmonary surfactant system. *Chem Phys Lipids.* 2006;141(1–2):105–118.

183. Matsumura Y, Ban N, Inagaki N. Aberrant catalytic cycle and impaired lipid transport into intracellular vesicles in ABCA3 mutants associated with nonfatal pediatric interstitial lung disease. *Am J Physiol Lung Cell Mol Physiol.* 2008;295(4):L698–L707.

184. Matsumura Y, Ban N, Ueda K, Inagaki N. Characterization and classification of ATP-binding cassette transporter ABCA3 mutants in fatal surfactant deficiency. *J Biol Chem.* 2006;281(45):34503–34514.

185. Cheong N, Madesh M, Gonzales LW, et al. Functional and trafficking defects in ATP binding cassette A3 mutants associated with respiratory distress syndrome. *J Biol Chem.* 2006;281(14):9791–9800.

186. Trapnell BC, Whitsett JA, Nakata K. Pulmonary alveolar proteinosis. *N Engl J Med.* 2003;349(26):2527–2539.

187. Prakash UB, Barham SS, Carpenter HA, Dines DE, Marsh HM. Pulmonary alveolar phospholipoproteinosis: experience with 34 cases and a review. *Mayo Clin Proc.* 1987;62(6):499–518.

188. Goldstein LS, Kavuru MS, Curtis-McCarthy P, Christie HA, Farver C, Stoller JK. Pulmonary alveolar proteinosis: clinical features and outcomes. *Chest.* 1998;114(5):1357–1362.

189. Seymour JF, Presneill JJ. Pulmonary alveolar proteinosis: progress in the first 44 years. *Am J Respir Crit Care Med.* 2002;166(2):215–235.

190. Kitamura T, Tanaka N, Watanabe J, et al. Idiopathic pulmonary alveolar proteinosis as an autoimmune disease with neutralizing antibody against granulocyte/macrophage colony-stimulating factor. *J Exp Med.* 1999;190(6):875–880.

191. Bonfield TL, Russell D, Burgess S, Malur A, Kavuru MS, Thomassen MJ. Autoantibodies against granulocyte macrophage colony-stimulating factor are diagnostic for pulmonary alveolar proteinosis. *Am J Respir Cell Mol Biol.* 2002;27(4):481–486.

192. Lin FC, Chang GD, Chern MS, Chen YC, Chang SC. Clinical significance of anti-GM-CSF antibodies in idiopathic pulmonary alveolar proteinosis. *Thorax.* 2006;61(6):528–534.

193. Inoue Y, Trapnell BC, Tazawa R, et al. Characteristics of a large cohort of patients with autoimmune pulmonary alveolar proteinosis in Japan. *Am J Respir Crit Care Med.* 2008;177(7):752–762.

194. Carey B, Trapnell BC. The molecular basis of pulmonary alveolar proteinosis. *Clin Immunol.* 2010;135(2):223–235.

195. Uchida K, Beck DC, Yamamoto T, et al. GM-CSF autoantibodies and neutrophil dysfunction in pulmonary alveolar proteinosis. *N Engl J Med.* 2007;356(6):567–579.

196. Uchida K, Nakata K, Trapnell BC, et al. High-affinity autoantibodies specifically eliminate granulocyte-macrophage colony-stimulating factor activity in the lungs of patients with idiopathic pulmonary alveolar proteinosis. *Blood.* 2004;103(3):1089–1098.

197. Hansen G, Hercus TR, McClure BJ, et al. The structure of the GM-CSF receptor complex reveals a distinct mode of cytokine receptor activation. *Cell.* 2008;134(3):496–507.

198. Suzuki T, Sakagami T, Rubin BK, et al. Familial pulmonary alveolar proteinosis caused by mutations in CSF2RA. *J Exp Med.* 2008;205(12):2703–2710.

199. Suzuki T, Sakagami T, Young LR, et al. Hereditary pulmonary alveolar proteinosis: pathogenesis, presentation, diagnosis, and therapy. *Am J Respir Crit Care Med.* 2010;182(10):1292–1304.

200. Tanaka T, Motoi N, Tsuchihashi Y, et al. Adult-onset hereditary pulmonary alveolar proteinosis caused by a single-base deletion in CSF2RB. *J Med Genet.* 2011;48(3):205–209.

201. Dranoff G, Crawford AD, Sadelain M, et al. Involvement of granulocyte-macrophage colony-stimulating factor in pulmonary homeostasis. *Science.* 1994;264(5159):713–716.

202. Stanley E, Lieschke GJ, Grail D, et al. Granulocyte/macrophage colony-stimulating factor-deficient mice show no major perturbation of hematopoiesis but develop a characteristic pulmonary pathology. *Proc Natl Acad Sci USA.* 1994;91(12):5592–5596.

203. Nishinakamura R, Nakayama N, Hirabayashi Y, et al. Mice deficient for the IL-3/GM-CSF/IL-5 beta c receptor exhibit lung pathology and impaired immune response, while beta IL3 receptor-deficient mice are normal. *Immunity.* 1995;2(3):211–222.

204. Robb L, Drinkwater CC, Metcalf D, et al. Hematopoietic and lung abnormalities in mice with a null mutation of the common beta subunit of the receptors for granulocyte-macrophage colony-stimulating factor and interleukins 3 and 5. *Proc Natl Acad Sci USA.* 1995;92(21):9565–9569.

205. Hadchouel A, Wieland T, Griese M, et al. Biallelic mutations of methionyl-tRNA synthetase cause a specific type of pulmonary alveolar proteinosis prevalent on reunion island. *Am J Hum Genet.* 2015;96(5):826–831.

206. van Meel E, Wegner DJ, Cliften P, et al. Rare recessive loss-of-function methionyl-tRNA synthetase mutations presenting as a multi-organ phenotype. *BMC Med Genet.* 2013;14:106.

207. Armanios MY, Chen JJ, Cogan JD, et al. Telomerase mutations in families with idiopathic pulmonary fibrosis. *N Engl J Med.* 2007;356(13):1317–1326.

208. Tsakiri KD, Cronkhite JT, Kuan PJ, et al. Adult-onset pulmonary fibrosis caused by mutations in telomerase. *Proc Natl Acad Sci USA.* 2007;104(18):7552–7557.

209. Cronkhite JT, Xing C, Raghu G, et al. Telomere shortening in familial and sporadic pulmonary fibrosis. *Am J Respir Crit Care Med.* 2008;178(7):729–737.

210. Diaz de Leon A, Cronkhite JT, Katzenstein AL, et al. Telomere lengths, pulmonary fibrosis and telomerase (TERT) mutations. *PLoS One.* 2010;5(5):e10680.

211. Armanios M. Telomerase and idiopathic pulmonary fibrosis. *Mutat Res.* 2012;730(1–2):52–58.

212. Yamaguchi H, Calado RT, Ly H, et al. Mutations in TERT, the gene for telomerase reverse transcriptase, in aplastic anemia. *N Engl J Med.* 2005;352(14):1413–1424.

213. Calado RT, Brudno J, Mehta P, et al. Constitutional telomerase mutations are genetic risk factors for cirrhosis. *Hepatology.* 2011;53(5):1600–1607.

214. Hartmann D, Srivastava U, Thaler M, et al. Telomerase gene mutations are associated with cirrhosis formation. *Hepatology.* 2011;53(5):1608–1617.

215. Diaz de Leon A, Cronkhite JT, Yilmaz C, et al. Subclinical lung disease, macrocytosis, and premature graying in kindreds with telomerase (TERT) mutations. *Chest.* 2011;140(3):753–763.

216. Calado RT, Regal JA, Hills M, et al. Constitutional hypomorphic telomerase mutations in patients with acute myeloid leukemia. *Proc Natl Acad Sci USA.* 2009;106(4):1187–1192.

217. Kirwan M, Vulliamy T, Marrone A, et al. Defining the pathogenic role of telomerase mutations in myelodysplastic syndrome and acute myeloid leukemia. *Hum Mutat.* 2009;30(11):1567–1573.

218. Newton C, Batra K, Torrealba J, et al. Telomere-related lung fibrosis is diagnostically heterogeneous but uniformly progressive. *Eur Respir J.* 2016;48(6):1710–1720.

219. Silhan LL, Shah PD, Chambers DC, et al. Lung transplantation in telomerase mutation carriers with pulmonary fibrosis. *Eur Respir J.* 2014;44(1):178–187.

220. Borie R, Kannengiesser C, Hirschi S, et al. Severe hematologic complications after lung transplantation in patients with telomerase complex mutations. *J Heart Lung Transplant.* 2014.

221. Tokman S, Singer JP, Devine MS, et al. Clinical outcomes of lung transplantation in patients with telomerase mutations. *J Heart Lung Transplant.* 2015;34(10):1318–1324.

222. Cogan JD, Kropski JA, Zhao M, et al. Rare variants in RTEL1 are associated with familial interstitial pneumonia. *Am J Respir Crit Care Med.* 2015;191(6):646–655.

223. Stuart BD, Choi J, Zaidi S, et al. Exome sequencing links mutations in PARN and RTEL1 with familial pulmonary fibrosis and telomere shortening. *Nat Genet.* 2015;47(5):512–517.

224. Kannengiesser C, Borie R, Menard C, et al. Heterozygous RTEL1 mutations are associated with familial pulmonary fibrosis. *Eur Respir J.* 2015.

225. Kropski JA, Mitchell DB, Markin C, et al. A novel dyskerin (DKC1) mutation is associated with familial interstitial pneumonia. *Chest.* 2014;146(1):e1–e7.

226. Alder JK, Stanley SE, Wagner CL, Hamilton M, Hanumanthu VS, Armanios M. Exome sequencing identifies mutant TINF2 in a family with pulmonary fibrosis. *Chest.* 2015;147(5):1361–1368.

226a. Stanley SE, Gable DL, Wagner CL, et al. Loss-of-function mutations in the RNA biogenesis factor *NAF1* predispose to pulmonary fibrosis–emphysema. *Sci Transl Med.* 2016;8(351):351ra107.

227. Wang Y, Kuan PJ, Xing C, et al. Genetic defects in surfactant protein A2 are associated with pulmonary fibrosis and lung cancer. *Am J Hum Genet.* 2009;84(1):52–59.

228. van Moorsel CH, Ten Klooster L, van Oosterhout MF, et al. SFTPA2 mutations in familial and sporadic idiopathic interstitial pneumonia. *Am J Respir Crit Care Med.* 2015;192(10):1249–1252.

229. Nathan N, Giraud V, Picard C, et al. Germline SFTPA1 mutation in familial idiopathic interstitial pneumonia and lung cancer. *Hum Mol Genet.* 2016.

230. Maitra M, Wang Y, Gerard RD, Mendelson CR, Garcia CK. Surfactant protein A2 mutations associated with pulmonary fibrosis lead to protein instability and endoplasmic reticulum stress. *J Biol Chem.* 2010;285(29):22103–22113.

231. Seibold MA, Wise AL, Speer MC, et al. A common MUC5B promoter polymorphism and pulmonary fibrosis. *N Engl J Med.* 2011;364(16):1503–1512.

232. Fingerlin TE, Murphy E, Zhang W, et al. Genome-wide association study identifies multiple susceptibility loci for pulmonary fibrosis. *Nat Genet.* 2013;45(6):613–620.

233. Hunninghake GM, Hatabu H, Okajima Y, et al. MUC5B promoter polymorphism and interstitial lung abnormalities. *N Engl J Med.* 2013;368(23):2192–2200.

234. Schroeder BW, Verhaeghe C, Park SW, et al. AGR2 is induced in asthma and promotes allergen-induced mucin overproduction. *Am J Respir Cell Mol Biol.* 2012;47(2):178–185.

235. Zhao F, Edwards R, Dizon D, et al. Disruption of Paneth and goblet cell homeostasis and increased endoplasmic reticulum stress in Agr2-/- mice. *Dev Biol.* 2010;338(2):270–279.

236. Tsuru A, Fujimoto N, Takahashi S, et al. Negative feedback by IRE1beta optimizes mucin production in goblet cells. *Proc Natl Acad Sci USA.* 2013;110(8):2864–2869.

237. Mushiroda T, Wattanapokayakit S, Takahashi A, et al. A genome-wide association study identifies an association of a common variant in TERT with susceptibility to idiopathic pulmonary fibrosis. *J Med Genet.* 2008;45(10):654–656.

238. Calado RT, Young NS. Telomere diseases. *N Engl J Med.* 2009;361(24):2353–2365.

239. Levy D, Neuhausen SL, Hunt SC, et al. Genome-wide association identifies OBFC1 as a locus involved in human leukocyte telomere biology. *Proc Natl Acad Sci USA.* 2010;107(20):9293–9298.

240. Codd V, Nelson CP, Albrecht E, et al. Identification of seven loci affecting mean telomere length and their association with disease. *Nat Genet.* 2013;45(4):422–427. 427e421–e422.

241. Castellana G, Lamorgese V. Pulmonary alveolar microlithiasis. World cases and review of the literature. *Respiration.* 2003;70(5):549–555.

242. Sosman MC, Dodd GD, Jones WD, Pillmore GU. The familial occurrence of pulmonary alveolar microlithiasis. *Am J Roentgenol Radium Ther Nucl Med.* 1957;77(6):947–1012.

243. Ucan ES, Keyf AI, Aydilek R, et al. Pulmonary alveolar microlithiasis: review of Turkish reports. *Thorax.* 1993;48(2):171–173.

244. Melamed JW, Sostman HD, Ravin CE. Interstitial thickening in pulmonary alveolar microlithiasis: an underappreciated finding. *J Thorac Imaging.* 1994;9(2):126–128.

245. Helbich TH, Wojnarovsky C, Wunderbaldinger P, Heinz-Peer G, Eichler I, Herold CJ. Pulmonary alveolar microlithiasis in children: radiographic and high-resolution CT findings. *AJR Am J Roentgenol.* 1997;168(1):63–65.

246. Corut A, Senyigit A, Ugur SA, et al. Mutations in SLC34A2 cause pulmonary alveolar microlithiasis and are possibly associated with testicular microlithiasis. *Am J Hum Genet.* 2006;79(4):650–656.

247. Huqun, Izumi S, Miyazawa H, et al. Mutations in the SLC34A2 gene are associated with pulmonary alveolar microlithiasis. *Am J Respir Crit Care Med.* 2007;175(3):263–268.

248. Wang H, Yin X, Wu D. Novel human pathological mutations. SLC34A2. Pulmonary alveolar microlithiasis. *Hum Genet.* 2010;127(4):471.

249. Dogan OT, Ozsahin SL, Gul E, et al. A frame-shift mutation in the SLC34A2 gene in three patients with pulmonary alveolar microlithiasis in an inbred family. *Intern Med.* 2010;49(1):45–49.

250. Ishihara Y, Hagiwara K, Zen K, Huqun, Hosokawa Y, Natsuhara A. A case of pulmonary alveolar microlithiasis with an intragenetic deletion in SLC34A2 detected by a genome-wide SNP study. *Thorax.* 2009;64(4):365–367.

251. Hashimoto M, Wang DY, Kamo T, et al. Isolation and localization of type IIb Na/Pi cotransporter in the developing rat lung. *Am J Pathol.* 2000;157(1):21–27.

252. Feild JA, Zhang L, Brun KA, Brooks DP, Edwards RM. Cloning and functional characterization of a sodium-dependent phosphate transporter expressed in human lung and small intestine. *Biochem Biophys Res Commun.* 1999;258(3):578–582.

253. Traebert M, Hattenhauer O, Murer H, Kaissling B, Biber J. Expression of type II Na-P(i) cotransporter in alveolar type II cells. *Am J Physiol.* 1999;277(5 Pt 1):L868–L873.

254. Saito A, Nikolaidis NM, Amlal H, et al. Modeling pulmonary alveolar microlithiasis by epithelial deletion of the Npt2b sodium phosphate cotransporter reveals putative biomarkers and strategies for treatment. *Sci Transl Med.* 2015;7(313):313ra181.

255. Mulugeta S, Nureki S, Beers MF. Lost after translation: insights from pulmonary surfactant for understanding the role of alveolar epithelial dysfunction and cellular quality control in fibrotic lung disease. *Am J Physiol Lung Cell Mol Physiol.* 2015;309(6): L507–L525.

256. Tanjore H, Blackwell TS, Lawson WE. Emerging evidence for endoplasmic reticulum stress in the pathogenesis of idiopathic pulmonary fibrosis. *Am J Physiol Lung Cell Mol Physiol.* 2012;302(8):L721–L729.

257. Stuart BD, Lee JS, Kozlitina J, et al. Effect of telomere length on survival in patients with idiopathic pulmonary fibrosis: an observational cohort study with independent validation. *Lancet Respir Med.* 2014;2(7):557–565.

258. Dai J, Cai H, Li H, et al. Association between telomere length and survival in patients with idiopathic pulmonary fibrosis. *Respirology.* 2015;20(6):947–952.

# CHAPTER 2

# Pathobiology of Novel Approaches to Treatment

SILVIA PUGLISI • CARLO VANCHERI

---

**KEY POINTS**

- By virtue of basic research and new clinical observations, the amount of information and data on the pathobiology of IPF is growing day by day, offering new and more ample opportunities to either develop new therapies or reposition known drugs for IPF.
- A number of preclinical and clinical studies are currently under way with the aim of finding new and more potent drugs or effective cell-based treatments for IPF and possibly to personalize treatments, identifying subcategories of patients on the basis of genetic backgrounds and response to treatment.
- This will certainly be possible in a future not so distant, provided that the tree of knowledge for the pathobiology of IPF continues to grow florid and robust.

---

An understanding of the pathogenesis of any disease is crucial to identifying those cellular and molecular mechanisms through which a disease arises and evolves. This may lead to the discovery and development of new compounds and drugs that, acting on specific targets, may be effective in slowing or stopping the disease. Unfortunately, the pathogenesis of many complex diseases caused by the combination of genetic, environmental, and lifestyle factors is still not clear. Idiopathic pulmonary fibrosis (IPF) is no exception to this rule, and its pathogenesis represents the perfect example of a complex disease due to the combination of genetic predisposition and exogenous risk factors. Nevertheless, during the last few years, we have gathered useful information about some of the cellular and molecular pathways involved in the origin and progression of this dreadful disease. However, it must be admitted that some of the data collected derive either from diagnostic biopsies and explanted lung tissues or from in vitro and in vivo animal studies, and for this reason they may have some limitations.

Lung tissue from biopsy, and even more explanted tissue, mirrors disease in specific moments and very often when it is in an advanced stage, whereas in vitro and in vivo studies, although very suggestive and extremely useful, need to be confirmed in the context of the human disease. In spite of these objective limitations, there is scientific agreement in considering IPF the result of the interaction between the individual genetic background, the chronic action of different exogenous risk factors such as smoking, and the relentless action of aging. In susceptible and aged individuals, chronic damage caused by risk factors elicits an abnormal response of alveolar–bronchiolar cells that subsequently leads to the activation of fibroblasts and ultimately to tissue fibrosis. During the last 10 years some of these pathobiologic mechanisms, involved in the abnormal response to damage of epithelial cells and fibroblasts, have been disclosed, and today the overall picture of the pathogenesis of IPF seems less obscure. Based on these considerations this chapter will review some aspects of IPF pathobiology that have inspired research studies that emerged into clinical trials leading to the development of new drugs. The pathobiologic foundations of some ongoing trials will be also reviewed.

## THE APPROACH TO TREATMENT IN THE OLD DAYS

For many years lung fibrosis was considered the result of a chronic inflammatory process of the alveolar tissue that could evolve into fibrosis. Based on this belief and a long empiric experience (not supported by scientific evidence), the treatment of IPF was built for decades on high doses of steroids associated with immunosuppressants, such as azathioprine. This approach was also endorsed by the ATS/ERS statement published in 2000, although two Cochrane reviews[1] underlined the lack of randomized controlled trials exploring the effect of steroids and immunosuppressants in IPF. Both reviews concluded that there was very little evidence supporting the role of these drugs for the treatment of IPF. This is not surprising considering that the presence of inflammatory and immune cells is not a dominant feature of IPF lung tissue.[2] In addition, even if it is difficult to conceive, fibrosis may take place without being preceded by chronic inflammation. It has been demonstrated that it is possible to induce a fibrotic reaction in a lung culture system free of blood cells and soluble mediators. This model of "washed lung" suggested that the disruption of the normal epithelial–fibroblast interaction, induced by hyperoxia as the fibrogenic stimulus, may be sufficient, in the absence of the classical inflammatory cells, to induce epithelial damage and to promote fibroblast growth and collagen deposition, in other words, to create tissue fibrosis.[3] This is possible because epithelial cells and fibroblasts, commonly considered structural cells, are not merely bystander cells forming the scaffold of the lung, but are instead able to produce and release mediators, to proliferate and differentiate into more active and aggressive phenotypes, and eventually to affect the behavior of the surrounding microenvironment. The turning point in defining the real nature of the pathogenesis of IPF was made by Selman in 2002; he described IPF as a noninflammatory fibroproliferative disorder triggered by an unknown stimulus responsible for alveolar epithelial cell (AEC) injury. According to this hypothesis, epithelial damage and the subsequent altered crosstalk between fibroblasts and epithelium caused the release of growth factors and cytokines involved in the recruitment and differentiation of mesenchymal cells into myofibroblasts.[4]

In spite of the clear evidence showing a limited role for inflammation in the pathogenesis of IPF, the treatment of this disease remained based on steroids and immunosuppressants. This was likely due to at least three reasons: (1) In the recent past the diagnosis of IPF was not as accurate as today, and in some patients, with other forms of lung fibrosis such as nonspecific interstitial pneumonia (NSIP), the "traditional treatment" with steroids and immunosuppressants could be effective. (2) There is a complete lack of any other alternative treatment with the exception of lung transplantation. (3) Controlled clinical trials demonstrating whether or not this treatment was effective are lacking. This final gap was eventually filled in 2012 with the

PANTHER study, a clinical trial designed to assess the efficacy and safety of triple therapy (prednisone, azathioprine, and N-acetylcysteine [NAC]) in IPF patients. Quite surprisingly, this trial was stopped before its conclusion because of an excessive number of deaths, hospitalizations, and adverse events in the treated group,[5] and the absence of any efficacy. The PANTHER study put an end to the "traditional therapy" with steroids and immunosuppressants for the treatment of IPF.

In the meantime, additional experimental data had confirmed the marginal role of inflammation in IPF showing instead the key role of AECs and fibroblasts. According to more recent studies, the inception of tissue fibrosis is due to the exposure of AECs to chronic microinjuries, such as those caused by smoking or environmental and/or professional exposures that may damage the epithelium, causing, in susceptible individuals, the activation of incorrect repair mechanisms and stress response pathways that eventually promote fibroblast recruitment and proliferation.[6] During normal tissue repair processes, when wound healing is over, the activity of fibroblasts ends, and they undergo apoptosis. However, in some circumstances, and IPF is one of those, fibroblast functions are altered resulting in their permanence into the tissue, ongoing deposition of extracellular matrix (ECM) proteins, parenchymal distortion, and ultimately fibrosis. Starting from this pathogenic evidence, new preclinical studies and clinical trials have been designed, shifting their focus from antiinflammatory molecules to targeting components of the wound healing cascade and fibrogenesis.

## THE ADVENT OF PIRFENIDONE

Pirfenidone (5-methyl-1-phenyl-2-[1H]-pyridone) is an orally available synthetic pyridone compound that has been shown to inhibit the progression of fibrosis in animal models and in in vitro systems. Pirfenidone has been used for the treatment of different models of fibrotic diseases, including liver, renal, and cardiac fibrosis, all situations characterized by the abnormal deposition of collagen. The mechanism of action is still not fully understood, but preclinical studies suggest that pirfenidone combines antiinflammatory, antioxidant, and above all antifibrotic properties. Pirfenidone exerts its antiinflammatory action mainly through the regulation of tumor necrosis factor alpha and beta (TNF-α and TNF-β) pathways,[7,8] whereas its antioxidant activity is exerted through the reduction of lipid peroxidation and partly because of its scavenger activity for toxic hydroxyl radicals.[9] However, pirfenidone is best known for its antifibrotic properties.

Fibroblasts are normally quiescent cells unless tissue injury occurs. In this situation they undergo a phenotypic transition into myofibroblasts acquiring contractile and secretory properties and synthesizing collagen and ECM proteins. This is an important step in the pathogenesis of IPF, and many studies have proposed TGF-β as the key fibrogenic cytokine responsible for fibroblast differentiation.[10] The major signaling pathway of TGF-β is through its transmembrane receptor serine/threonine kinases that in turn activate the cytoplasmic Smad proteins, and more specifically Smad3, inducing alpha smooth muscle actin (SMA) gene expression and subsequently fibroblast differentiation.[11] It has been also demonstrated that Smad-independent molecular pathways such as phosphatidylinositol-3-kinase/protein kinase B (PI3K/Akt) might be involved in myofibroblast differentiation induced by TGF-β.[12]

A number of in vitro and in vivo animal studies have demonstrated that pirfenidone inhibits collagen synthesis and ECM deposition and reduces fibroblast proliferation and, most important, their differentiation into myofibroblasts.[13] Other studies have shown that pirfenidone also decreases TGF-β–induced α-SMA and procollagen (Col) I at mRNA and protein levels. These "antifibrotic" effects are likely related to the inhibition exerted by pirfenidone on the phosphorylation induced by TGF-β of Smad3, p38, and Akt, key factors for the regulation of this pathway.[14] Other studies performed on the bleomycin model of lung fibrosis have described a diminished presence of profibrotic factors such as TGF-β in the bronchoalveolar lavage fluid (BALF) of pirfenidone-treated animals and a concurrent reduction of the accumulation of hydroxyproline, Col I, and Col III in BAL and lung tissue.[15]

Even if the exact mechanisms through which pirfenidone acts were only partially known, the identification of its antioxidant and antiinflammatory properties along with a surprising antifibrotic activity redefined the clinical interest for this pleiotropic drug. In spite of that, it took a few years to have the first double-blind randomized clinical trial testing the efficacy of pirfenidone in IPF patients. This was a Japanese Phase II study that was stopped after only 9 months because it was considered unethical to continue the study considering the increased number of acute exacerbations in the placebo group compared with the group treated with pirfenidone. The primary endpoint of the study was not achieved—there was no difference in the saturation of peripheral oxygen under exertion between the placebo and the pirfenidone arm, but a significant reduction in the decline of vital capacity was described in the

pirfenidone group.[16] These encouraging results led to another study in Japan, whose primary endpoint was the change in vital capacity from baseline at 52 weeks. This time the study met its primary endpoint showing that the loss in vital capacity was significantly higher in the placebo group. It was also proved that pirfenidone increased the progression-free survival (PFS) defined as the time until death and 10% or more decline in vital capacity from baseline.[17]

In the meantime two multinational randomized double-blind placebo-controlled Phase III trials (004 and 006) named CAPACITY started in Europe, Australia, and North America to test the efficacy of pirfenidone in patients affected by mild to moderate IPF. The primary endpoint, common to both studies, was defined as the change in forced vital capacity (FVC) percentage from baseline to 72 weeks. In study 004, pirfenidone significantly reduced FVC decline at week 72 but did not reduce decline in 6-min walk test (6MWT) distance, while study 006 failed to meet its primary endpoint but reduced the decline in 6MWT distance.[18] Based on the positive results of the one CAPACITY and Japanese studies, pirfenidone was approved in 2011 by the European Medicines Agency (EMA) for the treatment of mild to moderate IPF. The Food and Drug Administration (FDA) required an additional trial to approve the use of pirfenidone in the United States; this was called the ASCEND trial. In ASCEND, pirfenidone significantly reduced the proportion of patients who experienced a decline of 10% or more in FVC and the relative risk of death or disease progression.[19] All patients randomized to pirfenidone 2403 mg/day or placebo in the CAPACITY and ASCEND trials were included in a pooled analysis aimed to assess safety and efficacy of pirfenidone at 1 year of treatment. This study suggested that pirfenidone reduces the risk of death by 48% and improves PFS by 38% in IPF patients compared to placebo.[20]

As already underlined in this chapter, the understanding of the pathogenic mechanisms of a disease can be important to developing new drugs. Similarly, the comprehension of the mechanisms of action of a drug is useful to better understand its potential therapeutic effect as well as to predict and possibly avoid side effects. For this reason, preclinical and clinical studies thoroughly evaluated the safety profile of pirfenidone.

To further evaluate the long-term safety and tolerability of the drug, patients who participated in five different clinical trials were analyzed: three Phase III multinational trials (CAPACITY 004, 006, and ASCEND) and the two ongoing open label studies RECAP (002, 012). This study collected data from a large and well-defined cohort of IPF patients who were treated with pirfenidone and followed for up to 9.9 years. The major adverse events were gastrointestinal (GI) events [nausea (37.6%), diarrhea (28.1%), dyspepsia (18.4%), and vomiting (15.9%)] and rash (25.0%). Elevations in blood levels of aminotransferase greater than three times the upper limit of normal occurred in 3.1% of patients. All of these events were mild to moderate in severity, transient with dose modification, and without clinical long-term consequences.[21]

Many studies have been conducted to explain the molecular mechanism responsible for GI events. Animal studies showed that pirfenidone reduces the rate of gastric emptying and small intestinal transit, and this effect can be relieved by the administration of prokinetic drugs. It was demonstrated that the concomitant administration of mosapride and splitting pirfenidone doses during meals improve the decrease in gastric emptying rate caused by pirfenidone.[22]

Rubino et al. studied the pharmacokinetic features of pirfenidone in a group of healthy volunteers and described the effects of the simultaneous assumption with food. The combination of pirfenidone with food caused a reduction and delay in the absorption of the drug and a reduced plasma concentration of both drug and metabolites. These results have an important clinical repercussion because a correlation between plasma concentration and the risk of adverse events has been demonstrated, suggesting that food may reduce the incidence of GI events.[23]

On the basis of these previous studies, it is suggested that patients take the drug during or at the end of the meal, start with a longer initial dosing titration, and take a prokinetic drug if necessary to reduce the incidence of GI events. If GI events occur, it is suggested to reduce the dose and, if the adverse event persists, temporarily discontinue treatment until the symptoms become tolerable.[24]

Photosensitivity is the second most common adverse event that may be caused by pirfenidone. A study performed on guinea pigs demonstrated that pirfenidone is photoreactive, which means that it can absorb ultraviolet B and A (UVB, UVA) radiation, causing the generation of reactive oxygen species (ROS) and lipid peroxidations that may be responsible for sunburn. After oral administration, pirfenidone distribution to the UV-exposed tissue (skin) is even higher than in lung tissue.[25] Based on these findings, it is suggested that patients avoid sun exposure, protect skin with sunscreen active against both UVA and UVB radiation, and to wear protective clothes. Photosensitivity reaction is also related to pirfenidone dose, so that dosage adjustment or temporary discontinuation is indicated if the

side effect does not resolve spontaneously. Pharmacologic treatment with oral and/or topical steroids and antihistamines is suggested in cases of persistence of the skin reaction.

On one hand, it is helpful to reduce the dose of pirfenidone to reduce the risk of adverse events, but on the other it is necessary to maintain the correct serum concentration of the drug to maximize its effectiveness. It is important to adjust the dose of pirfenidone carefully in each patient to balance tolerability with expected efficacy.

It has been estimated that 70–80% of pirfenidone is metabolized by cytochrome CYP1A2 and by CYP2C9, 2C19, 2D6, and 2E1. Thus the concomitant use of inhibitors of CYP1A2, such as grapefruit and fluvoxamine, should be avoided during the treatment with pirfenidone because they could increase the exposure to the drug and the risk of side effects. Conversely, strong inducers of CYP1A2, such as cigarette smoke, should be avoided because they may accelerate drug clearance reducing its effectiveness.

The oral administration of pirfenidone is followed by a rapid degradation of the molecule in two metabolites, 5-hydroxypirfenidone and 5-carboxypirfenidone, and their elimination in the urine.[26] These two metabolites still have antifibrotic properties, as demonstrated by Togami et al., and their distribution in lung tissue is low if compared with the liver and kidneys because of a low affinity between metabolites and lung tissue.[27] The direct consequence of this observation is the intriguing idea that pirfenidone and its metabolites could reach higher concentrations in the lung when administered by inhalation instead of the traditional oral route.

## THE STORY OF NINTEDANIB

Based on its prognosis, IPF has been generically compared to malignant disease. Similar to cancer, IPF is associated with risk factors such as smoking and/or environmental or professional exposure, and the presence of a specific genetic background is considered fundamental for the occurrence of the disease. In addition, IPF and cancer share a number of pathogenic pathways such as genetic and epigenetic alterations, abnormal expression of miRNAs, cellular and molecular aberrance including an altered response to regulatory signals, delayed apoptosis, reduced cell-to-cell communication, and above all the activation of specific signal transduction pathways.[28] These signaling pathways are fundamental to translate any extracellular signal in an equivalent cell response and action. In this process, an extracellular signaling molecule stimulates a specific receptor inside the cell or on its surface, producing a series of intracellular events that lead, depending on the cellular type, to gene activation, metabolism alterations, or in general, changes in cell behavior.

A large variety of signal transduction pathways are activated both in cancer and in IPF, and many studies have demonstrated their involvement in the pathogenesis of these two diseases. It has been largely demonstrated that alterations of the Wnt signaling transduction pathway have clinical relevance in the pathogenesis of cancer.[29] Indeed, the Wnt/β-catenin signaling pathway regulates the expression of molecules involved in tissue invasion such as matrilysin, laminin, and cyclin-D1, and it is also involved in a biologically relevant crosstalk with TGF-β. It is interesting to note that the Wnt/β-catenin pathway is also strongly activated in IPF lung tissue as evidenced by extensive nuclear accumulation of β-catenin at different involved sites such as bronchiolar proliferative lesions, damaged alveolar structures, and fibroblast foci.[30] The functional significance of β-catenin has been well demonstrated by the description of an intense immunoreactivity for β-catenin and by the subsequent expression of high levels of cyclin-D1 and matrilysin. Caraci et al. have demonstrated that the Wnt/β-catenin pathway may also be activated by TGF-β through the induction of α-SMA expression via extracellular-regulated kinases (ERK)1/2 activation, glycogen synthase kinase-3beta (GSK-3beta) inhibition, and nuclear β-catenin translocation that leads to fibroblast activation and collagen production in human lung fibroblasts.[31]

Several studies are currently exploring the anticancer effect of specific inhibitors of the Wnt pathway such as ICG-001. It is interesting that the same compound has already been used with success in an animal model of lung fibrosis. Another key process not only described in carcinogenesis but also likely involved in causing IPF is the altered regulation of apoptosis. In this case the PI3K/Akt signaling pathway plays an important role. This pathway is involved in the regulation of cell growth, proliferation, and survival. Phosphoinositol-3-kinase (PI3K) stimulates the synthesis of phosphatidylinositol-3,4,5-triphosphate, which causes the activation of Akt-modulated cellular processes such as protection from apoptosis.[32] Based on its primary structure and in vitro lipid substrate specificity, it is possible to recognize three different classes of PI3K: classes I, II, and III. Recently, Conte et al. assessed the expression of class I PI3K p110 isoform in IPF lung tissue as well as in tissue-derived fibroblast cell lines and evaluated the effect of the selective inhibition of p110 isoforms on the proliferation and fibrogenic activity of the IPF

fibroblast. The expression of PI3K p110, alpha, beta, and delta isoforms does not differ between normal and IPF tissue–derived fibroblasts, whereas immune reactivity for p110 gamma was much stronger in both IPF lung homogenates and ex vivo fibroblast cell lines. Furthermore, both p110 gamma pharmacologic inhibition and gene silencing significantly inhibited the proliferation rate as well as α-SMA expression in IPF fibroblasts. These data strongly suggest that this isoform of PI3K may have a role in the pathogenesis of IPF, representing a novel specific pharmacologic target.[33]

In this regard, a recent study has demonstrated that oral administration of a p110 gamma inhibitor prevents bleomycin-induced pulmonary fibrosis in rats. More recently researchers have focused their attention on another signal transduction pathway activated in IPF and frequently altered in many cancers: the JAK–STAT signaling pathway. This system is a major signaling alternative to the second messenger system such as cyclic AMP, cyclic GMP, inositol triphosphate, diacylglycerol, and calcium. It transmits chemical signals from outside the cell, through the cell membrane toward the cytoplasm, and then into the nucleus. Here, it affects the activity of gene promoter regions, causing DNA transcription and cell activation. One of the regulatory mechanisms of the JAK-STAT signaling pathway is represented by the SOCS family (suppressor of cytokine signaling proteins). Bao et al. have demonstrated that in IPF patients there is a lower expression of SOCS1 and this finding has been related to more severe manifestations of the disease and to a worse prognosis.[34]

One of the most studied signaling pathways, strongly activated not only in many cancers, but also in IPF, is the tyrosine kinase pathway. Tyrosine kinase is an enzyme that acts as a sort of "on" or "off" switch that regulates many cellular functions. Mutations can turn tyrosine kinases in a nonstop functional state that, under specific circumstances, may lead to the initiation or progression of cancer. More recently this pathway has also been studied in the context of the wound healing process and fibrosis.[35] Indeed, tyrosine kinases catalyze the phosphorylation of tyrosine residues in proteins such as platelet-derived growth factor (PDGF), fibroblast growth factor (FGF), or vascular endothelial growth factor (VEGF), regulating a wide array of cellular functions, including cell growth, differentiation, adhesion, motility, and regulation of cell death.

PDGF, a ligand of tyrosine kinase receptor, is a heterodimeric molecule expressed in different cells, including fibroblasts. Binding of PDGF to its receptor (PDGFr) leads to autophosphorylation of the receptor and activates intracellular pathways, such as Ras, Raf, and MEK, and extracellular ones such as ERK and PI3K. PDGF is a potent growth factor for fibroblasts in vitro, and some mediators such as TGF-β and basic FGF have PDGF-dependent profibrotic activities. PDGF is more highly expressed in epithelial cells and alveolar macrophages in the lungs of patients with IPF.[36] Moreover, high levels of PDGF have been shown in irradiated mice, and the use of a PDGFr inhibitor has attenuated the development of pulmonary fibrosis in animal models induced by radiation.[37]

In addition to PDGF, FGF is involved not only in carcinogenesis but also in fibrogenesis. FGF receptors (FGFrs) are present on epithelial cells and fibroblasts and mediate epithelial–mesenchymal transition and fibroblast transition into myofibroblasts.[38] FGF and more specifically two members of this family of growth factors such as FGF1 and FGF2 are potent activators of fibroblast proliferation and collagen production. The binding of FGF to FGFr causes autophosphorylation and activation of downstream signaling via PI3K/Akt, ERK1/2, and Ras/Raf/MAPK pathways.[39] Interestingly, TGF-β regulates the FGFr cascade, inducing the upregulation of FGFr-1 and the release of FGF2 in human lung fibroblasts.[40,41] In animal models of pulmonary fibrosis FGFr-1 is strongly upregulated, whereas it is not expressed in control animals, suggesting its involvement in the fibrotic process.[42] This is substantiated by the observation that inhibition of FGF signaling ameliorates bleomycin-induced pulmonary fibrosis.[43] In addition, increased levels of FGF have been detected in lung cells of patients affected by IPF.[44]

If the role of VEGF in cancer is well recognized, its involvement in IPF is less clear. VEGF is produced by alveolar and bronchial epithelial cells, airway smooth muscle cells, fibroblasts, and endothelial cells. VEGFr is characterized by the typical intracellular domain that undergoes autophosphorylation as a consequence of the binding VEGF-VEGFr, activating different signaling pathways (p38, PI3K, Ras) involved in cell proliferation and migration. In IPF patients, VEGF expression is low in fibroblasts and leukocytes in fibrotic lesions, but increased in endothelial cells and AECs.[45] Parkas et al. reported direct effects of VEGF-A in lung fibroblasts, enhancing collagen I expression induced by β.[46] More recently, high VEGF serum concentration in IPF patients was related to a worse 5-year survival rate.[47] The precise role of VEGF-VEGFr signaling in IPF is controversial, and further studies are required to clarify its exact role. Nevertheless, VEGF and even more PDGF and FGF have a potent effect on fibroblast activation and proliferation, and their inhibition is expected to reduce fibrosis in IPF.

Based on the previous discussion, tyrosine kinases receptor inhibitors, widely used in non–small cell lung

carcinoma and other cancers, have been tested for the treatment of IPF. Imatinib mesylate, a specific inhibitor of PDGFr, was evaluated for its potential antifibrotic effects in preclinical and clinical studies. It was able to inhibit fibroblast proliferation and collagen deposition in vitro and in vivo, but when it was evaluated in a clinical trial, no benefit in slowing disease progression was found.[48] To achieve a more potent antifibrotic effect, other compounds able to exert an inhibition of multiple receptors were tested. BIBF 1000, an inhibitor of PDGFr, VEGFr, and FGFr, was first evaluated in a mice model of bleomycin-induced pulmonary fibrosis and in an ex vivo fibroblast differentiation assay. It was found to attenuate fibrosis by reducing the expression of profibrotic factors and by decreasing collagen deposition.[49]

Along the same lines, BIBF1120 (nintedanib), a triple kinase inhibitor, with potent suppressing effects on VEGFr, PDGFr, and FGFr, was also evaluated. Nintedanib exerts its inhibitory effect on PDGF, FGF, and VEGF through the occupation of the intracellular ATP-binding pocket of the tyrosine kinases.[50] This drug interferes with fibroblast proliferation as well as with the secretion and deposition of ECM. It has been shown in a mice model that nintedanib reduces TIMP1 and TIMP2, which in turn inhibit matrix metalloproteinases responsible for the degradation of collagen type I and II. It also reduces collagen deposition and inhibits the transformation of fibroblasts into myofibroblasts in human lung fibroblasts of IPF patients[51] by TGF-β.[52]

More recently, nintedanib was studied in clinical trials as a potential antifibrotic therapy in IPF, demonstrating that treatment with this drug may reduce the decline in lung function of IPF patients by about 50%. Based on these results, nintedanib has been approved as a new therapy in patients with IPF. This is relevant, because for the first time, based on the observation of the pathogenic similarities between IPF and cancer, a drug "borrowed" from another field, in this case oncology, has been "repositioned" for IPF. "Drug repositioning" is an interesting and convenient strategy that may save time and reduce costs in the development of a specific drug. The safety profile of the explored drug is already known so that the risk of adverse events is reduced. In addition, the mechanism of action of a repositioned drug is known and can be used in those diseases where a similar mechanism is involved. Today, computational strategies are available to explore the mechanisms of action of approved drugs and to match them with cellular and/or molecular targets involved in the pathogenesis of virtually any disease.

The first randomized, double-blind, placebo-controlled, Phase II trial conducted to evaluate the efficacy of nintedanib in IPF patients (TOMORROW study) demonstrated, in the group receiving BIBF1120, a reduction of 68.4% in the annual rate of decline in FVC and a lower incidence of acute exacerbations compared with placebo.[53] Following the results of this clinical trial, two other randomized double-blind Phase III trials (INPULSIS-1, INPULSIS-2) were performed. A total of 1066 IPF patients were randomized in a 3:2 ratio to receive placebo or BIBF1120. This treatment reduced the rate of decline in FVC over the 52-week study period in both INPULSIS trials. The secondary endpoints were represented by the time to the first exacerbation and the change in total St. George's Respiratory Questionnaire (SGRQ) score, but no consistent differences were found between the placebo and the nintedanib groups.[54] Recently, pooled analyses of data from the three trials (TOMORROW, INPULSIS 1 and 2) were performed to obtain an overall estimate of the clinical efficacy of nintedanib in 1231 IPF patients. Nintedanib consistently slowed disease progression, reducing the annual rate decline in FVC compared with the placebo group and causing a modest change in SGRQ total score from the baseline. This analysis also demonstrated a positive trend toward a reduction in risk for all-cause and respiratory mortality.[55]

Nintedanib, after its oral administration, is rapidly metabolized by hepatocytes into metabolite BIBF1202. This metabolite is eliminated through the liver and feces, while the excretion in the urine is minimal.[56] The hepatic metabolism of nintedanib is CYP450 independent; therefore, the drug interactions are very limited if compared with pirfenidone. Particular care should be used in patients affected by coagulopathy at risk of bleeding because nintedanib, as an inhibitor of VEGF, can theoretically cause bleeding. The most frequent adverse events recorded during the studies were GI events, especially diarrhea, which occurred in 61.5% of patients in INPULSIS-1 and 63.2% in INPULSIS-2, and increased liver enzymes levels, which occurred in 4.9% of patients in INPULSIS-1 and 5.2% of patients in INPULSIS-2, respectively. In the pooled data analysis, diarrhea was the most frequent adverse event in the nintedanib group (61.5% of patients treated with nintedanib vs. 17.9% of patients treated with placebo). In general, adverse events are reversible with reducing the dose of nintedanib or stopping the treatment, without clinically significant consequences.[55]

Diarrhea was described as the most frequent adverse event following nintedanib assumption. The pathophysiologic mechanism of drug-induced diarrhea is still not completely understood, but some studies conducted for oncologic tyrosine kinase inhibitors could be helpful to understand the molecular mechanisms through which

diarrhea develops. It has been supposed that patients treated with tyrosine kinase inhibitors that are directed against EGFR experience diarrhea because of the excessive chloride secretion and deficient sodium absorption. In the normal colon, sodium absorption and chloride secretion are stimulated directly by intracellular messengers such as c-AMP and intracellular calcium. EGFR is a negative regulator of chloride secretion and is expressed in GI normal mucosa. EGFR inhibitors could increase chloride secretion, inducing a secretory diarrhea.[57] Diarrhea following imatinib has also been related to c-Kit inhibition, highly expressed in the interstitial cells of Cajal, which have a pacemaker function in the intestine, so that c-Kit inhibition can cause an alteration in the intestinal motility resulting in diarrhea.[58]

Nintedanib dose reduction rapidly lowers the incidence and severity of diarrhea. Sometimes the addition of loperamide is indicated as a useful treatment to decrease intestinal motility.

## NAC (*N*-ACETYLCYSTEINE) OR NOT NAC, THAT IS THE QUESTION

The use of antioxidants in the treatment of IPF is based on the hypothesis that the disease can develop from an oxidant-antioxidant imbalance responsible for repeated AEC injuries followed by fibrotic repair. ROS play an important role in the fibrotic process as demonstrated by the reduced levels of glutathione (GSH) in BAL of IPF patients.[59] NAC is a precursor of GSH and a powerful antioxidant scavenger of ROS. The first clinical trial to test oral NAC combined with prednisone and azathioprine was the IFIGENIA study, which showed that NAC combination therapy given for 1 year significantly reduced the functional decline of IPF in terms of vital and diffusing capacity compared to prednisone and azathioprine alone. In spite of these encouraging results it took several years to have additional information on the therapeutic role of NAC in IPF. In 2011 a specific study, named "PANTHER," was initiated to assess the efficacy of the triple therapy (prednisone, azathioprine, and NAC) compared to NAC alone and placebo in a 1:1:1 ratio. It is well known that the trial failed, showing an increase in the number of deaths and hospitalizations in the group treated with the triple therapy. The study was continued to explore the difference between NAC monotherapy and placebo. This part of the PANTHER study showed quite clearly that NAC alone was not superior to placebo in reducing FVC decline.[60]

A noteworthy recent observation suggests that a single nucleotide polymorphism in the TOLLIP gene, known to be involved in lung host defense, may influence the effect of antioxidant therapy in IPF patients. These data suggest that IPF patients with the rs3750920 TOLLIP TT genotype may respond to NAC treatment.[61] Inhaled NAC in monotherapy has also been tested in a multicenter, perspective, randomized, controlled clinical trial in Japanese patients with early-stage IPF. This study demonstrated a possible beneficial effect of the drug in patients with early-stage IPF.[62] Recently, a retrospective observational study involving 22 Japanese patients affected by early untreated IPF was conducted to assess the efficacy on FVC and GSH levels. This study suggested that patients with higher oxidative stress could develop a better response to NAC treatment, likely because NAC replenishes GSH levels, correcting the oxidant–antioxidant imbalance.[63] Thus oxidative stress can be a possible marker of response to NAC treatment. These results support new perspective clinical trials to test the efficacy of either oral NAC based on genotypic stratification of IPF patients or inhaled NAC based on oxidative stress levels of patients with an early-stage disease. These approaches will allow for identifying subgroups of patients responding to NAC, hopefully opening a fascinating view on the first attempt of personalized therapy for IPF. As things stand, the real effectiveness of NAC is still debated and more studies are needed.

## ANTACID TREATMENT: MORE DOUBTS THAN CERTAINTIES

Gastroesophageal reflux is highly prevalent in patients with IPF compared with patients affected by other interstitial lung diseases and healthy people.[64] It has been proposed that in some predisposed patients, gastroesophageal reflux disease (GERD) and repetitive microaspiration of acid in the airways can cause continuous AEC injury, triggering those pathogenic mechanisms underlying IPF.[65] Microaspiration also may be involved in acute exacerbations of IPF as suggested by the discovery of high levels of pepsin in BALF of IPF patients with acute exacerbations. The logical consequence of these observations was to investigate the role of proton pump inhibitors (PPI) in IPF. Indeed in the literature there is some evidence showing a positive role for antacid treatment in IPF.

It has been also demonstrated that PPI could also have antifibrotic and antiinflammatory properties through the direct suppression of proinflammatory cytokines (such as TNF-α, IL1-β, IL-6) and via the downregulation of TGF-β receptors involved in fibroblast proliferation.[66]

In a noncontrolled retrospective study of 204 IPF patients, Lee et al. observed a lower radiologic fibrosis score and longer survival in those patients receiving antacid treatment.[67] It was also reported that medication for GERD and Nissen fundoplication were independent predictors of longer survival for IPF. A more recent study has demonstrated a slower decline of functional capacity in IPF patients affected by GERD and treated with antacid therapy suggesting, once again, a possible benefit for antacid treatment.[68] More recently, Lee et al. have reported in a cohort of 786 IPF patients a protective effect of PPI used for at least 4 months.[69] Based on these results the current guidelines for IPF treatment provide a conditional recommendation for the use of PPIs in IPF patients.[70] Recently, a post hoc analysis from the placebo groups of three trials of pirfenidone (CAPACITY and ASCEND) showed that antacid therapy is not related to a clinical significant improvement in outcomes after 52 weeks of treatment in either PFS or mortality.[71] According to this study IPF patients with advanced disease (defined as FVC <70%) receiving antacid treatment had a higher infection rate than patients who did not receive antacid treatment. New studies are required to assess the real efficacy of antacid treatment, especially in advanced IPF stages.

## CURRENT CLINICAL TRIALS: THE FUTURE IS COMING

The pathobiology of IPF is complex; several cellular and molecular mechanisms are involved in its occurrence and progression. Some of these mechanisms are obscure, some others are partially clear, and some of them are well understood and are being used to develop new therapeutic strategies. By virtue of this, a great deal of preclinical and clinical work has been performed in the last few years, and much more is currently under way to explore novel treatments and therapeutic strategies for IPF. All of them are obviously inspired by the new pathogenic knowledge that comes every day from the research field. Recently, there has been interest in novel agents that target type 2 T-helper cell (Th2) inflammatory pathways such as interleukin 13 (IL-13). Phase II randomized, double-blind, placebo-controlled trials of two monoclonal antibodies against IL-13, lebrikizumab and tralokinumab, are currently under way. The rationale for the use of antimonoclonal antibodies against IL-13 is based on some studies that nicely showed that IL-13, a cytokine secreted by Th2 cells, is a strong stimulator of fibroblast proliferation, acting through multiple mechanisms, including interaction with TG-beta and CCL2, thus inducing fibrosis.[72] However, the exact mechanism whereby IL-13 promotes pulmonary fibrosis has not been completely defined, with studies showing either a TGF-β–dependent[73] or a TGF-β–independent pathway.[74] IL-13 signals through its respective receptor subunits via JAK2–STAT6–dependent and AP1-dependent pathways,[75] but some studies have suggested that IL-13 Ra2 also has a role in the signaling mechanisms.[76] Thus, it has been suggested that IL-13 and its receptor subunits are involved in the pathogenesis of pulmonary fibrosis, and even if the correct mechanism is still not completely understood, they are considered targetable. In this regard Murray et al. studied biopsy samples from IPF patients who experimented a rapidly progressing form of IPF, demonstrating that the IL-13 pathway was enhanced compared to IPF patients with a slower decline in FVC. It has also been suggested that the inhibition of IL-13 promotes lung repair and helps to restore epithelial integrity; therefore, targeting IL-13 inhibits fibrotic processes and promotes the repairing process in the lung.[77]

According to the recent evidence, fibroblasts in IPF lungs could partially derive from circulating monocytes that leave the circulation, reach the lung, and then differentiate into fibrocytes through a process mediated by a family of proteins named pentraxins.[78] There are three main systemic pentraxins in humans: SAP (serum amyloid P component), CRP (C-reactive protein), and PTX3. It has been demonstrated that PTX3 promotes fibrocyte differentiation, whereas injections of SAP in a mouse model of pulmonary fibrosis inhibit fibrosis.[79] A previous study has also showed the potential for pentraxin SAP to inhibit bleomycin-induced lung fibrosis through the inhibition of monocyte differentiation in fibrocytes in vitro and in vivo.[80] On the basis of these evidences, a new drug PRM-151 (recombinant human pentraxin 2, known as serum amyloid P) was tested in IPF patients in a randomized, double-blind, placebo-controlled trial that assessed safety, tolerability, and pharmacokinetics of single ascending intravenous doses of this drug administered to healthy subjects and IPF patients. The drug was well tolerated, and just transient skin reactions were observed as adverse events. A 30–40% decrease in the number of fibrocytes 24 h post dose was also registered, suggesting that drug administration may be associated with a reduction of these cells in IPF. Interestingly, FVC showed a trend toward improvement in the treated group.[81] However, the number of patients of this preliminary, although very interesting, study was very low. Further and larger studies are needed to test the real efficacy of this molecule. A clinical trial exploring the efficacy of pentraxin 2 on a larger population of patients with IPF is currently under way.

Connective tissue growth factor (CTGF) is a matricellular protein that connects cell surfaces and ECM. Lung fibroblasts are dependent on CTGF that regulates their attachment to the matrix and subsequently their migration, differentiation, and apoptosis.[82] CTGF is upregulated in tissues subjected to mechanical stress as may happen in lung fibrosis,[83] and it is believed that activation of fibroblasts by TGF-β also induces CTGF expression. Increased levels of CTGF have been recorded in BALF and lung tissue of IPF patients.[84] It has also been proven in animal models that targeting CTGF diminishes fibrosis.[85] Raghu et al. for the first time studied the efficacy of anti-CTGF monoclonal antibodies for the treatment of IPF patients in a Phase II clinical trial,[86] and following these results a new phase II clinical trial was started to assess efficacy and safety of this new molecule.[87]

In parallel to the numerous pharmacological investigations, cell-based strategies have been explored as a possible alternative to pharmacologic treatments. Cell-based therapies represent an innovative possibility to treat patients with lung fibrosis because transplanted cells could be potentially able to proliferate and differentiate into alveolar cells replacing the damaged epithelial alveolar cells and some benefits could be obtained from the paracrine properties of the newly administered cells. Different kinds of cells have been proposed for a possible new IPF treatment, including not only AECs, but also lung mixed epithelial cells, mesenchymal cells, stem cells, and circulating endothelial progenitor cells.

Serrano-Mollar et al. have reported that transplanting AECsII, obtained by in vitro differentiation of healthy organs, in bleomycin-induced pulmonary fibrosis lung could reverse the fibrotic process.[88] Stem cells also represent a promising option for therapeutic application in IPF and because of their capacity to differentiate into different cell lines and to exert both antiproliferative and antiinflammatory effects. Stem cell properties have been investigated in murine models of lung fibrosis in different studies, showing that murine bone marrow–derived mesenchymal stem cells are able to target damaged pulmonary areas and to reduce inflammation and collagen deposition in the lung.[89] Similar results were achieved using transplanted placenta-derived stem cells, demonstrating neutrophil infiltration decrease and a significative reduction in the severity of fibrosis.[90]

The most important issues, concerning the type of cells used, regard cell recruitment to the lung, the induction of differentiation in epithelial lung cells, and the risk of cancer, especially teratoma. Different routes of cell administration were tested, intravenously or through intraperitoneal or intratracheal instillation, showing different capacity to reach the lung, but it is still debatable which is the more effective. Other issues are unsolved such as the effective cell dose equivalent for cell therapy, defined as the minimum cell number required to have a significant result. Few clinical trials have been conducted so far on cell-based therapy in IPF, and only some of these have been published, with limited results mainly focused on safety. Safety and tolerability are the most important issues because of the risk of teratoma and other risks associated with isolation, culture, and storage of cells. The most commonly used cells are mesenchymal cells, which are characterized by low immunogenicity and low risk of teratoma. The future development of cell therapy is fascinating and possibly realistic using bioengineering approaches that according to recent studies will make it possible to use decellularized whole lungs as a scaffold for subsequent cellular implantation.[91]

## CONCLUSION: IS PATHOBIOLOGY IMPORTANT FOR NOVEL APPROACHES TO TREATMENT?

Is the understanding of the pathobiology of IPF really important for exploring novel approaches to treatment? The answer to this question is simple and obvious: yes. In spite of that, and against any clinical and pathobiologic evidence, IPF has been treated with steroids and immunosuppressants for many years. As already discussed in this chapter, this was mainly due to the absence of other effective medical treatments, to some diagnostic inaccuracy that considered as IPF/UIP some forms of NSIP responding to steroids, and to the incomprehensible lack of proper studies showing the exact position of steroids and immunosuppressants in the therapeutic "scenario" of IPF. From this point of view the PANTHER study did justice to the "noninflammatory hypothesis" confirming that antiinflammatory treatment with steroids is not effective in IPF and even harmful. Fortunately, in other cases the potential drugs studied were more in tune with the pathobiology of IPF. Today, IPF is considered an epithelial-driven process triggered by an abnormal response of these cells to chronic injuries likely caused by specific risk factors such as smoking or environmental exposures. Genetic predisposition and aging play a fundamental role in altering the response of epithelial cells to chronic damage. The final result of all this is the activation of fibroblasts, and their recruitment, proliferation, and differentiation into myofibroblasts, resulting in scar formation and loss of lung function.

For these reasons, during the last few years the scientific attention has focused on some steps of the fibrogenic process, characterized by the activation of multiple and different pathways that may represent specific therapeutic targets. Indeed, pirfenidone was tested for its pleiotropic properties, as a drug able to act in different pathways of the fibrogenic process, and its efficacy has been proved in several preclinical and clinical studies that have made pirfenidone the first drug approved for the treatment of IPF. The story of nintedanib, a drug born to be used in oncology for non–small cell lung cancer, is also interesting. By virtue of the observation of some pathobiologic similarities between cancer and IPF, such as the activation of the same signaling transduction pathways, nintedanib has been repositioned and eventually approved for the treatment of IPF. The approval of pirfenidone first and then of nintedanib represents a fundamental if not historic moment for patients affected by IPF and their families. The opportunity to have a treatment slowing down the progression of the disease or reducing the risk of death has helped to attenuate the fatalism that for a long time has been associated with the diagnosis of IPF. The current approach to treatment is based on sequential therapy, so that one of the two approved drugs is started and when it is believed to be ineffective or side effects due to the drug are severe, it is possible to switch to the alternative drug. Similar to cancer, for the first time exists the possibility to have a first-line and, as alternative, a second-line of treatment. Two different clinical trials are currently under way exploring the safety of the association of pirfenidone and nintedanib, and hopefully, as in other diseases, there will be the possibility to use in the same patients a combination of drugs. The mechanisms of action of the two drugs seem different, so it is reasonable to think of a possible increase in their efficacy without necessarily having a sum of side effects.

By virtue of basic research and new clinical observations, the amount of information and data on the pathobiology of IPF is growing day by day, offering new and more ample opportunities to either develop new therapies or reposition known drugs for IPF. A number of preclinical and clinical studies are currently under way with the aim of finding new and more potent drugs or effective cell-based treatments for IPF and possibly to personalize treatments, identifying subcategories of patients on the basis of genetic backgrounds and response to treatment. This will certainly be possible in a future not so distant, provided that the tree of knowledge for the pathobiology of IPF continues to grow florid and robust.

# REFERENCES

1. Richeldi L, Davies HR, Ferrara G, et al. Corticosteroids for idiopathic pulmonary fibrosis. *Cochrane Database Syst Rev.* 2003;3:CD002880.
2. Funke M, Geiser T. Idiopathic pulmonary fibrosis: the turning point is now! *Swiss Med Wkly.* 2015;145:w14139.
3. Adamson IY, Young L, Bowden DH. Relationship of alveolar epithelial injury and repair to the induction of pulmonary fibrosis. *Am J Pathol.* 1988;130(2):377–383.
4. Pardo A, Selman M. Idiopathic pulmonary fibrosis: new insights in its pathogenesis. *Int J Biochem Cell Biol.* 2002;34(12):1534–1538.
5. Idiopathic Pulmonary Fibrosis Clinicl Research Network, Raghu G, Anstrom KJ, et al. Prednisone, azathioprine, and N-acetylcysteine for pulmonary fibrosis. *N Engl J Med.* 2012;366(21):1968–1977.
6. Ward HE, Nicholas TE. Alveolar type I and type II cells. *Aust N Z J Med.* 1984;14(5, suppl 3):731–734.
7. Oku H, Nakazato H, Horikawa, et al. Pirfenidone suppresses tumor necrosis factor-alpha, enhances interleukin-10 and protects mice from endotoxic shock. *Eur J Pharmacol.* 2002;446:167–176.
8. Iyer SN, Gurujeyalakshmi G, Giri SN. Effects of pirfenidone on transforming growth factor-beta gene expression at the transcriptional level in bleomycin hamster model of lung fibrosis. *J Pharmacol Exp Ther.* 1999;291:367–373.
9. Misra HP, Rabideau C. Pirfenidone inhibits NADPH-dependent microsomal lipid peroxidation and scavenges hydroxyl radicals. *Mol Cell Biochem.* 2000;204:119–126.
10. Raghu G, Masta S, Meyers D, Narayanan AS. Collagen synthesis by normal and fibrotic human lung fibroblasts and the effect of transforming growth factor-beta. *Am Rev Respir Dis.* 1989;140(1):95–100.
11. Shi J, Massague J. Mechanisms of TGFbeta signaling from cell membrane to the nucleus. *Cell.* 2003;113:685–700.
12. Gu L, Zhu YJ, Yang X, et al. Effect of TGF-beta/Smad signaling pathway on lung myofibroblast differentiation. *Acta Pharmacol Sin.* 2007;28(3):382–391.
13. Conte E, Gili E, Fagone E, et al. Effect of pirfenidone on proliferation, TGf-beta-induced myofibroblast differentiation and fibrogenic activity of primary human lung fibroblasts. *Eur J Pharm Sci.* 2014;58:13–19.
14. Conte E, Fruciano M, Fagone E, et al. Inhibition of PI3K prevents the proliferation and differentiation of human lung fibroblasts into myofibroblasts: the role of class I P110 isoforms. *PLoS One.* 2011;6(10):e24663.
15. Nakayama S, Mukae H, Sakamoto N, et al. Pirfenidone inhibits the expression of HSP47 in TGF-beta1-stimulated human lung fibroblasts. *Life Sci.* 2008;82(3,4):210–217.
16. Azuma A, Nukiwa T, Tsuboi E, et al. Double-blind, placebo-controlled trial of pirfenidone in patients with idiopathic pulmonary fibrosis. *Am J Respir Crit Care Med.* 2005;171(9):1040–1047.
17. Taniguchi H, Ebina M, Kondoh Y, et al. Pirfenidone in idiopathic pulmonary fibrosis. *Eur Respir J.* 2010;35(4):821–829.
18. Noble PW, Albera C, Bradford WZ, et al. Pirfenidone in patients with idiopathic pulmonary fibrosis (CAPACITY): two randomised trials. *Lancet.* 2011;377(9779):1760–1769.
19. King Jr TE, Bradford WZ, Castro-Bernardini S, et al. A phase 3 trial of pirfenidone in patients with idiopathic pulmonary fibrosis. *N Engl J Med.* 2014;370(22):2083–2092.
20. Noble PW, Albera C, Williamson Z, et al. Pirfenidone for idiopathic pulmonary fibrosis: analysis of pooled data from three multinational phase 3 trials. *Eur Respir J.* 2016;47:243–253.
21. Lancaster L, Albera C, Williamson Z, et al. Safety of pirfenidone in patients with idiopathic pulmonary fibrosis: integrated analysis of cumulative data from 5 clinical trials. *BMJ Open Resp Res.* 2016;3:e000105.
22. Itoh T, Koyabu K, Morimoto A, et al. Ameliorative effects of mosapride or Rikkunshi-to on the suppression of gastrointestinal motility by pirfenidone in rats. *Jpn Pharmacol Ther.* 2012;40:405–411.
23. Rubino CM, Bhavnani SM, Ambrose PG, et al. Effect of food and antacids on the pharmacokinetics of pirfenidone in older healthy adults. *Pulm Pharmacol Ther.* 2009;22:279–285.
24. Costabel U, Bendstrup E, Cottin V, et al. Pirfenidone in idiopathic pulmonary fibrosis: expert panel discussion on the management of drug-related adverse events. *Adv Ther.* 2014;31:375–391.
25. Seto Y, Inoue R, Kato M, et al. Photosafety assessments on pirfenidone: photochemical, photobiological, and pharmacokinetic characterization. *J Photochem Photobiol B.* 2013;120:44–51.
26. Huang NY, Ding L, Wang J, et al. Pharmacokinetics, safety and tolerability of pirfenidone and its major metabolite after single and multiple oral doses in healthy Chinese subjects under fed conditions. *Drug Res (Stuttg).* 2013;63:388–395.
27. Togami K, Kanehira Y, Tada H. Pharmacokinetic evaluation of tissue distribution of pirfenidone and its metabolites for idiopathic pulmonary fibrosis therapy. *Biopharm Drug Dispos.* 2015;36:205–215.
28. Vancheri C. Idiopathic pulmonary fibrosis and cancer: do they really look similar? *BMC Med.* 2015;13:220.
29. Konigshoff M, Balsara N, Pfaff EM, et al. Functional Wnt signalling is increased in idiopathic pulmonary fibrosis. *PLoS One.* 2008;3(5):e2142.
30. Chilosi M, Poletti V, Zamò A, et al. Aberrant Wnt/beta-catenin pathway activation in idiopathic pulmonary fibrosis. *Am J Pathol.* 2003;162(5):1495–1502.
31. Caraci F, Gili E, Calafiore M, et al. TGF-beta1 targets the GSK-3beta/beta-catenin pathway via ERK activation in the transition of human lung fibroblasts into myofibroblasts. *Pharmacol Res.* 2008;57(4):274–282.
32. Bowley E, O'Gorman DB, Gan BS. Beta-catenin signalling in fibro-proliferative disease. *J Surg Res.* 2014;138(1):141–150.

33. Conte E, Gili E, Fruciano M, et al. PI3Kp110gamma over-expression in idiopathic pulmonary fibrosis lung tissue and fibroblast cells: in vitro effects of its inhibition. *Lab Invest.* 2013;93(5):566–576.

34. Bao Z, Zhang Q, Wan H, et al. Expression of suppressor of cytokine signalling 1 in the peripheral blood of patient with idiopathic pulmonary fibrosis. *Chin Med J.* 2014;127(11):2117–2120.

35. Grimminger F, Günther A, Vancheri C. The role of tyrosine kinases in the pathogenesis of idiopathic pulmonary fibrosis. *Eur Respir J.* 2015;45(5):1426–1433.

36. Antoniades HN, Bravo MA, Avila RE, et al. Platelet-derived growth factor in idiopathic pulmonary fibrosis. *J Clin Invest.* 1990;86:1055–1064.

37. Abdollahi A, Li M, Ping G, et al. Inhibition of platelet-derived growth factor signalling attenuates pulmonary fibrosis. *J Exp Med.* 2005;201(6):925–935.

38. Zou H, Nie XH, Zhang T, et al. Effect of basic fibroblast growth factor on the proliferation, migration and phenotypic modulation of airway smooth muscle cells. *Chin Med J.* 2008;121:424–429.

39. Wollin L, Wex E, Pautsch A, et al. Mode of action of nintedanib in the treatment of idiopathic pulmonary fibrosis. *Eur Respir J.* 2015;45:1434–1445.

40. Thannickal VJ, Aldweib KD, Rajan T, et al. Upregulated expression of fibroblast growth factor (FGF) receptors by transforming growth factor beta 1(TGF beta1) mediates enhanced mitogenic responses to FGFs in cultured human lung fibroblasts. *Biochem Biophys Res Commun.* 1998;251:437–441.

41. Khalil N, Xu YD, O'Connor R, et al. Proliferation of pulmonary interstitial fibroblasts is mediated by transforming growth factor-beta1-induced release of extracellular fibroblast growth factor 2 and phosphorylation of p38 MAPK and JNK. *J Biol Chem.* 2005;280:43000–43009.

42. Barrios R, Pardo A, Ramos C, et al. Upregulation of acid fibroblast growth factor during development of experimental lung fibrosis. *Am J Physiol.* 1997;273:L451–L458.

43. Inoue Y, King Jr TE, Barker E, et al. Basic fibroblast growth factor and its receptors in idiopathic pulmonary fibrosis and lymphangioleiomyomatosis. *Am J Respir Crit Care Med.* 2002;166:765–773.

44. Yu ZH, Wang DD, Zhou ZY, et al. Mutant soluble ectodomain of fibroblast growth factor receptor-2 III c attenuates bleomycin induced pulmonary fibrosis in mice. *Biol Pharm Bull.* 2012;35:731–736.

45. Ebina M, Shimizukawa M, Shibata N, et al. Heterogeneous increase in CD 43 positive alveolar capillaries in idiopathic pulmonary fibrosis. *Am J Respir Crit Care Med.* 2004;169:1203–1208.

46. Farkas L, Farkas D, Ask K, et al. VEGF ameliorates pulmonary hypertension through inhibition of endothelial apoptosis in experimental lung fibrosis in rats. *J Clin Invest.* 2009;119:1298–1311.

47. Ando M, Miyazaki E, Ito T, et al. Significance of serum vascular endothelial growth factor level in patients with idiopathic pulmonary fibrosis. *Lung.* 2010;188:247–252.

48. Daniels CE, Lasky JA, Limper AH, et al. Imatinib treatment for idiopathic pulmonary fibrosis: randomized placebo-controlled trial results. *Am J Respir Crit Care Med.* 2010;181(6):604–610.

49. Chaudhary NI, Roth GJ, Hilberg F, et al. Inhibition of PDGF, VEGF and FGF signalling attenuates fibrosis. *Eur Respir J.* 2007;29:976–985.

50. Hostettler KE, Zhong J, Papakonstantinou E, et al. Antifibrotic effects of nintedanib in lung fibroblasts derived from patients with idiopathic pulmonary fibrosis. *Respir Res.* 2014;15:157.

51. Pardo A, Cabrera S, Maldonado M, et al. Role of matrix metallopreotinases in idiopathic pulmonary fibrosis. *Respir Res.* 2016;17:23.

52. Wollin L, Maillet I, Quesniaux V, et al. Anti fibrotic and antiinflammatory activity of the tyrosine kinase inhibitor nintedanib in experimental models of lung fibrosis. *J Pharmacol Exp Ther.* 2014;349:209–220.

53. Richeldi L, Costabel U, Selman M, et al. Efficacy of a tyrosine kinase inhibitor in idiopathic pulmonary fibrosis. *N Engl J Med.* 2011;365(12):1079–1087.

54. Richeldi L, du Bois RM, Raghu G, et al. Efficacy and safety of nintedanib in idiopathic pulmonary fibrosis. *N Engl J Med.* 2014;370(22):2071–2082.

55. Richeldi L, Cottin V, du Bois RM, et al. Nintedanib in patients with idiopathic pulmonary fibrosis: combined evidence from the TOMORROW and INPULSIS trials. *Respir Med.* 2016;113:74–79.

56. Woodcock HV, Molyneaux PL, Maher TM, et al. Reducing lung function decline in patients with idiopathic pulmonary fibrosis: potential of nintedanib. *Drug Des Devel Ther.* 2013;7:503–510.

57. Uribe JM, Keely SJ, Traynor-Kaplan AE, et al. Phosphatidylinositol 3-kinase mediates the inhibitory effect of epidermal growth factor on calcium-dependent chloride secretion. *J Biol Chem.* 1996;271:26588–26595.

58. Deininger MWN, O'Brien SG, For JM, et al. Practical management of patients with chronic myeloid leukemia receiving imatinib. *J Clin Oncol.* 2003;21:1637–1647.

59. Behr J, Degenkolb B, Krombach F, et al. Intracellular glutathione and bronchoalveolar cells in fibrosing alveolitis: effects of N-acetylcysteine. *Eur Respir J.* 2002;19:906–911.

60. Martinez FJ, de Andrade JA, Anstrom KJ, et al. Randomized trial of acetylcysteine in idiopathic pulmonary fibrosis. *N Engl J Med.* 2014;370(22):2093–2101.

61. Oldham JM, Ma SF, Martinez FJ, et al. TOLLIP, MUC5B and the response to N-acetylcysteine among individuals with idiopathic pulmonary fibrosis. *Am J Respir Crit Care Med.* 2015;192(12):1475–1482.

62. Homma S, Azuma A, Taniguchi H, et al. Efficacy of inhaled N-acetylcysteine monotherapy in patients with early stage idiopathic pulmonary fibrosis. *Respirology.* 2012;17:467–477.

63. Muramatsu Y, Sugino K, Ishida F, et al. Effect of inhaled N-acetylcysteine monotherapy on lung function and redox balance in idiopathic pulmonary fibrosis. *Respir Invest.* 2016;54:170–178.

64. Morehead RS. Gastro-oesophageal reflux disease and non-asthma lung disease. *Eur Respir Rev.* 2009;18(114):233–243.

65. Schachter LM, Dixon J, Pierce RJ, et al. Severe gastroesophageal reflux is associated with reduced carbon monoxide diffusing capacity. *Chest.* 2003;123(6):1932–1938.

66. Ghebremariam YT, Cooke JP, Gerhart W, et al. Pleiotropic effect of the proton pump inhibitor esomeprazole leading to suppression of lung inflammation and fibrosis. *J Transl Med.* 2015;13:249.

67. Lee JS, Ryu JH, Elicker BM, et al. Gastroesophageal reflux therapy is associated with longer survival in patients with idiopathic pulmonary fibrosis. *Am J Respir Crit Care Med.* 2011;184:1390–1394.

68. Lee JS, Collard HR, Anstrom KJ, et al. Anti-acid therapy and disease progression in idiopathic pulmonary fibrosis: an analysis of data from three randomized controlled trials. *Lancet Respir Med.* 2013;1(5):369–376.

69. Lee CM, Lee DH, Ahn BK, et al. Protective effect of proton pump inhibitor for survival in patients with gastroesophageal reflux disease and idiopathic pulmonary fibrosis. *J Neurogastroenterol Motil.* 2016:15–192.

70. Raghu G, Rochwerg B, Zhang Y, et al. An official ATS/ERS/JRS/ALAT clinical practice guideline:treatment of idiopathic pulmonary fibrosis: executive summary. An update of the 2011 clinical guideline. *Am J Respir Crit Care Med.* 2015;192(2):e3–e19.

71. Kreuter M, Wuyts W, Renzoni E, et al. Antiacid therapy and disease outcomes in idiopathic pulmonary fibrosis: a pooled analysis. *Lancet Respir Med.* 2016;4(5):381–389.

72. Murray LA, Argentieri RI, Farrel FX, et al. Hyperresponsiveness of IPF/UIP fibroblasts: interplay between TGF beta1, IL13 and CCl2. *Int J Biochem Cell Biol.* 2008;10:2174–2182.

73. Lee CG, Homer RJ, Zhu Z, et al. Interleukin-13 induces tissue fibrosis by selectively stimulating and activating transforming growth factor beta(1). *J Exp Med.* 2001;194:809–821.

74. Kaviratne M, Hesse M, Leusink M, et al. IL-13 activates a mechanism of tissue fibrosis that is completely TGF-beta independent. *J Immunol.* 2004;173:4020–4029.

75. Nishimura Y, Nitto T, Inoue T, Node K. IL-13 attenuates vascular tube formation via JAK2-STAT6 pathway. *Circ J.* 2008;72:469–475.

76. Zheng T, Liu W, Oh SY, et al. IL-13 receptor alpha2 selectively inhibits IL-13-induced responses in the murine lung. *J Immunol.* 2008;180:522–529.

77. Murray LA, Zhang H, Oak SR, et al. Targeting interleukin-13 with tralokinumab attenuates lung fibrosis and epithelial damage in a humanized SCID idiopathic pulmonary fibrosis model. *Am J Respir Cell Mol Biol.* 2014;50(5):985–994.

78. Pilling D, Cox N, Vakil V, et al. The Long pentraxin PTX3 promotes fibrocyte differentiation. *PLoS One.* 2015;10(3):e0119709.

79. Pilling D, Buckley CD, Salmon M, et al. Inhibition of fibrocyte differentiation by serum amyloid P. *J Immunol.* 2003;171:5537–5546.

80. Pilling D, Gomer RH. Persistent lung inflammation and fibrosis in serum amyloid P component (APCs-/-) knock-out mice. *PLoS One.* 2014;9(4):e93730.

81. Van den Blink B, Dillingh MR, Ginns LC, et al. Recombinant human pentraxin-2 therapy in patients with idiopathic pulmonary fibrosis: safety, pharmacokinetics and exploratory efficacy. *Eur Respir J.* 2016;47(3):889–897.

82. Leask A, Abraham DJ. All in the CCN family: essential matricellular signaling modulators emerge from the bunker. *J Cell Sci.* 2006;119:4803–4810.

83. Liu F, Mih JD, Shea BS, et al. Feedback amplification of fibrosis through matrix stiffening and COX-2 suppression. *J Cell Biol.* 2010;190:693–706.

84. Pan LH, Yamauchi K, Uzuki M, et al. Type II alveolar epithelial cells and interstitial fibroblasts express connective tissue growth factor in IPF. *Eur Respir J.* 2001;17:1220–1227.

85. Lipson KE, Wong C, Teng Y, et al. CTGF is a central mediator of tissue remodelling and fibrosis and its inhibition can reverse the process of fibrosis. *Fibrog Tissue Repair.* 2012;5(suppl 1):S24.

86. Raghu G, Scholand MB, De Andrade J, et al. Safety and efficacy of anti-CTGF monoclonal antibody FG-3019 for the treatment of idiopathic pulmonary fibrosis (IPF): results of phase II clinical trial two years after initiation. *Am J Respir Crit Care Med.* 2014;189:A1426.

87. Raghu G, Scholand MB, De Andrade J, et al. FG-3019 anti-connective tissue growth factor monoclonal antibody: results of an open-label clinical trial in IPF. *Eur Respir J.* 2016;47(5):1481–1491.

88. Serrano-Mollar A, Nacher M, Gay-Jordi G, et al. Intratracheal transplantation of alveolar type II cells reverses bleomycin-induced lung fibrosis. *Am J Resp Crit Care.* 2007;176:1261–1268.

89. Ortiz LA, Gambelli F, McBride C, et al. Mesenchymal stem cell engraftment in lung is enhanced in response to bleomycin exposure and ameliorates its fibrotic effects. *Proc Natl Acad Sci USA.* 2003;100:8407–8411.

90. Cargnoni A, Gibelli L, Tosini A, et al. Transplantation of allogeneic and xenogeneic placenta-derived cells reduces bleomycin-induced lung fibrosis. *Cell Transplant.* 2009;18:405–422.

91. Mendez JJ, Ghaedi M, Steinbacher D, et al. Epithelial cell differentiation of human mesenchymal stromal cells in decellularized lung scaffolds. *Tissue Eng.* 2014;20:1735–1746.

# CHAPTER 3

# Smoking-Related Interstitial Lung Diseases

ROBERT VASSALLO • JAY H. RYU

---

**KEY POINTS**

- Substantial evidence implicates cigarette smoking as the principal etiologic factor responsible for the development of respiratory bronchiolitis–interstitial lung disease (RB-ILD), desquamative interstitial pneumonia (DIP), and pulmonary Langerhans cell histiocytosis (PLCH).
- Cigarette smoking is an important precipitant of acute eosinophilic pneumonia (AEP) and pulmonary hemorrhage in patients with Goodpasture syndrome, and smokers are at higher risk of developing idiopathic pulmonary fibrosis (IPF) and rheumatoid arthritis (RA)-associated ILD.
- It is important to recognize and continue to investigate the role of cigarette smoke in the pathogenesis and clinical course of these diverse diffuse parenchymal lung diseases.
- Although relatively uncommon, these diseases are a significant health burden and frequently affect young adults in their most productive years.

---

Cigarette smoke is a complex mixture of more than 4000 chemicals, many of which exert toxic effects on cellular function. In addition to chronic obstructive pulmonary disease (COPD) and cancer, cigarette smokers may develop diffuse parenchymal lung diseases (Box 3.1).[1-4] These diffuse parenchymal lung diseases are referred to as "smoking-related interstitial lung diseases," a term that recognizes the suspected causal association with cigarette smoking. Novel insights regarding the relationship between smoking and interstitial lung disease (ILD) are highlighted in this updated chapter.

## SMOKING AND INTERSTITIAL LUNG DISEASE

Cigarette smoking is now widely accepted as the primary cause of certain ILDs, namely respiratory bronchiolitis–interstitial lung disease (RB-ILD), desquamative interstitial pneumonia (DIP), and pulmonary Langerhans cell histiocytosis (PLCH).[1-6] Cigarette smoking is also a risk factor for the development of idiopathic pulmonary fibrosis (IPF)[7] and rheumatoid arthritis (RA)–associated ILD,[8,9] and has been reported to cause some cases of acute eosinophilic pneumonia (AEP)[10] and pulmonary hemorrhage syndromes. Paradoxically, cigarette smoking may confer protection from developing some other ILDs such as hypersensitivity pneumonitis (HP).[11] We have described a classification scheme (Box 3.1) outlining these subgroups and their relationship to smoking.[12] This classification illustrates the highly complex effects of smoking on the lung parenchyma.

The Group 1 diseases (Box 3.1) include the three diffuse lung diseases classically regarded as smoking-related ILDs. This designation is supported by several lines of clinical, epidemiologic, and investigative evidence showing a direct role for cigarette smoking as witnessed in the temporal relationship to disease onset and progression, resolution on smoking cessation, and recurrence or progression on resumption of smoking.[13-17] Several case series have reported a history of smoking in the overwhelming majority of Group 1 patients, with the prevalence being highest in RB-ILD[4,18] and PLCH,[2,5,19,20] and less common in DIP (Table 3.1).[4,21,22] The reported coexistence of all three lesions in the same patient,[13] the potential for disease remission with smoking cessation,[4] the recurrence of disease in transplanted lungs,[23,24] and the description of analogous lesions in mice exposed to high doses of cigarette smoke[15] all provide support to the designation of RB-ILD, DIP, and PLCH as smoking-induced ILDs.

For diseases allocated to Group 2 (Box 3.1) the association with cigarette smoking is less robust than for Group 1 diseases. Cigarette smoking, particularly during the relatively early phase after initiation of smoking, seems to be an important precipitating factor in some but not in all cases of Group 2 diseases. The most relevant conditions in this category include AEP and certain pulmonary hemorrhage syndromes.[10,25–28] AEP deserves particular attention because a number

of recent studies have implicated recent-onset exposure to cigarette smoke as a principal inducer of this disease in some patients diagnosed to have this disorder.[26,27,29–32] In addition, increase in the number of cigarettes smoked per day in chronic smokers has been described to induce AEP.[32,33] Of particular interest is the response of certain subjects with resolved AEP to a rechallenge with cigarette smoke exposure that triggers peripheral eosinophilia and other associated pathophysiologic abnormalities, suggesting that exposure to cigarette smoke to induce certain responses is relevant to the development of acute diffuse lung disease in susceptible hosts.[27]

Diseases included in Group 3 (Box 3.1) are chronic diffuse lung diseases that are statistically more likely to develop in cigarette smokers.[34,35] For instance, cigarette smoking is known to increase the relative risk of RA-associated ILD, possibly by triggering RA-specific immune reactions to citrullinated proteins.[9,34,36] Similarly, smokers have a higher risk of developing IPF than nonsmokers.[35] The precise significance of these observations has been a topic of substantial debate, but there is limited evidence that smoking itself is directly fibrogenic to the lung.[37,38] It is not appropriate to consider smoking as an inducer of these diseases, but rather a disease modifier or potentially a cofactor that facilitates the development of profibrotic responses that lead to these diffuse fibrotic lung diseases.

The fourth and final group consists of diseases that are less prevalent in smokers compared with

---

**BOX 3.1**
**Proposed Classification of Smoking-Related Interstitial lung Diseases (ILDs)**

Group 1—Chronic ILDs that are very likely caused by cigarette smoking[4–6,13,21,50]
    Respiratory bronchiolitis–associated ILD
    Desquamative interstitial pneumonia
    Adult pulmonary Langerhans cell histiocytosis
Group 2—Acute ILDs that may be precipitated by cigarette smoking[25,27–29,160]
    Acute eosinophilic pneumonia
    Pulmonary hemorrhage syndromes
Group 3—ILDs that are statistically more prevalent in smokers[7,8,34–36]
    Idiopathic pulmonary fibrosis
    Rheumatoid arthritis–associated ILD
Group 4—ILDs that are less prevalent in smokers[39–42,159]
    Hypersensitivity pneumonitis
    Sarcoidosis

---

**TABLE 3.1**
**Key Characteristics of Group 1 Chronic Smoking-Related Diffuse Lung Diseases**

| | RB-ILD | DIP | PLCH |
|---|---|---|---|
| Association with cigarette smoking | 95% | 60–90% | 95% |
| Clinical features | Chronic cough and dyspnea, inspiratory crackles | Chronic cough and dyspnea, inspiratory crackles | Chronic cough and dyspnea Pneumothorax in 15% |
| High-resolution CT findings | Centrilobular nodules and ground-glass opacities | Ground-glass and reticular opacities | Peribronchiolar nodules, cavitated nodules, and cysts with relative sparing of lung bases |
| Key histologic findings | Pigment-laden macrophages in the respiratory bronchioles, and alveolar ducts | Diffuse alveolar filling with pigment-laden macrophages | Bronchiolocentric nodules, stellate lesions, CD1a-positive Langerhans cells |
| Response to corticosteroids | Modest, variable | Modest, variable | Modest, variable |

*DIP*, desquamative interstitial pneumonia; *PLCH*, pulmonary Langerhans cell histiocytosis; *RB-ILD*, respiratory bronchiolitis–associated interstitial lung disease.

nonsmokers and includes sarcoidosis and HP.[39-42] Cigarette smoking seems to provide certain "protective" effects that diminish the potential development of these granulomatous inflammatory lung diseases, possibly by inhibiting certain immunologic responses in the lung that are required for granuloma formation or the development of T-helper 1 (Th1)–polarized immune responses following exposure to inhaled antigens.[43,44] Epidemiologic studies demonstrate that levels of circulating IgG antibodies to pigeon antigens are higher among nonsmokers than smokers.[45] A similar study in farmers showed that nonsmokers and previous smokers had a higher prevalence of serum precipitin levels to various farmer's lung antigens, compared with current smokers.[46] Lung macrophages from cigarette smokers also have lower levels of costimulatory molecules than those of controls.[44] Because costimulatory molecules play a critical role in shaping the immune response to inhaled antigens, it is possible that smokers are hyporesponsive to inhaled antigens by virtue of diminished antigen-presenting capacity in the lung. Cigarette smoking and nicotine have also been demonstrated to inhibit the production of the potent Th1-polarizing cytokine interleukin-12 (IL-12).[43] It is conceivable that the diminished capacity of smokers' macrophages and dendritic cells to generate IL-12 may impede the development of hypersensitivity response to inhaled antigens and granuloma formation in the context of sarcoidosis. The observation that smoking is associated with a lower prevalence of sarcoidosis and HP should not be construed as an indication to promote smoking in patients with these diseases. On the contrary, insight gained from dissecting mechanisms by which smoking suppresses Th1 immunity—an essential driver of the immunopathogenic processes that characterizes these diffuse lung diseases—is also relevant to the pathogenesis of smoking-related lung cancer and airway diseases, diseases that are more prevalent in smokers partly because of impaired Th1 immunity.

The fact that some cases of RB-ILD or DIP may be induced by factors other than cigarette smoke exposure, and that some patients with PLCH are nonsmokers, had been interpreted as implying that these diseases do not necessarily represent specific smoking-induced lung diseases. However, it is well recognized that a number of specific histopathologic entities can be induced by heterogeneous etiologies, potentially a reflection that the lung has only a limited number of ways of responding to various insults. For example, the lesion of usual interstitial pneumonia (UIP) may be induced by asbestos exposure and be seen in patients with chronic HP, as well as in the context of autoimmune diseases such as RA-associated ILD.[47-49] Cigarette smoking is the most well-defined etiologic factor associated with the development of RB-ILD, DIP, and PLCH; however, the histopathologic lesions of RB, DIP, and PLCH do not exclusively occur in smokers and may occasionally be idiopathic or encountered in the context of other exposures or etiologies.[5,21,49,50]

Defining the relationship between smoking and specific ILDs has important clinical implications. Smoking cessation is imperative for all the diseases listed under Groups 1–3 in Box 3.1. It is our practice to use aggressive tobacco cessation strategies in these patients and have a low threshold for referral to nicotine dependence counselors. It is our practice to explicitly refer to diseases in Group 1 as "smoking-induced" to underscore the importance of smoking cessation and encourage removal of all tobacco products from the vicinity of the patient, including secondhand tobacco smoke exposure. Similarly, all current smokers with diseases in Groups 2 and 3 should be counseled regarding the emerging and compelling data implicating a direct pathogenic role for cigarette smoke exposure as a potential inducer or cofactor in disease induction and progression. The methods that should be considered in smoking cessation therapy include counseling and behavior therapy, nicotine replacement therapy, and pharmacotherapy, including the use of bupropion, varenicline, and clonidine in selected patients.[51,52]

## MECHANISMS BY WHICH TOBACCO SMOKE MAY PROMOTE INTERSTITIAL LUNG DISEASE

Even in smokers without clinically detectable lung disease, cigarette smoking induces inflammatory cell recruitment, consisting primarily of macrophages, neutrophils, and Langerhans cells (a subtype of the myeloid dendritic cell family expressing surface CD1a receptors), to small airways.[53-55] Although all smokers have some degree of inflammation in the airways, only a small minority of smokers develop clinically significant diffuse lung disease. The relative rarity of smoking-related ILDs compared with the overall prevalence of cigarette smoking suggests that cigarette smoke is not the only factor responsible for the induction of these diseases and implies that additional factors (endogenous such as genetic factors or exogenous such as infectious pathogens or allergens) are required for the induction of disease.

A characteristic morphologic feature of all Group 1 smoking-related ILDs is prominent bronchiolar inflammation.[13,38,56–58] In addition, Group 1 diseases demonstrate increased macrophages in the interstitium and the alveolar spaces.[38,56,57,59] Pigmented macrophage accumulation in small airways, interstitium, and distal airspaces is a key feature of many smoking-related ILDs. Specific mechanisms by which exaggerated macrophage accumulation occurs in Group 1 diseases are not fully defined, but likely involve exaggerated generation of macrophage recruiting and differentiating factors by airway epithelial cells, enhanced macrophage survival locally, and/or diminished apoptosis of recruited macrophages.[55,60] In these patients, lung epithelial cells have been demonstrated to aberrantly produce excessive granulocyte-macrophage colony stimulating factor (GM-CSF), a cytokine that provides proliferative and activation signals to both macrophages and dendritic cells.[61,62] Cigarette smoke extracts have also been shown to induce transforming growth factor beta (TGF-β) production by lung epithelial cells, a cytokine that is involved in Langerhans cell development, immune modulation, and fibrogenic responses in the airways.[63]

Cigarette smoking induces several abnormalities in immune and other lung cells that are likely relevant to the pathogenesis of smoking-related ILDs.[43,55,64,65] Certain constituents in cigarette smoke are known to activate epithelial cells, macrophages, neutrophils, and dendritic cells in vitro, promoting generation of chemokines and cytokines that lead to inflammation by promoting immune cell recruitment.[66,67] It is reasonable to speculate that smokers in whom ILD develops have an amplified inflammatory cascade associated with activation of multiple immune cell types that promote a vicious cycle of inflammatory cell recruitment. Whether failure of endogenous antiinflammatory mechanisms or additional exogenous insults such as viral infections have a role in promoting smoking-related ILDs is unknown but should be an important area of future research.

## RESPIRATORY BRONCHIOLITIS-ASSOCIATED INTERSTITIAL LUNG DISEASE

Niewoehner described RB as a histopathologic finding of pigmented macrophage accumulation centering on respiratory bronchioles and neighboring alveoli, a finding that was ubiquitous in cigarette smokers at autopsy.[68] Subsequent case series described similar findings on lung biopsy specimens from cigarette smokers.[1,13,50] RB can thus be considered a histologic marker of smoking and must be distinguished from

RB-ILD, a term coined by Myers and colleagues to recognize the clinicopathologic ILD occurring in cigarette smokers in whom surgical lung biopsy revealed only RB.[58] In patients with RB-ILD, the lesion of RB is not felt to be a mere indicator of exposure to smoking, but rather constitutes the primary and only histopathologic lesion accountable for the observed ILD. Following the original description by Myers and colleagues, other reports described in greater detail clinical and radiologic features of RB-ILD as a specific interstitial and bronchiolar process occurring in smokers and defined by the presence of RB as the only definable pathologic abnormality present on lung biopsy.[1,50,69]

The true prevalence of RB-ILD is difficult to estimate as many patients with this disorder may be asymptomatic.[4] The duration of exposure to cigarette smoke need not be lengthy or severe, although many have substantial cumulative tobacco exposures.[1] Most patients present in the fourth and fifth decade of life, and there is no gender predilection.[3,4,18] A clinicopathologic syndrome indistinguishable from RB-ILD can occasionally be encountered following exposure to solder fumes,[50] diesel smoke, and fiberglass.[1]

RB-ILD usually presents in a nonspecific fashion with chronic cough and exertional dyspnea; rarely, acute presentation may occur (Table 3.1).[70] The physical examination reveals inspiratory crackles in approximately half of patients, but digital clubbing is infrequent.[3,4,18] Pulmonary function testing yields various patterns, including normal, obstructive, restrictive, or mixed abnormalities.[4,18] The severity of physiologic impairment, if present, is usually mild to moderate.[4]

Chest radiography reveals bilateral, fine reticular, or reticulonodular opacities in about 60–70% of patients but may appear normal in some patients.[4,18,50] The main findings on chest high-resolution CT (HRCT) include bronchial wall thickening, fine centrilobular nodules, and patchy areas of ground-glass attenuation.[4,18,50] The ground-glass changes are typically bilateral and affect both upper and lower lung fields (Fig. 3.1).[59,71] Coexisting emphysematous changes are frequently noted, but honeycombing, traction bronchiectasis, and parenchymal fibrosis are not.

The differential diagnosis of RB-ILD includes not only consideration of other bronchiolar diseases, including infectious bronchiolitis, follicular bronchiolitis, and diffuse aspiration bronchiolitis, but also ILDs characterized by ground-glass opacities, particularly HP and nonspecific interstitial pneumonia (NSIP). Although surgical lung biopsy is often required for a definitive diagnosis, in clinical practice a provisional diagnosis may be established in many patients on the

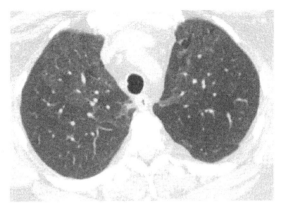

FIG. 3.1   High-resolution CT of the chest showing patchy areas of ground-glass attenuation in upper lung fields in a smoker with respiratory bronchiolitis–associated interstitial lung disease.

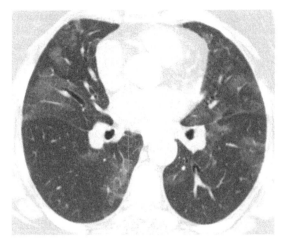

FIG. 3.2   High-resolution CT of the chest showing more extensive ground-glass opacities in a smoker with desquamative interstitial pneumonia.

basis of epidemiologic, clinical, and radiologic features, and reasonable exclusion of other potential diagnoses.[50] Bronchoscopic lung biopsy has a low yield, and bronchoalveolar lavage (BAL) findings are nonspecific in RB-ILD, but may be diagnostically helpful in distinguishing RB-ILD from other conditions such as HP that are associated with more specific features.

The histopathologic findings required for the diagnosis of RB-ILD are those of RB and include the presence of yellow-brown–pigmented macrophages in the lumens of respiratory bronchioles, alveolar ducts, and peribronchiolar alveolar spaces without significant associated interstitial pneumonia.[4,72] At low power, these features are patchy and are generally confined to peribronchiolar regions (bronchiolocentric distribution). Mild peribronchiolar fibrosis can be seen, but honeycombing is unusual.[50,71]

As in all of the Group 1 diseases, smoking cessation is a key component of RB-ILD management. Smoking cessation may lead to improvement in radiologic abnormalities and lung function.[4,73] The degree of improvement following smoking cessation appears to be limited in some patients, and abnormalities may persist for years.[1,18] For patients with significant lung impairment, corticosteroids or other immunosuppressive medications have been used in an attempt to limit progression of lung disease; however, evidence of their effectiveness is lacking.[18,74] Most patients with RB-ILD have a relatively good prognosis, and mortality from RB-ILD is uncommon.[4,18] Although smoking cessation may lead to disease remission in some patients with RB-ILD, longitudinal studies have shown that some patients remain symptomatic for years after smoking cessation.[18]

## DESQUAMATIVE INTERSTITIAL PNEUMONIA

DIP was originally believed to be a diffuse parenchymal lung disease resulting from desquamation of alveolar epithelial cells into the alveolar space but later was recognized as a process of alveolar filling from macrophage accumulation.[75] DIP is associated with cigarette smoking in at least two-thirds of cases[4,21,69] but can also be seen in nonsmokers, particularly in the context of autoimmune diseases,[47] some infections,[76] and drug exposures.[76,77] It has been reported to occur in children as well as adults.[4]

The clinical presentation of DIP is nonspecific with dyspnea and cough, and physical examination reveals inspiratory crackles in ~60% and digital clubbing in 25–50% of patients (Table 3.1).[4,69,78] Pulmonary function testing reveals restriction in one-third of cases, normal findings in 10–20%, and a mixed defect in the remainder.[4,69,78]

Chest radiography typically reveals patchy haziness or interstitial patterns with lower zone predominance.[4,79] The striking abnormality on HRCT is ground-glass opacities predominantly in the lower lung zones and often in a peripheral distribution (Fig. 3.2).[80,81] Irregular linear opacities are frequently present; however, honeycombing and significant architectural distortion are uncommon. In some instances, patients with DIP have been reported to develop HRCT findings suggestive of fibrotic NSIP (irregular linear opacities) on longitudinal follow-up.[3,82] Small parenchymal cysts and apical emphysematous changes may also be seen.[83]

On light microscopy, lung biopsies show characteristic filling of alveolar spaces with pigment-laden alveolar macrophages.[21] While both RB-ILD and DIP are associated with the accumulation of pigment-laden macrophages in alveolar spaces, the distribution of abnormality is more bronchiolocentric and patchy in RB, whereas in DIP it tends to be more diffuse.[13,49] The extent of interstitial fibrosis, lymphoid follicles, and eosinophilic infiltration has been reported to be more prevalent in DIP than in RB-ILD.[21,69] Fibroblast foci are not seen, and the DIP lesion appears temporally uniform.[49,72] A definitive diagnosis of DIP usually requires surgical lung biopsy, as it may be difficult to reliably differentiate DIP from NSIP or RB-ILD by clinical, radiologic, and bronchoscopic biopsy criteria.[13]

For those DIP patients who are smokers, smoking cessation is an essential component of therapy. Prolonged remission of DIP after smoking cessation has been described, but similar to all other smoking-related ILDs, the effect of smoking cessation on the natural history of DIP remains poorly characterized.[4,84] Although most DIP patients have a relatively good prognosis with a better than 90% 5-year survival,[4,78,85] some patients progress to respiratory failure and premature death within 5 to 10 years following the diagnosis.[4,21,69,78] Patients with DIP are frequently treated with corticosteroids, but the effectiveness of steroid therapy is variable and has not been evaluated in a prospective study.[4] Other immunosuppressants such as azathioprine and methotrexate have been used in anecdotal cases.[86] Lung transplantation is an option for patients with progressive disease, but DIP can recur in the transplanted lung.[87,88]

## PULMONARY LANGERHANS CELL HISTIOCYTOSIS

PLCH (also referred to as pulmonary Langerhans granulomatosis or pulmonary eosinophilic granuloma) is induced by cigarette smoke exposure in the majority of adult patients diagnosed to have this disorder and is characterized by accumulation of CD1a-expressing Langerhans cells in the lung, and occasionally in other organ systems.[89,90] Adult PLCH forms part of the spectrum of histiocytic diseases, which range from relatively benign processes such as unifocal LCH involving bone to disseminated multiorgan forms (more commonly in children) associated with significant morbidity and mortality.[91] Contrary to DIP and RB-ILD, which exclusively affect the lungs, ~15% of adult PLCH patients may have disease outside the thoracic cavity.[5,92] PLCH represents ~5% of the total number of diffuse parenchymal lung diseases diagnosed by lung biopsy.[92] PLCH tends to affect younger adults in their third and fourth decades.[5] PLCH appears to affect both men and women equally.

Approximately 95% of adults with PLCH are active or former smokers or have been exposed to substantial second-hand cigarette smoke.[2,20,57,92,93] While the pathogenesis remains poorly understood, it is likely that cigarette smoke constituents activate epithelial cells and other cell types in the airways to produce cytokines that promote recruitment, activation, and retention of Langerhans cells in the subepithelial regions of the airways.[61,62,94] Cigarette smoke also induces the production of cytokines with profibrotic functions, such as TGF-β; in turn, TGF-β and other cytokines such as GM-CSF may further promote local expansion of Langerhans cells and facilitate the development of tissue remodeling and fibrosis as is evident in more advanced PLCH cases.[95] It is possible that certain cigarette smoke constituents are taken up by immune or other cells and result in direct immune cell activation in peribronchiolar regions. Activated Langerhans cells and macrophages in peribronchiolar regions are likely to then promote secondary recruitment of T cells, plasma cells, and eosinophils, resulting in the formation of eosinophilic granulomatous inflammation from which the descriptive term "eosinophilic granuloma" is derived.

In recent years, somatic mutations leading to constitutive activation of the mitogen-activated protein kinase pathway, a key regulator of many cellular functions, including cell growth and proliferation, have been identified in LCH.[96,97] Similar mutations have been identified in a subset of cases of adult PLCH and include BRAF (usually BRAF-V600E), MAP2K1, and NRAS mutations.[98-101] Cumulatively, these data suggest that some cases of adult PLCH represent myeloid neoplastic processes rather than a reactive process induced by exposure to tobacco smoke. This observation raises the possibility of targeted therapy, such as vemurafenib in BRAF-V600E-positive cases, for patients who exhibit progressive disease despite smoking cessation, the cornerstone of management in adult PLCH.

As in other smoking-related ILDs, the clinical presentation tends to be nonspecific and includes dry cough and shortness of breath (Table 3.1). About one-third of patients are asymptomatic.[5] Constitutional symptoms occur in approximately 20–30% of patients, while few patients (around 10–15%) may present with a spontaneous pneumothorax that can be recurrent.[5,102] Rarely,

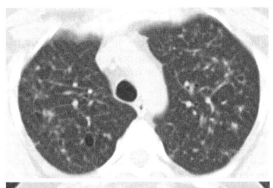

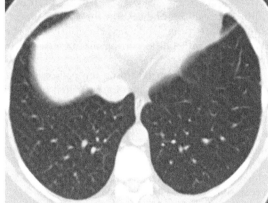

FIG. 3.3   High-resolution CT of the chest demonstrating a combination of nodular and cystic lesions in the upper lung fields and relative sparing of the lung bases in a smoker with pulmonary Langerhans cell histiocytosis.

patients may present with symptoms related to extrapulmonary manifestation, such as skin, lymph node, or bony involvement.

Pulmonary function testing demonstrates variable results and may show obstructive, restrictive, mixed, or nonspecific abnormalities; pulmonary function testing may at times be completely normal.[5] Physiologic studies reveal limitations in the exercise capacity that can occur even with relatively normal resting ventilatory function. Exercise limitation correlates with markers of pulmonary vascular dysfunction, implying vascular involvement as an important cause of exercise limitation in these patients.[103]

The chest radiograph is usually abnormal and shows reticulonodular opacities more prominent in the middle and upper lung zones.[104] The HRCT of the chest often reveals characteristic abnormalities that include nodules and cysts in varying combinations bilaterally with relative sparing of the lung bases (Fig. 3.3).

Nodules with or without cavitation predominate in early disease, whereas cystic changes predominate in more advanced disease.[104,105]

A bronchoscopic or surgically obtained lung biopsy is recommended to confirm the diagnosis but is not always necessary. Bronchoscopy is diagnostically useful if an elevated percentage of CD1a-positive cells is identified in the BAL fluid, with ≥5% being virtually diagnostic of PLCH.[106–108]

Histologic features of early PLCH include loosely formed nodules of mixed inflammatory cells centered on small airways in a bronchiolocentric pattern.[56,109] These bronchiolocentric lesions of pulmonary LCH typically form stellate lesions with central scarring.[72,109] Langerhans cells are abundant in early lesions and may be identified by immunohistochemical staining for the CD1a or Langerin (CD207) cell surface antigens or by the identification of intracellular Birbeck granules (pentalaminar rod-shaped intracellular structures) by electron microscopy.[57,72,107,109,110] Eosinophilic infiltration is often encountered and may be quite extensive earlier in the course of the disease.[57,72,107,109,110] Varying degrees of parenchymal infiltration with macrophages, lymphocytes, and eosinophils are noted, and in rare cases, extensive alveolar macrophage infiltration causes a "pseudo-DIP" reaction.[13,56] Some cases are associated with extensive vascular infiltration of inflammatory cells, resulting in a proliferative vasculopathy involving both arteries and veins.[111]

A critical component in the management of PLCH is smoking cessation. Smoking cessation often leads to stabilization of symptoms and radiologic abnormalities.[5,14,16,19,112] However, some individuals may show disease progression leading to respiratory failure despite smoking cessation.[5] There is no biomarker to predict which patient will improve and who will continue to get worse despite smoking cessation. For patients with severe disease, systemic pharmacotherapy is often considered in addition to smoking cessation. Corticosteroid therapy in the form of oral prednisone 40–60 mg daily with slow tapering over months has historically been used to treat patients with severe or progressive disease, but the data on therapeutic benefit of corticosteroids are limited.[92] Because of the perceived lack of effectiveness of corticosteroids, a number of other immunosuppressive agents, namely vinblastine, chlorodeoxyadenosine (also known as 2-CDA),[113] cyclophosphamide, and methotrexate, have been used to treat progressive PLCH.[92] Chlorodeoxyadenosine has been successfully used in the management of multisystem LCH involving the bone and skin, but its utility in the management of smoking-related PLCH is not well defined.[113,114] Whether immunosuppressive therapy is effective in the management of patients with progressive disease who continue to smoke is currently not known. As noted earlier, identification of somatic mutations in a subset of patients with PLCH raises the possibility of targeted therapy such as vemurafenib, a selective oral inhibitor of *BRAF* V600 kinase, in the treatment of *BRAF* V600E mutation-positive cases.[115]

Management of PLCH also includes treating associated complications and sequelae such as pneumothorax, pulmonary hypertension, and respiratory failure.[5,89,102,111] Pneumothorax is generally managed initially by chest tube drainage. Pleurodesis should be considered for most patients with spontaneous pneumothorax associated with PLCH because the recurrence rate of pneumothorax with conservative management only is ~60%.[102] Pulmonary hypertension is a complication that can be seen even in the absence of severe ventilatory impairment or hypoxemia in patients with PLCH and is present in nearly all patients with advanced disease.[92,111] The presence of pulmonary hypertension portends a poor prognosis.[92,111] We routinely perform a two-dimensional echocardiogram on patients with PLCH at the time of diagnosis and later in the clinical course if dyspnea or the degree of hypoxemia seems out of proportion to the severity of ventilatory impairment on pulmonary function testing.[92] If the patient has echocardiographic evidence of pulmonary hypertension, right-sided heart catheterization should be performed to confirm the presence, determine the severity, and assess response to vasomodulator therapy. The use of vasomodulators such as the endothelin antagonist bosentan and the phosphodiesterase inhibitor sildenafil should be considered in patients with moderate to severe pulmonary hypertension.[116,117]

Overall, most patients with PLCH have a relatively good prognosis, particularly if complete smoking cessation is achieved.[5,19,118] The overall median survival from time of diagnosis is ~13 years, with 5-year and 10-year survival rates of 75% and 64%, respectively.[5,92] Some individuals may progress to extensive pulmonary scarring and cystic changes leading to respiratory failure.[5,59,92] Lung transplantation is an option for patients with advanced PLCH. The overall survival of PLCH patients with lung transplants is comparable to that of individuals with other indications for lung transplantation.[24,119] Recurrence of PLCH in the transplanted lung, even after smoking cessation, has been described in a few cases.[23,24,120]

## ACUTE INTERSTITIAL LUNG DISEASES ASSOCIATED WITH SMOKING

AEP is an acute respiratory illness characterized by bilateral lung opacities, hypoxemia, and pulmonary eosinophilia.[121,122] While some cases of AEP are idiopathic, other cases have been linked to multiple etiologic factors including drugs,[123–127] toxin inhalation,[128] infections,[129–131] heavy metals,[128] and, more recently, cigarette smoke.[29,32,132,133] In 2004, 18 cases of AEP were documented among American military personnel deployed in the Iraq war.[10] The individuals affected were between the ages of 19 and 47 years; interestingly, all were smokers and 78% of them had begun smoking within 2 weeks to 2 months before the onset of illness.[10] Similar reports from Japan had previously described young adults with AEP occurring shortly after starting smoking.[25–27]

Very little is known regarding the pathogenesis of AEP. It is possible, although not proven, that acute cigarette smoke exposure coupled with other proallergic exposures may facilitate the generation of cytokines (e.g., interleukin-5) that enable massive recruitment and activation of eosinophils in the lungs.[134,135] Eosinophilic infiltration may subsequently promote direct damage to the lung tissue by release of soluble factors in eosinophilic granules.

The presentation of AEP may be mistaken for community-acquired pneumonia or acute respiratory distress syndrome depending on the severity of the illness. After initial presentation, the illness may progress rapidly over a 7- to 14-day period to diffuse pulmonary opacities and respiratory failure. Chest radiography typically shows bilateral alveolar opacities and small pleural effusions. Chest CT usually reveals patchy alveolar opacities of ground-glass and/or consolidative character, interlobular septal thickening, and pleural effusions (Fig. 3.4).[136]

Diagnosis rests on the identification of more than 20% eosinophils in the BAL fluid combined with the appropriate clinicoradiologic context.[122,137,138] The peripheral eosinophil count may be normal at presentation but is commonly elevated later in the clinical course.[122,137,138] Lung biopsy (bronchoscopic or surgical) is usually not required for diagnosis but, when performed, reveals marked eosinophilic infiltration in the interstitium and the alveoli.[139] The alveolar architecture is usually preserved.

The cornerstone in the treatment of smoking-related AEP is smoking cessation. In addition, corticosteroid therapy in varying doses has been used depending on the severity of respiratory manifestations. For example, prednisone 40–60 mg per day usually results

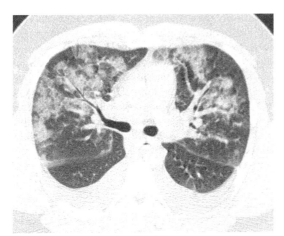

FIG. 3.4  High-resolution CT of the chest revealing bilateral consolidative and ground-glass opacities as well as pleural effusions in a 22-year-old man with acute eosinophilic pneumonia. He had begun smoking cigarettes 3 weeks before this evaluation for progressive dyspnea.

in relatively rapid improvement in those experiencing respiratory failure with diffuse pulmonary opacities and pleural effusions.[10,33] The prognosis in cases that are appropriately treated is generally excellent, although a few deaths have been reported caused by refractory respiratory failure.[10,33] After recovery, most patients have no long-term sequelae.[10,33]

Aside from AEP, cigarette smoking has also been implicated as an etiologic factor in acute pulmonary hemorrhage occurring in patients with Goodpasture syndrome, a pulmonary-renal syndrome associated with circulating anti–glomerular basement membrane (GBM) antibodies.[28,140] In a study of 51 patients with glomerulonephritis associated with anti-GBM antibodies, pulmonary hemorrhage occurred in all of the cigarette smokers compared with only 20% of the nonsmokers.[28] In addition, resumption of smoking was followed by recrudescence of pulmonary hemorrhage in one patient.[28]

## SMOKING AND PULMONARY FIBROSIS

There are other diffuse fibrotic lung diseases that occur at a higher frequency in cigarette smokers than in nonsmokers, but the cause-effect relationship is not well defined. For example, while there are a number of studies that have shown UIP, the histopathologic lesion in IPF, to be more common among smokers, there are limited data that cigarette smoking directly causes interstitial fibrosis.[7,35,141,142] It is conceivable

that cigarette smoke might act as a cofactor along with some other unknown environmental or endogenous profibrotic stimuli in susceptible individuals and promote interstitial fibrosis, or possibly UIP. Smoking has also been reported to influence the clinical course associated with UIP.[143] A study on survival in IPF patients showed that current smokers with IPF may have a survival advantage compared to IPF patients who quit smoking or never smoked. However, in multivariate analysis, this "protective effect" was lost, and both current and former smokers were observed to have a greater risk of death when compared with never-smokers.[143] The putative "protective effect" of smoking was also brought into question in a study of 249 patients with IPF in whom severity-adjusted survival was higher among never-smokers.[141] This study demonstrated that severity-adjusted survival was higher in nonsmokers when compared with either former smokers or the combined group of former and current smokers and showed that the presumed "protective" smoking effect is likely due to less severe disease at presentation in the smokers or former smokers.

Some smokers manifest a combination of emphysema with fibrosis, so-called combined pulmonary fibrosis and emphysema (CPFE) syndrome.[144-146] In such patients, spirometric values may underestimate the degree of pulmonary dysfunction because of counteracting physiologic processes.[147,148] However, severe impairment of gas exchange will be evident, including a low diffusing capacity. These patients with CPFE have a high prevalence of pulmonary hypertension and poor prognosis.[144,147-149]

Cigarette smokers are also at increased risk of developing RA, and individuals with established RA are at higher risk of developing ILD than nonsmokers with RA.[150,151] A study of 336 patients with RA found that those with a >25 pack-year smoking history were significantly more likely to have radiologic evidence of ILD (odds ratio of 3.76; 95% CI, 1.59–8.88).[8] Cigarette smoking likely represents the principal preventable risk factor for RA-associated ILD.[152]

The significance of interstitial opacities in smokers without clinically evident ILD is not well defined. Recently, Washko and colleagues[153] analyzed data from a large cohort of smokers included in the COPDGene study and reported interstitial radiographic abnormalities in 8% of this population. Interestingly, the presence of radiographic interstitial abnormalities correlated with less radiographic emphysema and a greater likelihood of spirometric restrictive impairment. The most frequently observed interstitial abnormalities on HRCT were centrilobular or peribronchial ground-glass opacities and subpleural reticular, nodular, or ground-glass opacities. While histopathologic findings were not available for this study population, centrilobular nodules and ground-glass opacities most likely represent RB, which is ubiquitous in smokers. It is tempting to speculate that the observed peripheral subpleural radiographic abnormality in older subjects is an early subclinical form of pulmonary fibrosis similar to that seen in IPF.[154]

## INTERSTITIAL LUNG DISEASES THAT ARE LESS COMMON IN SMOKERS

HP is an allergic immune-mediated interstitial and small airway disease that may be induced by exposure to many different types of antigens in the environment. HP has been reported to occur less frequently among smokers compared with nonsmokers.[155] Potential mechanisms by which cigarette smoking may decrease the risk of HP in individuals exposed to antigens include inhibition of macrophage and dendritic cell costimulatory capacity, suppression of cytokines such as interleukin-12 by activated dendritic cells, and suppression of T-cell function.[44,156] However, HP can and does occur in smokers.[157] In one study that compared the clinical features of HP in smokers and nonsmokers, recurrence of symptoms following diagnosis and vital capacity measurements were worse in smokers.[157]

Sarcoidosis is another ILD that is less common in smokers compared with nonsmokers.[39] In a large case-control study on etiologic factors in sarcoidosis, a history of cigarette smoking was less frequent among the 706 subjects with sarcoidosis compared with control subjects (OR 0.62, 95% CI, 0.50–0.77).[158] Although smoking reduces the prevalence of sarcoidosis, it does not confer any benefit to patients with established sarcoidosis, who may have a worse outcome than non-smokers with sarcoidosis.[159]

## SUMMARY

Substantial evidence implicates cigarette smoking as the principal etiologic factor responsible for the development of RB-ILD, DIP, and PLCH. Cigarette smoking is an important precipitant of AEP and pulmonary hemorrhage in patients with Goodpasture syndrome, and smokers are at higher risk of developing IPF and RA-associated ILD. It is important to recognize and continue to investigate the role of cigarette smoke in the pathogenesis and clinical course of these diverse diffuse parenchymal lung diseases. Although relatively uncommon, these diseases are a significant health burden and frequently affect young adults in their most productive years. With the global increase in the prevalence of cigarette smoking, particularly in developing countries, it is likely that the burden of tobacco-related diseases, including smoking-related ILDs, will become heavier. Practitioners should use and recognize smoking cessation strategies as a critical component of therapy for these patients, with corticosteroids and other immune modifying agents employed as adjunctive treatments.

## REFERENCES

1. Fraig M, Shreesha U, Savici D, Katzenstein AL. Respiratory bronchiolitis: a clinicopathologic study in current smokers, ex-smokers, and never-smokers. *Am J Surg Pathol*. 2002;26(5):647–653.
2. Friedman PJ, Liebow AA, Sokoloff J. Eosinophilic granuloma of lung: clinical aspects of primary histiocytosis in the adult. *Medicine*. November 1981;60(6): 385–396.
3. Ryu JH, Colby TV, Hartman TE, Vassallo R. Smoking-related interstitial lung diseases: a concise review. *Eur Respir J*. January 2001;17(1):122–132.
4. Ryu JH, Myers JL, Capizzi SA, Douglas WW, Vassallo R, Decker PA. Desquamative interstitial pneumonia and respiratory bronchiolitis-associated interstitial lung disease. *Chest*. January 2005;127(1):178–184.
5. Vassallo R, Ryu JH, Schroeder DR, Decker PA, Limper AH. Clinical outcomes of pulmonary Langerhans'-cell histiocytosis in adults. *N Engl J Med*. February 14, 2002;346(7): 484–490.
6. Margaritopoulos GA, Vasarmidi E, Jacob J, Wells AU, Antoniou KM. Smoking and interstitial lung diseases. *Euro Respir Rev*. 2015;24(137):428–435.
7. Miyake Y, Sasaki S, Yokoyama T, et al. Occupational and environmental factors and idiopathic pulmonary fibrosis in Japan. *Ann Occup Hyg*. April 2005;49(3):259–265.
8. Saag KG, Kolluri S, Koehnke RK, et al. Rheumatoid arthritis lung disease. Determinants of radiographic and physiologic abnormalities. *Arthritis Rheum*. October 1996;39(10):1711–1719.
9. Klareskog L, Stolt P, Lundberg K, et al. A new model for an etiology of rheumatoid arthritis: smoking may trigger HLA-DR (shared epitope)-restricted immune reactions to autoantigens modified by citrullination. *Arthritis Rheum*. January 2006;54(1):38–46.
10. Shorr AF, Scoville SL, Cersovsky SB, et al. Acute eosinophilic pneumonia among US Military personnel deployed in or near Iraq. *JAMA*. 2004;292(24):2997–3005.
11. Girard M, Israel-Assayag E, Cormier Y. Pathogenesis of hypersensitivity pneumonitis. *Curr Opin Allergy Clin Immunol*. April 2004;4(2):93–98.
12. Patel RR, Ryu JH, Vassallo R. Cigarette smoking and diffuse lung disease. *Drugs*. 2008;68(11):1511–1527.

13. Vassallo R, Jensen EA, Colby TV, et al. The overlap between respiratory bronchiolitis and desquamative interstitial pneumonia in pulmonary Langerhans cell histiocytosis: high-resolution CT, histologic, and functional correlations. *Chest*. October 2003;124(4):1199–1205.

14. Mogulkoc N, Veral A, Bishop PW, Bayindir U, Pickering CA, Egan JJ. Pulmonary Langerhans' cell histiocytosis: radiologic resolution following smoking cessation. *Chest*. May 1999;115(5):1452–1455.

15. Zeid NA, Muller HK. Tobacco smoke induced lung granulomas and tumors: association with pulmonary Langerhans cells. *Pathology*. July 1995;27(3):247–254.

16. Negrin-Dastis S, Butenda D, Dorzee J, Fastrez J, d'Odemont JP. Complete disappearance of lung abnormalities on high-resolution computed tomography: a case of histiocytosis X. *Can Respir J*. May–June 2007;14(4):235–237.

17. Bernstrand C, Cederlund K, Ashtrom L, Henter JI. Smoking preceded pulmonary involvement in adults with Langerhans cell histiocytosis diagnosed in childhood. *Acta Paediatr*. November 2000;89(11):1389–1392.

18. Portnoy J, Veraldi KL, Schwarz MI, et al. Respiratory bronchiolitis-interstitial lung disease: long-term outcome. *Chest*. March 2007;131(3):664–671.

19. Elia D, Torre O, Cassandro R, Caminati A, Harari S. Pulmonary Langerhans cell histiocytosis: a comprehensive analysis of 40 patients and literature review. *Euro J Inter Med*. 2015;26(5):351–356.

20. Mason RH, Foley NM, Branley HM, et al. Pulmonary Langerhans cell histiocytosis (PLCH): a new UK register. *Thorax*. 2014;69(8):766–767.

21. Craig PJ, Wells AU, Doffman S, et al. Desquamative interstitial pneumonia, respiratory bronchiolitis and their relationship to smoking. *Histopathology*. September 2004;45(3):275–282.

22. Godbert B, Wissler M-P, Vignaud J-M. Desquamative interstitial pneumonia: an analytic review with an emphasis on aetiology. *Euro Respir Rev*. 2013;22(128):117–123.

23. Etienne B, Bertocchi M, Gamondes JP, et al. Relapsing pulmonary Langerhans cell histiocytosis after lung transplantation. *Am J Respir Crit Care Med*. January 1998;157(1):288–291.

24. Dauriat G, Mal H, Thabut G, et al. Lung transplantation for pulmonary langerhans' cell histiocytosis: a multicenter analysis. *Transplantation*. March 15, 2006;81(5):746–750.

25. Nakajima M, Matsushima T. Acute eosinophilic pneumonia following cigarette smoking. *Intern Med*. October 2000;39(10):759–760.

26. Shiota Y, Kawai T, Matsumoto H, et al. Acute eosinophilic pneumonia following cigarette smoking. *Intern Med*. October 2000;39(10):830–833.

27. Watanabe K, Fujimura M, Kasahara K, et al. Acute eosinophilic pneumonia following cigarette smoking: a case report including cigarette-smoking challenge test. *Intern Med*. November 2002;41(11):1016–1020.

28. Donaghy M, Rees AJ. Cigarette smoking and lung haemorrhage in glomerulonephritis caused by autoantibodies to glomerular basement membrane. *Lancet*. December 17, 1983;2(8364):1390–1393.

29. Nakajima M, Manabe T, Niki Y, Matsushima T, Takashi S. A case of cigarette smoking-induced acute eosinophilic pneumonia showing tolerance. *Chest*. November 2000;118(5):1517–1518.

30. Alp H, Daum RS, Abrahams C, Wylam ME. Acute eosinophilic pneumonia: a cause of reversible, severe, noninfectious respiratory failure. *J Pediatr*. March 1998;132 (3 Pt 1):540–543.

31. Nakagome K, Kato J, Kubota S, Kaneko F, Hisatomi T, Horiuchi T. Acute eosinophilic pneumonia induced by cigarette smoking. *Nihon Kokyuki Gakkai Zasshi*. February 2000;38(2):113–116.

32. Rhee CK, Min KH, Yim NY, et al. Clinical characteristics and corticosteroid treatment of acute eosinophilic pneumonia. *Eur Respir J*. 2013;41(2):402–409.

33. Uchiyama H, Suda T, Nakamura Y, et al. Alterations in smoking habits are associated with acute eosinophilic pneumonia. *Chest*. May 2008;133(5):1174–1180.

34. Wolfe F. The effect of smoking on clinical, laboratory, and radiographic status in rheumatoid arthritis. *J Rheum*. March 2000;27(3):630–637.

35. Baumgartner KB, Samet JM, Stidley CA, Colby TV, Waldron JA. Cigarette smoking: a risk factor for idiopathic pulmonary fibrosis. *Am J Respir Crit Care Med*. 1997;155(1):242–248.

36. Luukkainen R, Saltyshev M, Pakkasela R, Nordqvist E, Huhtala H, Hakala M. Relationship of rheumatoid factor to lung diffusion capacity in smoking and non-smoking patients with rheumatoid arthritis. *Scand J Rheumatol*. 1995;24(2):119–120.

37. Katzenstein A-L, Mukhopadhyay S, Zanardi C, Dexter E. Clinically occult interstitial fibrosis in smokers: classification and significance of a surprisingly common finding in lobectomy specimens. *Hum Pathol*. March 2010;41(3):316–325.

38. Franks TJ, Galvin JR. Smoking-related "interstitial" lung disease. *Arch Pathol Lab Med*. 2015;139(8):974–977.

39. Valeyre D, Soler P, Clerici C, et al. Smoking and pulmonary sarcoidosis: effect of cigarette smoking on prevalence, clinical manifestations, alveolitis, and evolution of the disease. *Thorax*. July 1988;43(7):516–524.

40. Hance AJ, Basset F, Saumon G, et al. Smoking and interstitial lung disease. The effect of cigarette smoking on the incidence of pulmonary histiocytosis X and sarcoidosis. *Ann NY Acad Sci*. 1986;465:643–656.

41. Warren CP. Extrinsic allergic alveolitis: a disease commoner in non-smokers. *Thorax*. October 1977;32(5):567–569.

42. Douglas JG, Middleton WG, Gaddie J, et al. Sarcoidosis: a disorder commoner in non-smokers? *Thorax*. October 1986;41(10):787–791.

43. Vassallo R, Tamada K, Lau JS, Kroening PR, Chen L. Cigarette smoke extract suppresses human dendritic cell function leading to preferential induction of Th-2 priming. *J Immunol.* August 15, 2005;175(4):2684–2691.

44. Israel-Assayag E, Dakhama A, Lavigne S, Laviolette M, Cormier Y. Expression of costimulatory molecules on alveolar macrophages in hypersensitivity pneumonitis. *Am J Respir Crit Care Med.* June 1999;159(6):1830–1834.

45. Anderson K, Morrison SM, Bourke S, Boyd G. Effect of cigarette smoking on the specific antibody response in pigeon fanciers. *Thorax.* 1988;43(10):798–800.

46. Cormier Y, Belanger J, Durand P. Factors influencing the development of serum precipitins to farmer's lung antigen in Quebec dairy farmers. *Thorax.* February 1985;40(2):138–142.

47. Hakala M, Paakko P, Huhti E, Tarkka M, Sutinen S. Open lung biopsy of patients with rheumatoid arthritis. *Clin Rheumatol.* 1990;9(4):452–460.

48. Churg A, Muller NL, Flint J, Wright JL. Chronic hypersensitivity pneumonitis. *Am J Surg Pathol.* February 2006;30(2):201–208.

49. Travis WD, Costabel U, Hansell DM, et al. An official american thoracic society/european respiratory society statement: update of the international multidisciplinary classification of the idiopathic interstitial pneumonias. *Am J Respir Crit Care Med.* 2013;188(6):733–748.

50. Moon J, du Bois RM, Colby TV, Hansell DM, Nicholson AG. Clinical significance of respiratory bronchiolitis on open lung biopsy and its relationship to smoking related interstitial lung disease. *Thorax.* 1999;54(11):1009–1014.

51. Ranney L, Melvin C, Lux L, McClain E, Lohr KN. Systematic review: smoking cessation intervention strategies for adults and adults in special populations. *Ann Intern Med.* December 5, 2006;145(11):845–856.

52. Siu AL, Force USPST. Behavioral and pharmacotherapy interventions for tobacco smoking cessation in adults, including pregnant women: U.S. Preventive Services Task Force recommendation statement. *Ann Intern Med.* 2015;163(8):622–634.

53. Kuschner WG, D'Alessandro A, Wong H, Blanc PD. Dose-dependent cigarette smoking-related inflammatory responses in healthy adults. *Eur Respir J.* October 1996;9(10):1989–1994.

54. Casolaro MA, Bernaudin JF, Saltini C, Ferrans VJ, Crystal RG. Accumulation of Langerhans' cells on the epithelial surface of the lower respiratory tract in normal subjects in association with cigarette smoking. *Am Rev Respir Disease.* February 1988;137(2):406–411.

55. Crotty Alexander LE, Shin S, Hwang JH. Inflammatory diseases of the lung induced by conventional cigarette smoke: a review. *Chest.* 2015;148(5):1307–1322.

56. Colby TV, Lombard C. Histiocytosis X in the lung. *Hum Pathol.* October 1983;14(10):847–856.

57. Travis WD, Borok Z, Roum JH, et al. Pulmonary Langerhans cell granulomatosis (histiocytosis X). A clinicopathologic study of 48 cases. *Am J Surg Pathol.* 1993;17(10):971–986.

58. Myers JL, Veal Jr CF, Shin MS, Katzenstein AL. Respiratory bronchiolitis causing interstitial lung disease. A clinicopathologic study of six cases. *Am Rev Respir Dis.* 1987;135(4):880–884.

59. Remy-Jardin M, Remy J, Gosselin B, Becette V, Edme JL. Lung parenchymal changes secondary to cigarette smoking: pathologic-CT correlations. *Radiology.* March 1993;186(3):643–651.

60. Tomita K, Caramori G, Lim S, et al. Increased p21(CIP1/WAF1) and B cell lymphoma leukemia-x(L) expression and reduced apoptosis in alveolar macrophages from smokers. *Am J Respir Crit Care Med.* September 1, 2002;166(5):724–731.

61. Tazi A, Bonay M, Bergeron A, Grandsaigne M, Hance AJ, Soler P. Role of granulocyte-macrophage colony stimulating factor (GM-CSF) in the pathogenesis of adult pulmonary histiocytosis X. *Thorax.* June 1996;51(6):611–614.

62. Tazi A, Bouchonnet F, Grandsaigne M, Boumsell L, Hance AJ, Soler P. Evidence that granulocyte macrophage-colony-stimulating factor regulates the distribution and differentiated state of dendritic cells/Langerhans cells in human lung and lung cancers. *J Clin Invest.* February 1993;91(2):566–576.

63. Wang RD, Wright JL, Churg A. Transforming growth factor-beta1 drives airway remodeling in cigarette smoke-exposed tracheal explants. *Am J Respir Cell Mol Biol.* October 2005;33(4):387–393.

64. D'Hulst AI, Vermaelen KY, Brusselle GG, Joos GF, Pauwels RA. Time course of cigarette smoke-induced pulmonary inflammation in mice. *Eur Respir J.* August 2005;26(2):204–213.

65. Lu LM, Zavitz CC, Chen B, Kianpour S, Wan Y, Stampfli MR. Cigarette smoke impairs NK cell-dependent tumor immune surveillance. *J Immunol.* January 15, 2007;178(2):936–943.

66. Kode A, Yang SR, Rahman I. Differential effects of cigarette smoke on oxidative stress and proinflammatory cytokine release in primary human airway epithelial cells and in a variety of transformed alveolar epithelial cells. *Respir Res.* 2006;7:132.

67. Yang SR, Chida AS, Bauter MR, et al. Cigarette smoke induces proinflammatory cytokine release by activation of NF-kappaB and posttranslational modifications of histone deacetylase in macrophages. *Am J Physiol.* July 2006;291(1):L46–L57.

68. Niewoehner DE, Kleinerman J, Rice DB. Pathologic changes in the peripheral airways of young cigarette smokers. *N Engl J Med.* October 10, 1974;291(15):755–758.

69. Yousem SA, Colby TV, Gaensler EA. Respiratory bronchiolitis-associated interstitial lung disease and its relationship to desquamative interstitial pneumonia. *Mayo Clin Proc.* 1989;64(11):1373–1380.

70. Mavridou D, Laws D. Respiratory bronchiolitis associated interstitial lung disease (RB-ILD): a case of an acute presentation. *Thorax.* October 2004;59(10):910–911.

71. Hartman TE, Tazelaar HD, Swensen SJ, Muller NL. Cigarette smoking: CT and pathologic findings of associated pulmonary diseases. *Radiographics*. 1997;17(2): 377–390.

72. Aubry MC, Wright JL, Myers JL. The pathology of smoking-related lung diseases. *Clin Chest Med*. March 2000;21(1):11–35. vii.

73. Wells AU, Nicholson AG, Hansell DM, du Bois RM. Respiratory bronchiolitis-associated interstitial lung disease. *Sem Respir Crit Care Med*. October 2003;24(5):585–594.

74. Nadrous HF, Pellikka PA, Krowka MJ, et al. Pulmonary hypertension in patients with idiopathic pulmonary fibrosis. *Chest*. October 2005;128(4):2393–2399.

75. Liebow AA, Steer A, Billingsley JG. Desquamative interstitial pneumonia. *Am J Med*. September 1965;39:369–404.

76. Iskandar SB, McKinney LA, Shah L, Roy TM, Byrd Jr RP. Desquamative interstitial pneumonia and hepatitis C virus infection: a rare association. *South Med J*. September 2004;97(9):890–893.

77. Flores-Franco RA, Luevano-Flores E, Gaston-Ramirez C. Sirolimus-associated desquamative interstitial pneumonia. *Respiration*. 2007;74(2):237–238.

78. Carrington CB, Gaensler EA, Coutu RE, FitzGerald MX, Gupta RG. Natural history and treated course of usual and desquamative interstitial pneumonia. *N Engl J Med*. April 13, 1978;298(15):801–809.

79. Hansell DM, Nicholson AG. Smoking-related diffuse parenchymal lung disease: HRCT-pathologic correlation. *Sem Respir Crit Care Med*. August 2003;24(4): 377–392.

80. Heyneman LE, Ward S, Lynch DA, Remy-Jardin M, Johkoh T, Muller NL. Respiratory bronchiolitis, respiratory bronchiolitis-associated interstitial lung disease, and desquamative interstitial pneumonia: different entities or part of the spectrum of the same disease process? *Am J Roentgenol*. December 1999;173(6):1617–1622.

81. Hidalgo A, Franquet T, Gimenez A, Bordes R, Pineda R, Madrid M. Smoking-related interstitial lung diseases: radiologic-pathologic correlation. *Euro Radiol*. 2006; 16(11):2463–2470.

82. Hartman TE, Primack SL, Kang EY, et al. Disease progression in usual interstitial pneumonia compared with desquamative interstitial pneumonia. Assessment with serial CT. *Chest*. 1996;110(2):378–382.

83. Mueller-Mang C, Grosse C, Schmid K, Stiebellehner L, Bankier AA. What every radiologist should know about idiopathic interstitial pneumonias. *Radiographics*. May–June 2007;27(3):595–615.

84. Matsuo K, Tada S, Kataoka M, et al. Spontaneous remission of desquamative interstitial pneumonia. *Intern Med*. October 1997;36(10):728–731.

85. Bjoraker JA, Ryu JH, Edwin MK, et al. Prognostic significance of histopathologic subsets in idiopathic pulmonary fibrosis. *Am J Respir Crit Care Med*. January 1998;157(1):199–203.

86. Flusser G, Gurman G, Zirkin H, Prinslo I, Heimer D. Desquamative interstitial pneumonitis causing acute respiratory failure, responsive only to immunosuppressants. *Respiration*. 1991;58(5–6):324–326.

87. King MB, Jessurun J, Hertz MI. Recurrence of desquamative interstitial pneumonia after lung transplantation. *Am J Respir Crit Care Med*. 1997;156(6): 2003–2005.

88. Verleden GM, Sels F, Van Raemdonck D, Verbeken EK, Lerut T, Demedts M. Possible recurrence of desquamative interstitial pneumonitis in a single lung transplant recipient. *Eur Respir J*. 1998;11(4):971–974.

89. Vassallo R, Ryu JH, Colby TV, Hartman T, Limper AH. Pulmonary Langerhans'-cell histiocytosis. *N Engl J Med*. June 29, 2000;342(26):1969–1978.

90. Tazi A. Adult pulmonary Langerhans' cell histiocytosis. *Eur Respir J*. June 2006;27(6):1272–1285.

91. Favara BE, Feller AC, Pauli M, et al. Contemporary classification of histiocytic disorders. The WHO Committee on histiocytic/reticulum cell proliferations. Reclassification Working Group of the Histiocyte Society. *Med Pediatr Oncol*. September 1997;29(3):157–166.

92. Chaowalit N, Pellikka PA, Decker PA, et al. Echocardiographic and clinical characteristics of pulmonary hypertension complicating pulmonary Langerhans cell histiocytosis. *Mayo Clin Proc*. 2004;79(10):1269–1275.

93. Delobbe A, Durieu J, Duhamel A, Wallaert B. Determinants of survival in pulmonary Langerhans' cell granulomatosis (histiocytosis X). Groupe d'Etude en Pathologie Interstitielle de la Societe de Pathologie Thoracique du Nord. *Eur Respir J*. October 1996;9(10):2002–2006.

94. Aguayo SM, King Jr TE, Waldron Jr JA, Sherritt KM, Kane MA, Miller YE. Increased pulmonary neuroendocrine cells with bombesin-like immunoreactivity in adult patients with eosinophilic granuloma. *J Clin Invest*. September 1990;86(3):838–844.

95. Asakura S, Colby TV, Limper AH. Tissue localization of transforming growth factor-beta1 in pulmonary eosinophilic granuloma. *Am J Respir Crit Care Med*. November 1996;154(5):1525–1530.

96. Harmon CM, Brown N. Langerhans cell histiocytosis: a clinicopathologic review and molecular pathogenetic update. *Arch Pathol Lab Med*. 2015;139(10): 1211–1214.

97. Diamond EL, Durham BH, Haroche J, et al. Diverse and targetable kinase alterations drive histiocytic neoplasms. *Cancer Discovery*. February 2016;6(2):154–165.

98. Yousem SA, Dacic S, Nikiforov YE, Nikiforova M. Pulmonary langerhans cell histiocytosis: profiling of multifocal tumors using next-generation sequencing identifies concordant occurrence of BRAF V600E mutations. *Chest*. 2013;143(6):1679–1684.

99. Hervier B, Haroche J, Arnaud L, et al. Association of both Langerhans cell histiocytosis and Erdheim-Chester disease linked to the BRAFV600E mutation. *Blood*. 2014;124(7):1119–1126.

100. Roden AC, Hu X, Kip S, et al. BRAF V600E expression in langerhans cell histiocytosis: clinical and immunohistochemical study on 25 pulmonary and 54 extrapulmonary cases. *Am J Surg Pathol*. April 2014;38(4):548–551.

101. Mourah S, How-Kit A, Meignin V, et al. Recurrent NRAS mutations in pulmonary Langerhans cell histiocytosis. *Eur Respir J*. June 2016;47(6):1785–1796.

102. Mendez JL, Nadrous HF, Vassallo R, Decker PA, Ryu JH. Pneumothorax in pulmonary Langerhans cell histiocytosis. *Chest*. March 2004;125(3):1028–1032.

103. Crausman RS, Jennings CA, Tuder RM, Ackerson LM, Irvin CG, King Jr TE. Pulmonary histiocytosis X: pulmonary function and exercise pathophysiology. *Am J Respir Crit Care Med*. January 1996;153(1):426–435.

104. Moore AD, Godwin JD, Muller NL, et al. Pulmonary histiocytosis X: comparison of radiographic and CT findings. *Radiology*. July 1989;172(1):249–254.

105. Brauner MW, Grenier P, Mouelhi MM, Mompoint D, Lenoir S. Pulmonary histiocytosis X: evaluation with high-resolution CT. *Radiology*. July 1989;172(1):255–258.

106. Soler P, Chollet S, Jacque C, Fukuda Y, Ferrans VJ, Basset F. Immunocytochemical characterization of pulmonary histiocytosis X cells in lung biopsies. *Am J Pathol*. March 1985;118(3):439–451.

107. Chollet S, Soler P, Bernaudin JF, Basset F. Exploratory bronchoalveolar lavage. *Presse Med*. June 9, 1984;13(24):1503–1508.

108. Baqir M, Vassallo R, Maldonado F, Yi ES, Ryu JH. Utility of bronchoscopy in pulmonary langerhans cell histiocytosis. *J Bronchology Interv Pulmonol*. October 2013;20(4):309–312.

109. Roden AC, Yi ES. Pulmonary Langerhans cell histiocytosis: an update from the pathologists' perspective. *Arch Pathol Lab Med*. 2016;140(3):230–240.

110. Yousem SA, Colby TV, Chen YY, Chen WG, Weiss LM. Pulmonary Langerhans' cell histiocytosis: molecular analysis of clonality. *Am J Surg Pathol*. May 2001;25(5):630–636.

111. Fartoukh M, Humbert M, Capron F, et al. Severe pulmonary hypertension in histiocytosis X. *Am J Respir Crit Care Med*. January 2000;161(1):216–223.

112. Abbott GF, Rosado-de-Christenson ML, Franks TJ, Frazier AA, Galvin JR. From the archives of the AFIP: pulmonary Langerhans cell histiocytosis. *Radiographics*. May–June 2004;24(3):821–841.

113. Aerni MR, Christine Aubry M, Myers JL, Vassallo R. Complete remission of nodular pulmonary Langerhans cell histiocytosis lesions induced by 2-chlorodeoxyadenosine in a non-smoker. *Respir Med*. 2007;102(2)):316–319.

114. Pardanani A, Phyliky RL, Li CY, Tefferi A. 2-Chlorodeoxyadenosine therapy for disseminated Langerhans cell histiocytosis. *Mayo Clin Proc*. March 2003;78(3):301–306.

115. Hyman DM, Puzanov I, Subbiah V, et al. Vemurafenib in multiple nonmelanoma cancers with BRAF V600 mutations. *N Engl J Med*. 2015;373(8):726–736.

116. Kiakouama L, Cottin V, Etienne-Mastroianni B, Khouatra C, Humbert M, Cordier JF. Severe pulmonary hypertension in histiocytosis X: long-term improvement with bosentan. *Eur Respir J*. July 2010;36(1):202–204.

117. Le Pavec J, Lorillon G, Jaïs X, et al. Pulmonary Langerhans cell histiocytosis-associated pulmonary hypertension: clinical characteristics and impact of pulmonary arterial hypertension therapies. *Chest*. 2012;142(5):1150–1157.

118. Tazi A, de Margerie C, Naccache JM, et al. The natural history of adult pulmonary Langerhans cell histiocytosis: a prospective multicentre study. *Orphanet J Rare Dis*. 2015;10:30.

119. Saleem I, Moss J, Egan JJ. Lung transplantation for rare pulmonary diseases. *Sarcoidosis Vasc Diffuse Lung Dis*. December 2005;22(suppl 1):S85–S90.

120. Gabbay E, Dark JH, Ashcroft T, et al. Recurrence of Langerhans' cell granulomatosis following lung transplantation. *Thorax*. April 1998;53(4):326–327.

121. Philit F, Etienne-Mastroianni B, Parrot A, Guerin C, Robert D, Cordier JF. Idiopathic acute eosinophilic pneumonia: a study of 22 patients. *Am J Respir Crit Care Med*. November 1, 2002;166(9):1235–1239.

122. Allen J. Acute eosinophilic pneumonia. *Sem Respir Crit Care Med*. April 2006;27(2):142–147.

123. Yokoyama A, Mizushima Y, Suzuki H, Arai N, Kitagawa M, Yano S. Acute eosinophilic pneumonia induced by minocycline: prominent Kerley B lines as a feature of positive re-challenge test. *Jpn J Med*. March–April 1990;29(2):195–198.

124. Barnes MT, Bascunana J, Garcia B, Alvarez-Sala JL. Acute eosinophilic pneumonia associated with antidepressant agents. *Pharm World Sci*. October 1999;21(5):241–242.

125. Noh H, Lee YK, Kan SW, Choi KH, Ha DS, Lee HY. Acute eosinophilic pneumonia associated with amitriptyline in a hemodialysis patient. *Yonsei Med J*. June 2001;42(3):357–359.

126. McCormick M, Nelson T. Cocaine-induced fatal acute eosinophilic pneumonia: a case report. *WMJ*. April 2007;106(2):92–95.

127. Miller BA, Gray A, Leblanc TW, Sexton DJ, Martin AR, Slama TG. Acute eosinophilic pneumonia secondary to daptomycin: a report of three cases. *Clin Infect Dis*. June 1, 2010;50(11):e63–68.

128. Kawayama T, Fujiki R, Morimitsu Y, Rikimaru T, Aizawa H. Fatal idiopathic acute eosinophilic pneumonia with acute lung injury. *Respirology*. December 2002;7(4):373–375.

129. Takizawa H. Acute eosinophilic pneumonia: possible role of hyperreactivity of airway epithelial cells. *Intern Med*. November 2002;41(11):917.

130. Glazer CS, Cohen LB, Schwarz MI. Acute eosinophilic pneumonia in AIDS. *Chest*. November 2001;120(5):1732–1735.

131. Jeon EJ, Kim KH, Min KH. Acute eosinophilic pneumonia associated with 2009 influenza A (H1N1). *Thorax*. March 2010;65(3):268–270.

132. Miki K, Miki M, Okano Y, et al. Cigarette smoke-induced acute eosinophilic pneumonia accompanied with neutrophilia in the blood. *Intern Med.* November 2002;41(11):993–996.

133. Al-Saieg N, Moammar O, Kartan R. Flavored cigar smoking induces acute eosinophilic pneumonia. *Chest.* April 2007;131(4):1234–1237.

134. Rom WN, Weiden M, Garcia R, et al. Acute eosinophilic pneumonia in a New York City firefighter exposed to World Trade Center dust. *Am J Respir Crit Care Med.* September 15, 2002;166(6):797–800.

135. Nakahara Y, Hayashi S, Fukuno Y, Kawashima M, Yatsunami J. Increased interleukin-5 levels in bronchoalveolar lavage fluid is a major factor for eosinophil accumulation in acute eosinophilic pneumonia. *Respiration.* 2001;68(4):389–395.

136. Daimon T, Johkoh T, Sumikawa H, et al. Acute eosinophilic pneumonia: thin-section CT findings in 29 patients. *Eur J Radiol.* March 2008;65(3):462–467.

137. King MA, Pope-Harman AL, Allen JN, Christoforidis GA, Christoforidis AJ. Acute eosinophilic pneumonia: radiologic and clinical features. *Radiology.* June 1997;203(3):715–719.

138. Allen JN, Pacht ER, Gadek JE, Davis WB. Acute eosinophilic pneumonia as a reversible cause of noninfectious respiratory failure. *N Engl J Med.* August 31, 1989;321(9):569–574.

139. Tazelaar HD, Linz LJ, Colby TV, Myers JL, Limper AH. Acute eosinophilic pneumonia: histopathologic findings in nine patients. *Am J Respir Crit Care Med.* January 1997;155(1):296–302.

140. Benz K, Amann K, Dittrich K, Hugo C, Schnur K, Dotsch J. Patient with antibody-negative relapse of goodpasture syndrome. *Clin Nephrol.* April 2007;67(4):240–244.

141. Antoniou KM, Hansell DM, Rubens MB, et al. Idiopathic pulmonary fibrosis: outcome in relation to smoking status. *Am J Respir Crit Care Med.* January 15, 2008;177(2):190–194.

142. Katzenstein A-L. Smoking-related interstitial fibrosis (SRIF): pathologic findings and distinction from other chronic fibrosing lung diseases. *J Clin Pathol.* 2013;66(10):882–887.

143. King Jr TE, Tooze JA, Schwarz MI, Brown KR, Cherniack RM. Predicting survival in idiopathic pulmonary fibrosis: scoring system and survival model. *Am J Respir Crit Care Med.* 2001;164(7):1171–1181.

144. Cottin V, Nunes H, Brillet PY, et al. Combined pulmonary fibrosis and emphysema: a distinct underrecognised entity. *Eur Respir J.* October 2005;26(4):586–593.

145. Jankowich MD, Rounds S. Combined pulmonary fibrosis and emphysema alters physiology but has similar mortality to pulmonary fibrosis without emphysema. *Lung.* 2010;188(5):365–373.

146. Ryerson CJ, Hartman T, Elicker BM, et al. Clinical features and outcomes in combined pulmonary fibrosis and emphysema in idiopathic pulmonary fibrosis. *Chest.* 2013;144(1):234–240.

147. Cottin V, Le Pavec J, Prevot G, et al. Pulmonary hypertension in patients with combined pulmonary fibrosis and emphysema syndrome. *Eur Respir J.* January 2010;35(1):105–111.

148. Mejia M, Carrillo G, Rojas-Serrano J, et al. Idiopathic pulmonary fibrosis and emphysema: decreased survival associated with severe pulmonary arterial hypertension. *Chest.* July 2009;136(1):10–15.

149. Sugino K, Ishida F, Kikuchi N, et al. Comparison of clinical characteristics and prognostic factors of combined pulmonary fibrosis and emphysema versus idiopathic pulmonary fibrosis alone. *Respirology.* 2014;19(2):239–245.

150. Klareskog L, Padyukov L, Alfredsson L. Smoking as a trigger for inflammatory rheumatic diseases. *Curr Opin Rheumatol.* January 2007;19(1):49–54.

151. Kelly CA, Saravanan V, Nisar M, et al. Rheumatoid arthritis-related interstitial lung disease: associations, prognostic factors and physiological and radiological characteristics–a large multicentre UK study. *Rheumatology (Oxford).* September 2014;53(9):1676–1682.

152. Kallberg H, Ding B, Padyukov L, et al. Smoking is a major preventable risk factor for rheumatoid arthritis: estimations of risks after various exposures to cigarette smoke. *Ann Rheum Dis.* March 2011;70(3):508–511.

153. Washko GR, Hunninghake GM, Fernandez IE, et al. Lung volumes and emphysema in smokers with interstitial lung abnormalities. *N Engl J Med.* March 10, 2011;364(10):897–906.

154. King Jr TE. Smoking and subclinical interstitial lung disease. *N Engl J Med.* March 10, 2011;364(10):968–970.

155. Selman M. Hypersensitivity pneumonitis: a multifaceted deceiving disorder. *Clin Chest Med.* September 2004;25(3):531–547. vi.

156. Arima K, Ando M, Ito K, et al. Effect of cigarette smoking on prevalence of summer-type hypersensitivity pneumonitis caused by Trichosporon cutaneum. *Arch Environ Health.* July–August 1992;47(4):274–278.

157. Ohtsuka Y, Munakata M, Tanimura K, et al. Smoking promotes insidious and chronic farmer's lung disease, and deteriorates the clinical outcome. *Intern Med.* October 1995;34(10):966–971.

158. Newman LS, Rose CS, Bresnitz EA, et al. A case control etiologic study of sarcoidosis: environmental and occupational risk factors. *Am J Respir Crit Care Med.* December 15, 2004;170(12):1324–1330.

159. Peros-Golubicic T, Ljubic S. Cigarette smoking and sarcoidosis. *Acta Med Croatica.* 1995;49(4–5):187–193.

160. Kitahara Y, Matsumoto K, Taooka Y, et al. Cigarette smoking-induced acute eosinophilic pneumonia showing tolerance in broncho-alveolar lavage findings. *Intern Med.* October 2003;42(10):1016–1021.

# CHAPTER 4

# Management of Idiopathic Pulmonary Fibrosis

STEFANIA CERRI • PAOLO SPAGNOLO • FABRIZIO LUPPI •
GIACOMO SGALLA • LUCA RICHELDI

---

**KEY POINTS**

- Over the last few years two drugs have been shown unequivocally to be both safe and effective in reducing disease progression in idiopathic pulmonary fibrosis (IPF).
- This achievement represents both a point of arrival and a starting point toward even more effective treatments.
- Based on the current knowledge of IPF pathogenesis, it is easy to predict that the future treatment of IPF will be based on multiple drugs.
- IPF patients will keep leading the way in the discovery of therapies for lung fibrosis and, while achieving the important critical goal of the identification of more effective treatments, will also help the large number of patients with non-IPF fibrotic lung disorders.

---

Idiopathic pulmonary fibrosis (IPF) is one of the most challenging diseases for chest physicians for a number of reasons, including the complexity of the diagnostic process, which requires close interaction with different specialists, and the almost invariably poor prognosis, with a 5-year survival of ~20%.[1,2] Moreover, until recently, IPF has lacked effective therapies. Following two decades of clinical trials, most of which have produced negative results, pirfenidone, a compound with broad antifibrotic, antiinflammatory, and antioxidant properties, and nintedanib, an orally available, small-molecule tyrosine kinase inhibitor with selectivity for vascular endothelial growth factor (VEGF), platelet-derived growth factor (PDGF), and fibroblast growth factor (FGF) receptors, have proved equally effective in slowing down functional decline and disease progression with an acceptable safety profile.[3,4] However, neither pirfenidone nor nintedanib is a cure for IPF; neither drug improves lung function and the disease continues to progress in most patients despite treatment. Likewise, the modalities for the follow-up of IPF patients are poorly defined. Accordingly, all decisions related to patient management need to be extensively discussed and agreed upon with the patients and their families. As a result, few respiratory disorders require of chest physicians more interactive skills and more dedication than IPF.

## PHARMACOLOGIC TREATMENTS

Since the publication of the first evidence-based guidelines for the diagnosis and management of IPF in 2011, when the panel of experts involved could not find enough evidence to recommend the use of any pharmacological agent for IPF,[1] recently completed landmark clinical trials have reshaped the evidence for the treatment of IPF. These advances have culminated in the approval of pirfenidone and nintedanib, two compounds with pleiotropic mechanisms of action that are capable of slowing down the rate of functional decline and disease progression of IPF. Nevertheless, the need for a cure for patients with IPF remains unmet. Accordingly, pharmacologic development in this field is more thriving than ever, looking for compounds with novel, mechanistically driven actions to address the plethora of pathways that are believed to be involved in IPF pathogenesis.[5]

### Guidelines for Treatment of Idiopathic Pulmonary Fibrosis: The 2015 Update

The large amount of evidence generated over the last 5 years has led to a revision of the 2011 clinical practice guidelines, which were updated in a new joint statement in 2015.[6] Similar to the 2011 document, the GRADE (Grading of Recommendations, Assessment, Development and Evaluation) methodology[7] was

**TABLE 4.1**

Comparison of Recommendations on Therapeutic Interventions for Idiopathic Pulmonary Fibrosis (IPF) in the 2015 and 2011 Guidelines[a]

| Agent | 2015 Guidelines | 2011 Guidelines |
|---|---|---|
| **NEW RECOMMENDATIONS** | | |
| Nintedanib (multiple tyrosine kinase inhibitor) | Conditional recommendation for use | Not addressed |
| Ambrisentan (selective endothelin receptor antagonist) | Strong recommendation against use | Not addressed |
| Imatinib (single tyrosine kinase inhibitor) | Strong recommendation against use | Not addressed |
| Sildenafil (phosphodiesterase-5 inhibitor) | Conditional recommendation against use | Not addressed |
| **REVISED RECOMMENDATIONS** | | |
| Pirfenidone | Conditional recommendation for use | Weak recommendation against use |
| Dual endothelin receptor antagonists | Conditional recommendation against use | Strong recommendation against use |
| Anticoagulation (warfarin) | Strong recommendation against use | Weak recommendation against use |
| Combination prednisone, azathioprine, and N-acetylcysteine | Strong recommendation against use | Weak recommendation against use |
| **UNCHANGED RECOMMENDATIONS** | | |
| Antacid therapy | Conditional recommendation for use | Weak recommendation for use |
| N-Acetylcysteine monotherapy | Conditional recommendation against use | Weak recommendation against use |

Recommendations for antipulmonary hypertension therapy for IPF-associated pulmonary hypertension and lung transplantation (e.g., single vs. bilateral lung transplantation) were deferred.

adopted to rate the quality of available evidence and express recommendations *for* or *against* the use of the treatments evaluated, with only the substitution of the term "weak" with "conditional" as compared with the 2011 document. While no pharmacologic treatment received a strong recommendation for use in IPF, the original document was amended substantially based on the available evidence as summarized in the following text. Table 4.1 provides a comparison of the 2011 and 2015 recommendations.

The previously widely accepted "triple therapy" (consisting of the combination of prednisone, azathioprine, and N-acetylcysteine [NAC]), which received a weak recommendation against use in the 2011 guidelines, ultimately proved to be associated with increased mortality as compared with placebo and with NAC alone in the three-arm PANTHER-IPF study (Prednisone, Azathioprine, and N-Acetylcysteine: A Study That Evaluates Response in IPF), which was conducted by National Heart, Lung, and Blood Institute–sponsored IPFnet.[8]

In this trial, patients with mild to moderate lung function impairment were randomized in a 1:1:1 ratio to receive prednisolone, azathioprine, and NAC; NAC alone; or placebo over a 60-week period. Following a prespecified safety and efficacy interim analysis, the independent data and safety monitoring board recommended termination of the combination therapy arm at a mean follow-up of 32 weeks, following the observation that the combination therapy was associated with a statistically significant increase in all-cause mortality, all-cause hospitalizations, and treatment-related severe adverse events.[8] The evidence that the "triple therapy"—considered the standard of care in IPF for a decade—is actually harmful should be regarded as groundbreaking and demonstrates that, even if negative, a properly designed randomized-controlled trial (RCT) can importantly inform guidelines, clinical practice, and future trial design. The PANTHER trial, which continued as a two-arm only study, showed no difference between NAC and placebo in terms of change of percentage predicted forced vital capacity (FVC) at 60 weeks and the majority of the secondary outcome measures.[9] The combination of prednisone, azathioprine, and NAC received a strong recommendation against use in the 2015 document, whereas the recommendation for NAC monotherapy remained unchanged (conditional recommendation against use). Despite the negative results of the PANTHER trial, NAC continues to be widely used in clinical practice, mostly because of its good safety and tolerability profile and low cost. Nebulization of NAC via aerosol may represent a more efficient way of delivering the drug directly to the lung parenchyma.[10,11] A post hoc analysis of the PANTHER trial dataset looked at the influence of polymorphisms in *TOLLIP* and *MUC5B* genes (two well-established associations with IPF susceptibility and survival)[12,13] on response to NAC, the rationale being that such polymorphisms are linked to alteration in the lung immune response through oxidative signaling.[14] NAC treatment was associated with improved survival in patients homozygous for the T allele of the rs3750920 *TOLLIP* polymorphism, whereas those carrying the GG genotype had a worse prognosis. Although it remains unclear whether a mechanistic link between oxidative stress and *TOLLIP*-related signaling exists, these data suggest that NAC might be effective in a subset of patients.

Anticoagulation, considered for years a potential therapy for IPF based on a small study that showed survival benefit in hospitalized patients treated with warfarin,[15] was also ultimately associated with increased mortality in a recent, early discontinued RCT (ACE-IPF—AntiCoagulant Effectiveness in Idiopathic Pulmonary Fibrosis)[16] and received a strong recommendation against use in the 2015 treatment guidelines.

The dual endothelin receptor antagonists (ERAs) bosentan and macitentan were given a conditional recommendation against use, based on the results of two Phase II and one Phase III trials.[17–19] Conversely, ambrisentan, a selective ERA, received a strong recommendation against use because of the lack of benefit and high likelihood of harm observed in the ARTEMIS (a Randomized, Placebo-Controlled Study to Evaluate Safety and Effectiveness of Ambrisentan in IPF study) trial, which was prematurely discontinued.[20] Sildenafil is an oral phosphodiesterase-5 inhibitor that has been studied in IPF in two RCTs.[21,22] Sildenafil was given a conditional recommendation against use because of the lack of benefit in any outcome measures apart from a marginal improvement in quality of life.

The recommendation on antacid treatment (AAT) remained unchanged (conditional recommendation for use), although the only data suggesting a beneficial

effect of AAT in patients with IPF derive from retrospective analysis of longitudinal cohorts and pooled analyses of patients randomized to placebo in three RCTs of different pharmacologic therapies.[23,24] Indeed, the role of AAT in IPF remains a matter of intense debate.[25]

The antifibrotic drugs pirfenidone and nintedanib have been consistently demonstrated to slow down functional decline and disease progression in IPF[3,4] and have been approved worldwide. Accordingly, both pirfenidone, which had received a weak recommendation against use in 2011, and nintedanib, which had not been previously addressed, received a conditional recommendation for use in patients with IPF in the 2015 guideline document.

### Pirfenidone

Pirfenidone is an orally administered pyridine with pleiotropic antifibrotic, antiinflammatory, and antioxidant properties, although its precise mechanisms of action remain unknown. This drug, which is the first agent licensed for treatment of patients with mild to moderate IPF, was initially approved for clinical use in Japan, Europe, India, and Canada following regulatory appraisal of the data on safety and efficacy coming from two multicenter trials performed in Japan and two large international multicenter clinical trials (CAPACITY 1/PIPF-006 and CAPACITY 2/PIPF-004).[26–28] Conversely, the US Food and Drug Administration (FDA) denied approval and required a new placebo-controlled Phase III trial, because of concerns regarding inconsistent evidence of efficacy (study PIPF-006 met the primary endpoint of change in percentage predicted FVC at week 72, while study PIPF-004 did not) along with the lack of a clear survival benefit. The ASCEND (Assessment of pirfenidone to Confirm Efficacy and Safety in Idiopathic Pulmonary Fibrosis) study assessed the effect of pirfenidone on disease progression (defined as decline of 10% or more in percentage predicted FVC, or death from any cause) in 555 patients randomly assigned to receive either pirfenidone 2403 mg per day or placebo for 52 weeks.[3] In the pirfenidone group, there was a relative reduction of 47.9% in the proportion of patients who had disease progression. In addition, there was a relative increase of 132.5% in the proportion of patients with no functional decline in the pirfenidone as compared with the placebo arm. Rates of all-cause or IPF-related mortality did not differ significantly between the two groups, although in a prespecified pooled analysis incorporating results from three Phase III trials (CAPACITY 1, CAPACITY 2, and ASCEND) the between-group difference favoring pirfenidone was significant for both all-cause and IPF-related mortality.

Gastrointestinal and skin-related adverse events were more common in the pirfenidone group than in the placebo group, but they were generally of mild to moderate intensity. Indeed, a similar proportion of patients in the pirfenidone (14%) and placebo (10%) group discontinued the study drug because of adverse events. Based on these findings, in October 2014 the FDA approved pirfenidone for treatment of IPF.

Postauthorization data on the use of pirfenidone in clinical practice are available from both international collaborative studies and real-life experiences in Japan and Europe, where pirfenidone was approved in 2010 and 2011, respectively. Interim reports from RECAP, an open-label extension study that enrolled patients who completed the CAPACITY program[29] and from PASSPORT (Pirfenidone Post-Authorization Safety Registry),[30] which prospectively collected data from pirfenidone-treated patients from 10 different countries, confirmed the safety and tolerability of the drug. A number of studies have provided additional information, although most of them reflect single-center experience. A German study conducted at a tertiary referral center showed that the majority of IPF patients treated with pirfenidone (62%) remained stable during treatment, although the rate of functional decline did not differ significantly from the pretreatment period.[31] Interestingly, reports from both Europe and Japan showed that patients with a more pronounced functional decline tend to respond better to the drug.[32–34] These studies confirmed the good safety and tolerability profile of pirfenidone, although weight loss and fatigue occurred more frequently than in the RCT setting.

## Nintedanib

Nintedanib is an orally available inhibitor of different tyrosine kinase receptors, including PDGF receptors α and β; VEGF receptors 1, 2, and 3; and FGF receptors 1, 2, and 3.[35] Activation of these receptors has been implicated in lung fibrosis pathogenesis[36] and in the murine model of bleomycin-induced fibrosis nintedanib was shown to prevent the development of lung fibrosis.[37]

The safety and efficacy of nintedanib at four different oral doses (50 mg once a day, 50 mg, 100 mg, or 150 mg twice daily) have been evaluated in a 52-week Phase II randomized, double-blind, placebo-controlled trial (TOMORROW—To Improve Pulmonary Fibrosis With BIBF 1120).[38] The primary outcome was the annual rate of decline in FVC, while secondary endpoints included rate of acute exacerbations (AE-IPF), quality of life, and total lung capacity. Nintedanib at a dose of 150 mg twice daily showed a trend toward

reduction of the decline in lung function. Specifically, the adjusted annual rate of decline in FVC was 0.06 L/year in the group receiving nintedanib 150 mg twice daily and 0.19 L/year in the placebo group, corresponding to a reduction of 68.4% in the rate of FVC loss ($P = .06$ using a closed testing procedure for multiplicity correction [primary analysis] and $P = .01$ using hierarchical testing, both prespecified). In addition, compared with placebo, significantly fewer patients in the group receiving nintedanib 150 mg twice daily had a decline in mean FVC of ≥10% or ≥200 mL (23.8 vs. 44.0%, respectively; $P = .004$). The highest dose of nintedanib was also associated with fewer AE-IPF and improved quality of life as assessed by St. George's Respiratory Questionnaire (SGRQ). The most frequent adverse event in the group receiving 150 mg nintedanib twice daily was diarrhea (55.3% vs. 15.3% in the placebo group), followed by nausea (23.5% vs. 9.4%) and vomiting (12.9% vs. 4.7%). The adverse events most frequently leading to study discontinuation were also diarrhea, nausea, and vomiting, but the proportion of patients who discontinued the study medication because of adverse events did not differ between the group receiving nintedanib 150 mg twice daily and the placebo group. The INPULSIS-1 and INPULSIS-2 trials were two parallel 52-week, randomized, double-blind, placebo-controlled, Phase III studies designed to confirm the efficacy and safety of nintedanib compared with placebo in patients with IPF.[4] A total of 1066 patients were randomized 3:2 to nintedanib 150 mg twice daily (n = 309 in INPULSIS-1 and n = 329 in INPULSIS-2) or placebo (n = 204 in INPULSIS-1 and n = 219 in INPULSIS-2). Both trials met the primary endpoint (e.g., nintedanib significantly reduced the rate of decline in FVC over the 52-week study period). Specifically, the adjusted annual rate of change in FVC was −114.7 mL in the nintedanib arm and −239.9 mL in the placebo arm in INPULSIS-1 (between-group difference: 125.3 mL; $P < .001$) and −113.6 mL and −207.3 mL in INPULSIS-2 (between-group difference: 93.7 mL; $P < .001$). Moreover, a number of prespecified sensitivity analyses confirmed the robustness of the results of the primary analysis. As for the two key secondary endpoints (i.e., time to the first AE-IPF as reported by the site investigator and the change from baseline in the total score on the SGRQ), the two trials provided inconsistent results. In fact, at week 52 the time to the first AE-IPF was significantly increased in the nintedanib arm in INPULSIS-2 (HR: 0.38, $P = .005$) but not in INPULSIS-1 (HR: 1.15, $P = .67$); on the other hand, the increase in the total SGRQ score was significantly smaller in the nintedanib group than in the placebo group (consistent with less deterioration in health-related quality of life) in INPULSIS-2, whereas in INPULSIS-1 there was no significant between-group difference in the adjusted mean change in the SGRQ total score from baseline to week 52. Similar to the TOMORROW trial, the most frequent adverse event in the nintedanib groups in both INPULSIS-1 and INPULSIS-2 was diarrhea (~60% within the first 3 months of treatment), which overall led to premature discontinuation in 4.4% of patients in the nintedanib group.[4,39] However, in both trials, the proportion of patients with serious adverse events was similar in the nintedanib and placebo arms. Similar to pirfenidone, in October 2014 nintedanib was approved by the FDA for treatment of IPF and has become commercially available worldwide in 2016.

## Limitations of Pharmacologic Treatment

Having two drugs approved for IPF is an outstanding achievement. Yet, there are limitations to the current therapeutic approach, and a number of questions regarding the most appropriate management of individual patients with IPF remain unanswered. Neither pirfenidone nor nintedanib is a cure, and most patients continue to experience disease progression despite treatment; it is unclear whether and to what extent these drugs remain effective beyond 52 weeks; it remains to be determined whether the beneficial effect on functional decline translates to a longer survival (measuring this outcome appears prohibitive because of the number of patients and study duration required for an adequately powered study)[40]; neither of the drugs significantly improves symptoms or quality of life; finally, it is unknown whether the results of the pirfenidone and nintedanib trials, which have enrolled highly selected patients, are generalizable to the more general IPF population.

Pirfenidone and nintedanib are broadly comparable in their efficacy and safety and tolerability profiles.[3,4] In addition, they exhibit similar side effect profiles with regard to gastrointestinal effects (mainly nausea and diarrhea) and liver enzyme elevation. Hence, it remains unclear which of these drugs should be used first and in which patients, although the initial choice should be based on careful consideration of patient clinical features, comorbidities, side effect profiles of the two drugs, as well as patient personal preferences. Whatever the initial choice, physicians may consider switching from one drug to the other in the presence of intolerable side effects or clear evidence of "treatment failure" (e.g., FVC decline >10% over 6 months despite treatment). A small retrospective study, in which seven patients were switched to nintedanib based on clinical grounds because of adverse events (mainly asthenia) while on pirfenidone, suggested that nintedanib may be better tolerated.[41] On the other hand, there are no data on patients switched from nintedanib to pirfenidone.

Timing for treatment initiation is also controversial. As with any inexorably progressive disease such as IPF, once the diagnosis is established, treatment should be started as early as possible to prevent functional decline and prolong survival.[42] However, in asymptomatic patients with preserved or marginally impaired lung function it may not be unreasonable to opt for a close clinical/functional monitoring after careful evaluation of the risks and benefits of such approach as well as the high cost of both medications.[43] Conversely, it is unknown whether pirfenidone and nintedanib are safe and efficacious also in patients with severe functional impairment (e.g., FVC < 50%). Although there are concerns that patients with advanced disease may be less likely to respond to treatment (also because of the frequent coexistence of pulmonary hypertension) and may experience more frequent and severe adverse events, there are no convincing data in this regard.

## MANAGEMENT OF ACUTE EXACERBATION OF IDIOPATHIC PULMONARY FIBROSIS

The clinical course of IPF is usually chronic and slowly progressive, although some patients may experience a rapidly progressive disease course.[1] According to the recently published international working group report, AE-IPF is defined as an acute (typically within less than 1 month), clinically significant, respiratory deterioration characterized by evidence of new, widespread alveolar abnormality after exclusion of cardiac failure or fluid overload as well as extraparenchymal causes such as pulmonary embolism, pneumothorax, or pleural effusion.[44] The prognosis of AE-IPF is poor; mortality during hospitalization is as high as 65%, and those who survive have a >90% mortality rate in the 6 months following discharge.[45–47] If AE-IPF is suspected, initial management should include chest HRCT (high-resolution computed tomography), echocardiogram, bronchoalveolar lavage, and infection screen to identify potentially treatable causes of disease progression. The majority of patients with AE-IPF require intensive care treatment, particularly when respiratory failure is associated with hemodynamic instability, significant comorbidities, or severe hypoxemia requiring monitoring of arterial blood gases or mechanical ventilation.

Many patients with AE are treated with systemic corticosteroids (up to 1g/day of prednisone equivalent, with or without immunosuppressants), although the evidence supporting this approach comes from anecdotal reports and small case series. Accordingly, the 2011 guidelines make a weak recommendation for the use of corticosteroids in AE-IPF.[1] The management of AE-IPF should include supportive care, focused on palliation of symptoms and correction of hypoxemia with supplemental oxygen.[44] Conversely, the use of mechanical ventilation is highly debated, and the 2011 guidelines make a weak recommendation against the use of mechanical ventilation to treat respiratory failure in IPF, based on the high (up to 90%) in-hospital mortality in this patient population.[1]

Potential therapies evaluated for the treatment of AE-IPF include, among others, cyclosporine,[48,49] rituximab combined with plasma exchange and intravenous immunoglobulin,[50] oral tacrolimus,[51] polymyxin-B immobilized fiber column hemoperfusion,[52,53] and intravenous thrombomodulin,[54,55] but only in uncontrolled observational cohorts. AE-IPF was a key secondary outcome in all three clinical trials of nintedanib.[4,38] In the TOMORROW trial, nintedanib was associated with a significant delay in time to first investigator-reported AE,[38] but this finding was supported but not confirmed in the subsequent Phase III INPULSIS trials.[4] Similarly, while a Phase II Japanese trial of pirfenidone was prematurely stopped because of a statistically significant reduction in AE in the pirfenidone arm,[26] these results were not replicated in subsequent, larger Phase III studies,[3,27,28] although neither the CAPACITY trials nor the ASCEND trial reported AE-IPF as an endpoint.

At present, there are no proven, effective therapies for AE-IPF, and pharmacologic treatment of this devastating complication is largely empiric. Well-designed clinical studies to guide therapeutic decisions in this setting are urgently needed.

## NONPHARMACOLOGIC TREATMENTS

The 2015 update of IPF guidelines did not prioritize an update on the indication for supplemental oxygen in patients with IPF,[6] and high-quality data assessing the benefit of long-term oxygen therapy (LTOT) in patients with IPF are still lacking.[56] Nevertheless, in the previous guideline document[1] LTOT was recommended in patients with clinically significant resting hypoxemia, and in clinical practice it is commonly prescribed also to patients showing significant oxygen desaturation on exercise. Because of the progressive nature of IPF, high flow rates are likely to be required. Supplemental oxygen may be associated with an increase in exercise capacity as assessed by endurance time.[57] On the other hand, a recent Cochrane review did not find enough evidence to demonstrate the benefit of supplemental oxygen on health-related quality of life, survival, costs, or time to exacerbation or hospitalization.[56]

Patients with IPF commonly experience lack of energy and fatigue, which may significantly impact daily life activities, particularly in younger patients. Pulmonary rehabilitation (PR) programs (including exercise training, nutritional modulation, occupational therapy, education, and psychosocial counseling) are designed to alleviate symptoms and optimize functional status in patients with chronic respiratory diseases, by stabilizing and/or reversing the extrapulmonary consequences of the disease. Typical PR programs consist of an initial intense component (usually 6–10 weeks) followed by a maintenance one.[58] The existing evidence of a beneficial effect of PR on quality of life and functional mobility in patients with pulmonary emphysema has been the starting point to suggest that similar effects may be achieved in patients suffering from other chronic respiratory diseases leading to exercise intolerance and disability.[59] Exercise training in patients with IPF is associated with improvement in exercise tolerance, functional capacity, dyspnea, and quality of life at least in the short term.[60] However, these benefits are not maintained 6 months after intervention.[61] IPF patients tend with time to discontinue any routine exercise because of increasing dyspnea. Whenever possible, this should be discouraged. Indeed, exercise such as daily walks or the use of stationary bicycle improves muscle strength and increases the sense of well-being.

Along with physical disability, patients with IPF may experience significant psychological and emotional impact, because of the progressive nature of the disease and its consequences of the perceived quality of life. In a cross-sectional study, Ryerson and colleagues already reported that dyspnea is strongly associated with depression score, functional status (as assessed by 4-min walk time), as well as pulmonary function.[62] In particular it has been observed that the relationship between dyspnea and depression is independent of other clinical variables, thus suggesting that pharmacologic and nonpharmacologic interventions affecting the depression may improve dyspnea and quality of life. In a single-center pilot study in patients with interstitial lung disease (most of them with IPF) a mindfulness-based stress reduction program was shown to improve several stress-related negative domains,[63] the effect lasting up to 12 months after the intervention. Similar experiences or other interventions addressing the emotional component of the disease should be assessed in larger studies addressing also the impact on disease-specific outcome.

## LUNG TRANSPLANTATION

Single- and double-lung transplantations represent therapeutic options in patients with advanced lung diseases refractory to medical treatment, and pulmonary fibrosis represents the second most frequent disease for which lung transplantation is performed.[64] The number of lung transplants performed for IPF has steadily increased in recent years, particularly in the United States where IPF now represents the leading indication for lung transplantation.[65] Five-year survival rates after lung transplantation in IPF are comparable to those in other disease indications and are estimated at 50–56%.[66-67]

Since 2005, lung transplant allocation in the United States has been based on the Lung Allocation Score (LAS) organ allocation algorithm, which prioritizes medical need (e.g., risk factors associated with either wait list or posttransplantation mortality) rather than waiting time.[68] Analyses of early postlung transplantation survival have suggested similar outcomes before and after the LAS was introduced, despite the higher burden of comorbidities among lung transplant recipients following the LAS implementation.[65,69] Initial analyses of the International Society for Heart and Lung Transplantation and United Network for Organ Sharing (UNOS) registries suggested improved 10-year survival with double-lung transplantation in patients with IPF after adjusting for patient comorbidities, although the data used in these analyses were largely collected before the LAS implementation.[70] A more recent review of UNOS data has confirmed that at 5 years double-lung transplantation is associated with longer median graft survival in patients with IPF in both the unadjusted (70.7 months vs. 48.9 months; $P < .001$) and inverse probability of treatment weighting–adjusted group (65.2 months vs. 50.4 months; $P = .001$).[71]

## CLOSING REMARKS

Over the last few years, after decades of efforts to enroll patients in placebo-controlled clinical trials, finally two drugs have been shown unequivocally to be both safe and effective in reducing disease progression in IPF. This landmark achievement represents both a point of arrival and a starting point toward even more effective treatments. We should not forget that today treating IPF patients with either nintedanib or pirfenidone is challenging: patients will not feel better and their lung function will inexorably decline, even if at a slower rate. Moreover, many of them will experience side effects, which will need careful and expert management to maintain their quality of life. Although guidelines in 2011 were recommending enrollment in clinical trials as the standard of care for IPF patients, this is not true anymore because since 2015 pharmacologic treatment has been the new standard of care. Nonetheless, for the reasons described earlier, clinicians will still need to consider the option to enroll their patients in clinical trials. For example, trials combining the two approved drugs are already actively recruiting patients and many new promising molecules are in early phases of development: hopefully many of them will progress to the later phases of trials in placebo-controlled combination studies. Based on our current knowledge of IPF pathogenesis, it is easy to predict that the future treatment of IPF will be based on multiple drugs. Of utmost importance, the knowledge gained until now and that will be gained over the next few years will also form the basis to approach the vast and heterogeneous universe represented by the other fibrotic interstitial lung diseases, for which a systematic attempt to discover an effective pharmacological treatment was almost completely lacking until a few months ago. In this way, IPF patients will keep leading the way in the discovery of therapies for lung fibrosis and, while achieving the important critical goal of the identification of more effective treatments, will also help the large number of patients with non-IPF fibrotic lung disorders.

## REFERENCES

1. Raghu G, et al. An official ATS/ERS/JRS/ALAT statement: idiopathic pulmonary fibrosis: evidence-based guidelines for diagnosis and management. *Am J Respir Crit Care Med*. 2011;183(6):788–824.
2. Hutchinson J, et al. Global incidence and mortality of idiopathic pulmonary fibrosis: a systematic review. *Eur Respir J*. 2015;46(3):795–806.
3. King Jr TE, et al. A phase 3 trial of pirfenidone in patients with idiopathic pulmonary fibrosis. *N Engl J Med*. 2014;370(22):2083–2092.
4. Richeldi L, et al. Efficacy and safety of nintedanib in idiopathic pulmonary fibrosis. *N Engl J Med*. 2014;370(22):2071–2082.
5. Spagnolo P, Maher TM, Richeldi L. Idiopathic pulmonary fibrosis: Recent advances on pharmacological therapy. *Pharmacol Ther*. 2015;152:18–27.
6. Raghu G, et al. An Official ATS/ERS/JRS/ALAT Clinical Practice Guideline: treatment of idiopathic pulmonary fibrosis. An update of the 2011 Clinical Practice Guideline. *Am J Respir Crit Care Med*. 2015;192(2):e3–e19.

7. Schunemann HJ, et al. An official ATS statement: grading the quality of evidence and strength of recommendations in ATS guidelines and recommendations. *Am J Respir Crit Care Med.* 2006;174(5):605–614.

8. Raghu G, et al. Prednisone, azathioprine, and N-acetylcysteine for pulmonary fibrosis. *N Engl J Med.* 2012;366(21):1968–1977.

9. Martinez FJ, et al. Randomized trial of acetylcysteine in idiopathic pulmonary fibrosis. *N Engl J Med.* 2014;370(22):2093–2101.

10. Hagiwara SI, Ishii Y, Kitamura S. Aerosolized administration of N-acetylcysteine attenuates lung fibrosis induced by bleomycin in mice. *Am J Respir Crit Care Med.* 2000;162(1):225–231.

11. Yoko M, et al. Efficacy of inhaled N-acetylcysteine monotherapy on lung function and redox balance in idiopathic pulmonary fibrosis. In: *C55. Interstitial Lung Disease: Diagnostic and Therapeutic Considerations.* American Thoracic Society; 2012:A4589.

12. Noth I, et al. Genetic variants associated with idiopathic pulmonary fibrosis susceptibility and mortality: a genome-wide association study. *Lancet Respir Med.* 2013;1(4):309–317.

13. Seibold MA, et al. A common MUC5B promoter polymorphism and pulmonary fibrosis. *N Engl J Med.* 2011;364(16):1503–1512.

14. Oldham JM, et al. TOLLIP, MUC5B, and the response to N-acetylcysteine among individuals with idiopathic pulmonary fibrosis. *Am J Respir Crit Care Med.* 2015;192(12):1475–1482.

15. Kubo H, et al. Anticoagulant therapy for idiopathic pulmonary fibrosis. *Chest.* 2005;128(3):1475–1482.

16. Noth I, et al. A placebo-controlled randomized trial of warfarin in idiopathic pulmonary fibrosis. *Am J Respir Crit Care Med.* 2012;186(1):88–95.

17. King Jr TE, et al. BUILD-1: a randomized placebo-controlled trial of bosentan in idiopathic pulmonary fibrosis. *Am J Respir Crit Care Med.* 2008;177(1):75–81.

18. King Jr TE, et al. BUILD-3: a randomized, controlled trial of bosentan in idiopathic pulmonary fibrosis. *Am J Respir Crit Care Med.* 2011;184(1):92–99.

19. Raghu G, et al. Macitentan for the treatment of idiopathic pulmonary fibrosis: the randomised controlled MUSIC trial. *Eur Respir J.* 2013;42(6):1622–1632.

20. Raghu G, et al. Treatment of idiopathic pulmonary fibrosis with ambrisentan: a parallel, randomized trial. *Ann Intern Med.* 2013;158(9):641–649.

21. Jackson RM, et al. Sildenafil therapy and exercise tolerance in idiopathic pulmonary fibrosis. *Lung.* 2010;188(2):115–123.

22. Zisman DA, et al. A controlled trial of sildenafil in advanced idiopathic pulmonary fibrosis. *N Engl J Med.* 2010;363(7):620–628.

23. Lee JS, et al. Anti-acid treatment and disease progression in idiopathic pulmonary fibrosis: an analysis of data from three randomised controlled trials. *Lancet Respir Med.* 2013;1(5):369–376.

24. Lee JS, et al. Gastroesophageal reflux therapy is associated with longer survival in idiopathic pulmonary fibrosis. *Am J Respir Crit Care Med.* 2011;184(12):1390–1394.

25. Kreuter M, et al. Antacid therapy and disease outcomes in idiopathic pulmonary fibrosis: a pooled analysis. *Lancet Respir Med.* 2016;4(5):381–389.

26. Azuma A, et al. Double-blind, placebo-controlled trial of pirfenidone in patients with idiopathic pulmonary fibrosis. *Am J Respir Crit Care Med.* 2005;171(9):1040–1047.

27. Taniguchi H, et al. Pirfenidone in idiopathic pulmonary fibrosis. *Eur Respir J.* 2010;35(4):821–829.

28. Noble PW, et al. Pirfenidone in patients with idiopathic pulmonary fibrosis (CAPACITY): two randomised trials. *Lancet.* 2011;377(9779):1760–1769.

29. Costabel U, et al. Analysis of lung function and survival in RECAP: an open-label extension study of pirfenidone in patients with idiopathic pulmonary fibrosis. *Sarcoidosis Vasc Diffuse Lung Dis.* 2014;31(3):198–205.

30. Maher TM, et al. S11 pirfenidone post-authorisation safety registry (passport)–interim analysis of IPF treatment. *Thorax.* 2014;69(suppl 2):A8–A9.

31. Oltmanns U, et al. Pirfenidone in idiopathic pulmonary fibrosis: real-life experience from a German tertiary referral center for interstitial lung diseases. *Respiration.* 2014;88(3):199–207.

32. Loeh B, et al. Intraindividual response to treatment with pirfenidone in idiopathic pulmonary fibrosis. *Am J Respir Crit Care Med.* 2015;191(1):110–113.

33. Okuda R, et al. Safety and efficacy of pirfenidone in idiopathic pulmonary fibrosis in clinical practice. *Respir Med.* 2013;107(9):1431–1437.

34. Harari S, et al. Efficacy of pirfenidone for idiopathic pulmonary fibrosis: an Italian real life study. *Respir Med.* 2015;109(7):904–913.

35. Hilberg F, et al. BIBF 1120: triple angiokinase inhibitor with sustained receptor blockade and good antitumor efficacy. *Cancer Res.* 2008;68(12):4774–4782.

36. Allen JT, Spiteri MA. Growth factors in idiopathic pulmonary fibrosis: relative roles. *Respir Res.* 2002;3:13.

37. Chaudhary NI, et al. Inhibition of PDGF, VEGF and FGF signalling attenuates fibrosis. *Eur Respir J.* 2007;29(5):976–985.

38. Richeldi L, et al. Efficacy of a tyrosine kinase inhibitor in idiopathic pulmonary fibrosis. *N Engl J Med.* 2011;365(12):1079–1087.

39. Corte T, et al. Safety, tolerability and appropriate use of nintedanib in idiopathic pulmonary fibrosis. *Respir Res.* 2015;16:116.

40. King Jr TE, et al. All-cause mortality rate in patients with idiopathic pulmonary fibrosis. Implications for the design and execution of clinical trials. *Am J Respir Crit Care Med.* 2014;189(7):825–831.

41. Milger K, et al. Switching to nintedanib after discontinuation of pirfenidone due to adverse events in IPF. *Eur Respir J.* 2015;46(4):1217–1221.

42. King CS, Nathan SD. Practical considerations in the pharmacologic treatment of idiopathic pulmonary fibrosis. *Curr Opin Pulm Med.* 2015;21(5):479–489.

43. Spagnolo P, du Bois RM, Cottin V. Rare lung disease and orphan drug development. *Lancet Respir Med.* 2013;1(6):479–487.

44. Collard HR, et al. Acute exacerbation of idiopathic pulmonary fibrosis. An International Working Group report. *Am J Respir Crit Care Med.* 2016;194(3):265–275.

45. Hyzy R, et al. Acute exacerbation of idiopathic pulmonary fibrosis. *Chest.* 2007;132(5):1652–1658.

46. Agarwal R, Jindal SK. Acute exacerbation of idiopathic pulmonary fibrosis: a systematic review. *Eur J Intern Med.* 2008;19(4):227–235.

47. Luppi F, et al. Acute exacerbation of idiopathic pulmonary fibrosis: a clinical review. *Intern Emerg Med.* 2015;10(4):401–411.

48. Homma S, et al. Cyclosporin treatment in steroid-resistant and acutely exacerbated interstitial pneumonia. *Intern Med.* 2005;44(11):1144–1150.

49. Sakamoto S, et al. Cyclosporin A in the treatment of acute exacerbation of idiopathic pulmonary fibrosis. *Intern Med.* 2010;49(2):109–115.

50. Donahoe M, et al. Autoantibody-targeted treatments for acute exacerbations of idiopathic pulmonary fibrosis. *PLoS One.* 2015;10(6):e0127771.

51. Horita N, et al. Tacrolimus and steroid treatment for acute exacerbation of idiopathic pulmonary fibrosis. *Intern Med.* 2011;50(3):189–195.

52. Oishi K, et al. Association between cytokine removal by polymyxin B hemoperfusion and improved pulmonary oxygenation in patients with acute exacerbation of idiopathic pulmonary fibrosis. *Cytokine.* 2013;61(1):84–89.

53. Seo Y, et al. Beneficial effect of polymyxin B-immobilized fiber column (PMX) hemoperfusion treatment on acute exacerbation of idiopathic pulmonary fibrosis. *Intern Med.* 2006;45(18):1033–1038.

54. Isshiki T, et al. Recombinant human soluble thrombomodulin treatment for acute exacerbation of idiopathic pulmonary fibrosis: a retrospective study. *Respiration.* 2015;89(3):201–207.

55. Kataoka K, et al. Recombinant human thrombomodulin in acute exacerbation of idiopathic pulmonary fibrosis. *Chest.* 2015;148(2):436–443.

56. Sharp C, Adamali H, Millar AB. Ambulatory and short-burst oxygen for interstitial lung disease. *Cochrane Database Syst Rev.* 2016;7:CD011716.

57. Arizono S, et al. Benefits of supplemental oxygen on exercise capacity in IPF patients with exercise-induced hypoxemia. *Eur Respir J.* 2015;46(S59):OA4971.

58. Nici L, et al. American Thoracic Society/European Respiratory Society statement on pulmonary rehabilitation. *Am J Respir Crit Care Med.* 2006;173(12):1390–1413.

59. Spruit MA, et al. Rehabilitation and palliative care in lung fibrosis. *Respirology.* 2009;14(6):781–787.

60. Vainshelboim B, et al. Exercise training-based pulmonary rehabilitation program is clinically beneficial for idiopathic pulmonary fibrosis. *Respiration.* 2014;88(5):378–388.

61. Holland AE, et al. Short term improvement in exercise capacity and symptoms following exercise training in interstitial lung disease. *Thorax.* 2008;63(6):549–554.

62. Ryerson CJ, et al. Depression and functional status are strongly associated with dyspnea in interstitial lung disease. *Chest.* 2011;139(3):609–616.

63. Sgalla G, et al. Mindfulness-based stress reduction in patients with interstitial lung diseases: a pilot, single-centre observational study on safety and efficacy. *BMJ Open Respir Res.* 2015;2(1):e000065.

64. Kotloff RM, Thabut G. Lung transplantation. *Am J Respir Crit Care Med.* 2011;184(2):159–171.

65. Yusen RD, et al. Lung transplantation in the United States, 1999–2008. *Am J Transplant.* 2010;10(4 Pt 2):1047–1068.

66. Mason DP, et al. Lung transplantation for idiopathic pulmonary fibrosis. *Ann Thorac Surg.* 2007;84(4):1121–1128.

67. Keating D, et al. Lung transplantation in pulmonary fibrosis: challenging early outcomes counterbalanced by surprisingly good outcomes beyond 15 years. *Transplant Proc.* 2009;41(1):289–291.

68. Egan TM, et al. Development of the new lung allocation system in the United States. *Am J Transplant.* 2006;6(5 Pt 2):1212–1227.

69. Iribarne A, et al. Despite decreased wait-list times for lung transplantation, lung allocation scores continue to increase. *Chest.* 2009;135(4):923–928.

70. Thabut G, et al. Survival after bilateral versus single-lung transplantation for idiopathic pulmonary fibrosis. *Ann Intern Med.* 2009;151(11):767–774.

71. Schaffer JM, et al. Single- vs double-lung transplantation in patients with chronic obstructive pulmonary disease and idiopathic pulmonary fibrosis since the implementation of lung allocation based on medical need. *JAMA.* 2015;313(9):936–948.

# CHAPTER 5

# Nonpharmacologic Therapy for Idiopathic Pulmonary Fibrosis

LEANN L. SILHAN • SONYE K. DANOFF

---

**KEY POINTS**

- A patient with idiopathic pulmonary fibrosis (IPF) requires multidisciplinary care.
- Symptomatic hallmarks of IPF include dyspnea, often driven by hypoxemia, and cough.
- Proper integration of nonpharmacologic management is imperative to improve quality of life and potentially increases survival.
- Nonpharmacologic treatment of IPF is largely focused on symptom management and falls under the umbrella of palliative care.

---

Idiopathic pulmonary fibrosis (IPF) is a complex disease, for which there is currently no cure. There are exciting emerging new therapies that will hopefully change the prognosis of this devastating disease. However, at present, the medical community must treat the multiple symptoms, manage comorbidities, and guide patients through difficult decisions regarding lung transplantation and end of life. A multidisciplinary approach is essential in providing patient-centered care to improve quality of life and includes the physician, nurse, respiratory therapist, oxygen specialist, social worker, palliative care specialist, and, in certain circumstances, lung transplant team. Thus a multidisciplinary approach to the nonpharmacologic treatment of IPF is both a mainstay of care and essential to provide optimal patient outcomes. Nonpharmacologic treatment of IPF is largely focused on symptom management and, thus, falls under the umbrella of palliative care. Palliative care encompasses treating all the symptoms of IPF, including cough, dyspnea, depression, anxiety, and fatigue, as well as assisting the patient in identifying his/her individual goals and using those values to guide therapeutic decision-making.

Symptomatic hallmarks of IPF include dyspnea, often driven by hypoxemia, and cough. Treating hypoxemia with supplemental oxygen has been shown to improve exercise tolerance and quality of life in various pulmonary diseases, and these findings have been extrapolated to IPF in clinical practice. Dyspnea often improves with oxygen supplementation and, in some individuals, cough improves as well. Cough is a predominant symptom in patients with IPF and one of the most challenging to treat, but effective therapy can provide highly valued relief to patients. Pulmonary rehabilitation is a keystone of therapy for those with exercise intolerance who have become more sedentary as the disease progresses, allowing patients to become more active again. Gastroesophageal reflux disease (GERD) is a common comorbidity in patients with IPF and potentially plays a role in the disease pathophysiology as well.

Comorbidities in IPF include high rates of depression and anxiety. Similarly, fatigue, related both to the disease and to comorbid sleep-disordered breathing, ischemic heart disease and cardiac arrhythmias, emphysema/chronic obstructive pulmonary disease (COPD), and tobacco use disorder are common, all of which are important to manage to improve the patient's quality of life and life expectancy. It is valuable to establish resuscitative status with the patient when the patient is prepared to discuss it, as mechanical ventilation outcomes in IPF are dismal if not in the setting of bridge to transplantation. When the disease progresses to the end stage, hospice care is a critical service, which can be provided in the home or in-patient setting. Lung transplantation is a potential option for a subset of patients who do not have comorbidities that preclude it and is a potential life-saving therapy (Fig. 5.1).

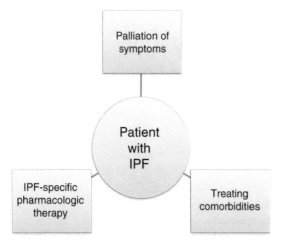

FIG. 5.1 A model for patient-centered care in idiopathic pulmonary fibrosis (IPF). The individual patient is central, and care includes palliation of symptoms, treating comorbidities, and IPF-specific pharmacologic therapy.

## PALLIATIVE CARE

Palliative care is defined in a recent ATS statement as interventions that "prevent and relieve suffering by controlling symptoms" as well as "to provide other support to patients and families in order to maintain and improve their quality of living."[1] In this context, virtually all of the care provided to patients with IPF can be considered palliative as, clearly, the goals are to control symptoms and maintain quality of life. Although palliative care was once considered synonymous with end of life, it is now more broadly considered as all interventions that focus on the symptoms of the patient as opposed to the disease. This reframing of palliative care is demonstrated by the schematics in Fig. 5.2 taken from this statement. In Fig. 5.2A and B, palliative care is shown as an alternative to disease-focused care engaged toward the end of life or as an incrementally increasing component of care in patients with progressive disease. An alternative concept illustrated in Fig. 5.2C is that of palliative care as a dynamic part of patient management, which varies dynamically based on the need of the patient and follows along from the earliest point of diagnosis to the end of life and beyond. This model most accurately reflects the typical engagement of symptom management in the care of patients with IPF, which might not have been explicitly considered to be palliation. The first component of palliative care is the management of symptoms directly related to IPF such as cough and dyspnea. However, the scope of symptoms experienced by patients with IPF may extend beyond these disease-specific symptoms to those more

broadly related to fatigue, decreased endurance, pain, depression, and anxiety (Fig 5.2). All of these areas are considered in detail in the following text. Several recent studies focused on perception of needs of the patient and the caregiver in IPF care have identified palliation as a critical deficiency.[2,3] Indeed, a recent statement by patients, caregivers, support networks, and providers in Europe entitled "The European IPF Patient Charter" lists the availability of palliative and end-of-life care as a critical "right" for all IPF patients.[4]

Integral to palliation is addressing the needs of the patient and his/her support system at the end of life. Because IPF is a progressive and often fatal disorder, it is critical to engage patients regarding their preferences and goals should the IPF lead to death. This may include the location of death, the availability of symptom control (hospice), as well as the desires/needs for family support after the death of the patient. A 2016 Swedish study of 285 patients with ILD on supplemental oxygen at the time of death found that only 41% of patients had engaged in end-of-life discussion before death. Nearly half of patients with ILD died in an acute hospital setting as opposed to about 30% in hospice. This contrasted with findings regarding patients with lung cancer on oxygen at the time of death where 59% had discussed end of life and 45% died in hospice. This highlights the importance of having not just a single but instead a series of conversations on end of life as a part of the continuum of care for IPF patients.[5]

## DYSPNEA

Dyspnea is the most common symptom reported by patients with IPF.[6] Although dyspnea may occur initially only with significant exertion, over time dyspnea becomes a frequent and disabling symptom. Typically, dyspnea on exertion in IPF is associated with hypoxemia. The use of supplemental oxygen has been studied primarily in pulmonary patients with COPD[7] and the benefits extrapolated to IPF. British Thoracic Society guidelines suggest supplemental long-term oxygen therapy is indicated in patients with chronic hypoxemia defined by $Pao_2 < 7.3$ kPa or between 7.3 and 8 kPa with polycythemia or evidence of pulmonary hypertension (PH). Current Medicare guidelines (http://www.medicare.gov/Pubs/pdf/11045.pdf) require evidence that the supplemental oxygen level is adequate to maintain an ambulatory saturation above 88%. Oxygen supplementation has been demonstrated to be beneficial in terms of increasing exercise capacity in IPF.[8] However, there have been

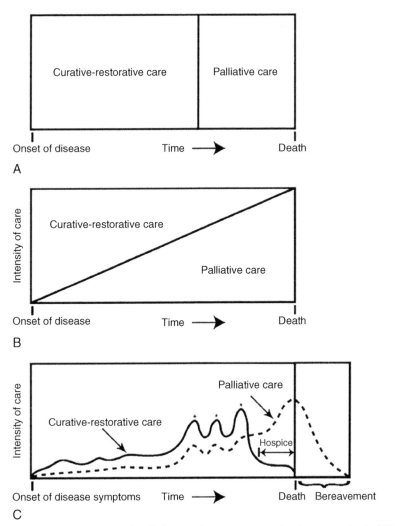

FIG. 5.2 Models of the integration of palliative care in management of pulmonary patients. (A) Traditional model of palliative care as an alternative to active medical care. (B) Alternative model of palliative care as a slowly, steadily increasing component of overall care as disease-specific therapy diminishes. (C) Dynamic integration of palliative care in the evolving disease pathway with changes in intensity associated with variation in the individual's need. (From Lanken PN, Terry PB, Delisser HM, et al. An official American Thoracic Society clinical policy statement: palliative care for patients with respiratory diseases and critical illnesses. *Am J Respir Crit Care Med.* 2008;177[8]:912–927, with permission.)

no systematic studies on the impact of supplemental oxygen use on the IPF patient's or caregiver's quality of life. The potential advantages of supplemental oxygen include relieving dyspnea and increasing activity. These benefits are balanced by a number of burdens associated with use of supplemental oxygen, including making the patient's disease public and need for extensive planning (to allow for adequate supply) as well as financial burden.

For some patients, dyspnea and hypoxemia will eventually exceed the capacity for oxygen at home. In this situation, the use of opiates to lower the perception of dyspnea has been shown to be effective.[9] Interestingly, a recent study of patients requiring oxygen at the end of life in Sweden showed that over 70% of ILD patients report dyspnea at or near the time of death.[5] This suggests that attention to this symptom may not be sufficient. However, further study in this area is clearly needed.

## COUGH

Cough is a very common and distressing symptom for patients with IPF and has been associated with disease progression and death, as well as decreased quality of life. The cough is typically persistent and nonproductive, often disabling, and occurs in up to 80% of patients with IPF.[10] By cough monitor data, it has been observed that the cough is predominantly a daytime symptom, with nocturnal cough being uncommon.[11] The cause of the cough is unknown, but studies have found a functional upregulation of sensory fibers within the respiratory tracts of patients with IPF and studies have also demonstrated a dysregulated and disrupted epithelium.[12] Other potential contributors to cough in IPF include postnasal drip, gastroesophageal reflux, and architectural distortion of the airways, known as traction bronchiectasis.

Treatment of cough in IPF is problematic for both patients and physicians, especially in the advanced stages of the disease when breathlessness can be significantly worsened by cough. There have been few studies demonstrating effective therapy, and there is no currently approved treatment for IPF-related cough. There are a number of options for treating chronic cough associated with IPF (Box 5.1). Benzonatate can be given up to four times per day and is well tolerated, but is not effective for many patients. Opiate-derived medications come in liquid or pill forms and may be coupled with guaifenesin in those who have a productive cough, but the use may be limited by side effects such as constipation and sedating effects. Corticosteroids have not been shown to be effective in treatment of IPF, but their use in the palliation of cough can be quite effective. A small, uncontrolled open-label study found that cough sensitivity to capsaicin and cough symptoms were reduced after 1 month of oral corticosteroids.[12] This is in line with clinical experience: some patients have significant improvement in cough with the use of oral corticosteroids, while others have little or no relief. The symptomatic benefits of corticosteroids have to be weighed with the risks of long-term use. Finally, airway nerve–active agents including thalidomide and gabapentin may provide relief from cough. A single-center study showed that the use of thalidomide for IPF-related cough over 24 months improved cough and respiratory quality of life.[13] However, there has not been a follow-up multicenter trial conducted, which limits the generalizability of the conclusions. The potential antitussive effects of thalidomide certainly warrant further investigation, but may be limited by potentially serious side effects, which include constipation, bradycardia, dizziness, and peripheral neuropathy.[14] Long-term use of thalidomide is often limited by these side effects. Gabapentin at a maximum tolerable dose of 1800 mg was found to be effective in treating refractory chronic cough in subjects without active respiratory disease in a randomized, double-blind, placebo-controlled trial, as measured by a significant difference in Leicester cough questionnaire score.[15] Although gabapentin may be effective for a minority of IPF patients, its use is often limited by side effects, especially fatigue, particularly given the high rates of preexisting fatigue in this population.

Other, less well-studied options can be helpful, with little downside, and include hot tea, menthol lozenges, which are a natural cough suppressant (range of 2–10 mg/lozenge of menthol; suggest the higher dose lozenge works best),[16] and clothing around the neck area such as a scarf. Some patients report the use of N-acetylcysteine (NAC)[17] and serrapeptase[18] in helping with cough. The use of NAC for treatment of IPF has not been found to be beneficial and may potentially be harmful in accelerating the rate of decline in FVC in the general population,[19] although there may be a subset of patients who may benefit.[20] There are no data to support the use of serrapeptase in IPF-related cough; however, there is some concern for safety. Serrapeptase has been reported in three cases of acute eosinophilic

---

**BOX 5.1**
**Treatment Options for Cough**

**COUGH–PHARMACOLOGIC OPTIONS**

Benzonatate

Opiate-containing medications (e.g., guaifenesin with codeine)

Corticosteroids

Airway nerve–acting medications (thalidomide, gabapentin)

Postnasal drip medication (nasal ipratropium, fluticasone)

Treatment of gastroesophageal reflux disease (lifestyle modification, protein pump inhibitors, H2-blockers)

**COUGH–OTHER OPTIONS**

Hot tea

Honey

Menthol lozenges

N-Acetycysteine

Number of other supplements

pneumonia and acute pneumonitis[21–23] and one case of acute granulomatous hepatitis.[24] It can decrease blood clotting, so it should be used with caution and avoided in those on anticoagulation medication or who have issues with bleeding. Other supplements have been suggested to help with cough, but there are limited data regarding their efficacy. The lack of regulation of herbal supplements makes it impossible to recommend one over another and adds concerns for safety profile and drug interactions.

## GASTROESOPHAGEAL REFLUX DISEASE

GERD can present with esophageal symptoms or with mucosal damage produced by the abnormal reflux of gastric contents into the esophagus or beyond, including the lung.[25] GERD is a common comorbidity in patients with IPF and potentially plays a role in the pathophysiology. Addressing GERD and microaspiration may be important in treating and controlling the progression of disease, both with medication and with lifestyle modification. However, who should be treated and how is not entirely clear, nor is evaluation standardized. Symptoms of heartburn and acid regurgitation have a very high specificity (89% and 95%, respectively), but low sensitivity (38% and 6%) for GERD, in the general population.[25] By contrast, patients with IPF are largely asymptomatic. In those with symptoms, resolution of symptoms with a trial of antacids provides additional evidence for pathologic esophageal acid exposure and essentially confirms a diagnosis of GERD.[26] Other testing available includes ambulatory pH monitoring, either by 24 h transnasal catheter with impedance to diagnose nonacidic reflux or by a wireless capsule. Upper endoscopy can diagnose the mucosal damage caused by esophageal acid exposure, but may, nevertheless, be normal in some with GERD.[25] Barium swallow study can diagnose a hiatal hernia, but is no longer recommended in the evaluation of GERD because of poor sensitivity and specificity.[27] Esophageal manometry is useful when esophageal dysmotility is suspected, but not recommended in the diagnosis of GERD.[28]

Gastroesophageal reflux is common in IPF, affecting 87–94% of patients.[29,30] The majority of IPF patients are asymptomatic, with "silent reflux," and the incidence of GERD is significantly higher than in the general population[31] and in patients with other advanced lung diseases.[32–34] The presence of hiatal hernias has also been found to be increased in those with IPF.[35] Laboratory models have demonstrated harmful effects when human alveolar epithelial cells are exposed to

gastric materials or its individual components leading to immune stimulation, airway inflammation, increased cell membrane permeability, and lung remodeling.[36–38] Several retrospective observational studies have shown favorable effects of proton pump inhibitors (PPIs) at improving or preventing deterioration of lung function.[39–42] Together, this evidence led to the 2015 ATS guideline recommendation that clinicians use regular antacid treatment for patients with IPF.[43] However, the expert panel did not unanimously agree, and it is currently a conditional recommendation, with low confidence. Reasonable options for medication therapy for GERD in IPF include PPIs as well as H2-blockers, although the PPIs may have appealing nonacid suppressant mechanisms that may be advantageous in IPF.[44,45] However, recent retrospective analysis of the pirfenidone trials does not support an effect of PPIs and suggests that their use increases risk of respiratory infections.[46] These studies have raised skepticism regarding the 2015 guidelines. Lifestyle modifications are a cornerstone to addressing gastroesophageal reflux in patients with IPF (Box 5.2). These include recommendations to elevate the head of the bed (e.g., risers placed under the feet of the headboard), weight and abdominal girth reduction, smoking cessation, and dietary modifications including not eating 3–4 h before bedtime and avoiding foods or drinks that cause distal esophageal sphincter relaxation such as coffee, wine, chocolate, high-fat foods, and citrus fruits. However, weight reduction has been the only therapy shown to consistently improve GERD in studies.[25] There is some evidence to support surgical correction of hiatal hernias and Nissen fundoplication, not only to correct acid reflux, but also to prevent the nonacid component of reflux, also known to be associated with lung injury; however, this is a retrospective observational study with

---

**BOX 5.2**
**Lifestyle Modifications for the Management of Gastroesophageal Reflux Disease (GERD)**

Weight loss[a]

Head of bed elevation[a]

Avoidance of recumbent position 3 h postprandially

Small meals, especially evening meal

Avoidance of trigger foods (chocolate, alcohol, caffeine)

[a]Shown to improve esophageal pH and/or GERD symptoms.

intrinsic selection bias.[47] Currently, a phase II clinical trial "WRAP-IPF" is recruiting patients to prospectively test the hypothesis that treatment with laparoscopic antireflux surgery in subjects with IPF and abnormal gastroesophageal reflux will slow the decline of forced vital capacity (FVC).[48]

## TREATING COMORBIDITIES

Depression and anxiety are prevalent in IPF and other interstitial lung diseases (ILDs), contribute to overall decreased quality of life, and do not resolve in the absence of treatment.[49] Most studies have been conducted in a mixed population of ILDs, including IPF, and have found depression prevalence of 21–49%.[49–53] Interestingly, there has been strong correlation of prevalence among multiple small studies. In the study by Holland et al., the prevalence of anxiety was 31% and depression 23% among 124 patients with ILD, 39% of whom had IPF. They also found a correlation between depression and higher MMRC score (more dyspnea) and number of comorbidities.[51] Given the high prevalence of depression and anxiety, patients should be routinely questioned regarding symptoms. However, treatments for depression and anxiety have not been specifically studied in IPF, and evidence must be extrapolated from other populations. Some patients may find pulmonary fibrosis–specific support groups helpful, both for having questions answered and for psychological health.[54] Cognitive behavioral therapy has been found to reduce symptoms of depression and anxiety in patients with COPD[55,56] and may be useful in those with IPF. Antidepressant medications improve depression in patients with chronic illnesses and have been found to be effective therapy in patients with depression and COPD.[57–59] In light of the strong association of depression and anxiety with symptoms of dyspnea, cough, and comorbidities, IPF-specific interventions may help and may include supplemental oxygen, pulmonary rehabilitation, and antifibrotic medication. Most studies that investigated prevalence of depression/anxiety were conducted before the availability of antifibrotic medications; thus some patients experienced feelings of hopelessness with no effective therapy. In the era of antifibrotic medications, there may be an additional benefit to these medications in lessening the sense of hopelessness.

Fatigue or exhaustion is a common symptom in IPF and negatively impacts quality of life.[52,60] The presence of this symptom should prompt screening and testing for sleep-disordered breathing, a highly prevalent comorbidity, with moderate to severe obstructive sleep apnea being found in up to 65% of patients with IPF.[61] Furthermore, improved quality of life has been demonstrated in patients with IPF and sleep apnea who are treated with continuous positive airway pressure.[61,62]

Pain has not been widely studied in IPF but is a symptom many patients experience. In a large national population-based study in Sweden, symptoms and treatment were examined during the last 7 days of life in patients with ILD and compared with those with lung cancer. While patients with lung cancer experienced more pain, 51% of patients with ILD had significant pain in their last 7 days of life.[5] If a patient has undergone a surgical lung biopsy, postthoracotomy pain syndrome may account for a source of pain. This occurs in approximately 50% of patients after thoracotomy and can persist in up to 30% of patients 5 years after surgery,[63] with lower rates in video-assisted thoracic surgery.[64] To improve quality of life in patients with IPF, we must be vigilant in screening for and treating pain, potentially involving pain management and palliative specialists.

PH is present in 20–40% of patients with IPF at the time of lung transplant referral[65] and is associated with increased risk of mortality.[66,67] Diagnosis with right-sided heart catheterization is the gold standard, but invasive. Echocardiogram and brain natriuretic peptide are other screening tests used to assist in diagnosing PH. Dyspnea out of proportion to fibrosis severity, exertional hypoxemia greater than expected with fibrosis severity, findings of right-sided heart dysfunction, and diffusion capacity (DLCO) diminished out of proportion to FVC are signs that a patient may have PH. Given increased mortality in patients with IPF who have comorbid PH, a rationale for treating PH with pulmonary vasodilators has been theorized, although trial outcomes have demonstrated poor results. While a trial of sildenafil in 180 subjects with IPF did not meet its primary endpoint (6-min walk distance improvement of 20% or more), secondary endpoints demonstrated improved dyspnea, oxygenation, DLCO, and quality of life, with borderline impact on survival in the extension phase of this study.[68] A subset of patients with IPF/PH may benefit from sildenafil, but further support is needed. Bosentan has not been shown to be effective, and ambrisentan and riociguat (RISE-IIP) were found to be harmful in randomized parallel trials,[69] so there is currently no evidence for endothelin receptor blockers in IPF, either with or without comorbid PH. Oxygen therapy for those who have resting, exertional, or nocturnal hypoxia is recommended.[43] Although the effect of oxygen on PH in IPF is not known, it has been found to reverse PH and cor pulmonale in COPD.[70]

Coronary artery disease (CAD) is present in up to 30% of patients with IPF[71,72] and is associated with increased mortality.[71] Symptoms of CAD can easily be attributed to symptoms of IPF; thus diagnosis may be delayed. Standard medical therapies for CAD are likely appropriate in most IPF patients. The need for platelet antagonists after coronary stenting may delay listing for lung transplantation, so these decisions must be made on a case-by-case basis.[73]

Other comorbidities in IPF include emphysema/COPD (combined pulmonary fibrosis and emphysema), lung cancer, and tobacco use disorder. Smoking cessation and treatment of comorbid pulmonary obstruction may improve prognosis and quality of life. The incidence of lung cancer is higher in patients with IPF than a control population,[74] and it shortens survival. Surgical and medical management of lung cancer is complicated by the risk of acute exacerbation from surgery or radiation, as well as some chemotherapeutic agents, and must be approached on an individual basis.[73]

## LUNG TRANSPLANTATION

A subset of patients with IPF are eligible for lung transplant. Since the implementation of the Lung Allocation Score in 2005, IPF has become the most common indication for lung transplant in the United States. These patients have a limited life expectancy and benefit from early referral for transplant.[75] For this population, lung transplant can increase the length and quality of their lives. Appropriate timing of referral is very important to allow management of modifiable comorbidities important for lung transplant success, recognition of previously unknown medical issues found in the lung transplant evaluation, and the establishment of the necessary trust between the patient and lung transplant team. In addition, given the unpredictable course and prognosis of IPF, early referral can avoid the difficult problem faced when a patient becomes too ill for transplant, or the haste of the evaluation leads to suboptimal candidate selection decisions.

In general, short- and long-term survival post lung transplant have continued to improve, but the median survival remains quite low at 5.6 years for all diseases and lower, 4.5 years, for IPF/ILD. The 1-year survival of all adults who undergo primary lung transplant is 84% in the 2009 to current era. However, the 1-year survival for IPF remains significantly lower at 73–76%.[75-78] The explanation for poorer outcomes is not completely understood. Possible factors include more advanced age (although worse outcomes compared with age-matched controls with COPD/emphysema), increased risk of primary graft dysfunction, smaller intrathoracic cavity space resulting from remodeling because of small fibrotic lungs, and possible differences in human leukocyte antigen sensitization. However, many patients do quite well, enjoying years of life, and a vast majority of them do not require continued oxygen supplementation. Studies show 22–38% of patients work post transplant, approximately one-half of those who worked pretransplant,[79,80] and over 90% of survivors report they would make the decision to undergo transplant again.[81-83] This is certainly balanced by the fact that patients have to take many medications, including immunosuppression, prophylactic antibiotics, various supplements, and medications to treat the many comorbid conditions, either preexisting or as a result of complications from immunosuppression. Solid organ transplant recipients receive 12 or more different medications per day,[84] and managing side effects requires much attention and affects quality of life.

The selection guidelines for lung transplant were updated in 2015 and include IPF-specific guidelines. In general, potential candidates include those with end-stage lung disease for which there are no further medical options, and in IPF, it is recommended that all patients who may be considered candidates are referred early, for reasons mentioned previously. Absolute contraindications for transplant include recent malignancy (except squamous or basal cell skin cancer), untreatable significant dysfunction of another organ system, uncorrected atherosclerotic disease, acute medical instability, uncorrectable bleeding, chronic infection with highly virulent/resistant microbes, tuberculosis infection, body mass index >35, nonadherence to medical therapy, psychiatric condition limiting ability to comply with complex medical therapy, absence of an adequate support system, limited functional status with poor rehabilitative potential, and substance abuse within the last 6 months.[85] A number of other relative contraindications are weighted differently among individual transplant centers. One that applies to IPF patients is age, with age >65 now considered a relative contraindication, although, typically, only when coupled with low physiologic reserve and other relative contraindications. Because of the higher risk of transplants for older patients, many centers will consider selected patients up to the age of 75 for lung transplantation who have few to no other comorbidities. Recommendations for the timing of referral include radiographic or histopathologic evidence of usual interstitial pneumonia or fibrosing nonspecific interstitial pneumonia regardless of lung function, abnormal lung function with FVC <80% predicted or $D_{LCO}$ <40%

predicted, dyspnea or functional limitation due to lung disease, or any oxygen requirement even if only with exertion.[85] Patients should also enroll in pulmonary rehabilitation before lung transplantation, both to maintain and to improve current health status, but also to prepare for major surgery, for maximal pretransplant robustness is essential for posttransplant success.[86,87] Many centers require enrollment and continued participation in a formal pulmonary rehabilitation program for patients to be actively listed for transplantation. Ultimately, lung transplant is an option for a small subset of patients with IPF, but remains a life-saving therapy for some.

## CONCLUSION
The patient with IPF requires multidisciplinary care. Proper integration of nonpharmacologic management is imperative to improve quality of life and potentially increase survival.

## REFERENCES
1. Lanken PN, Terry PB, Delisser HM, et al. An official American Thoracic Society clinical policy statement: palliative care for patients with respiratory diseases and critical illnesses. *Am J Respir Crit Care Med.* 2008;177(8):912–927.
2. Sampson C, Gill BH, Harrison NK, Nelson A, Byrne A. The care needs of patients with idiopathic pulmonary fibrosis and their carers (CaNoPy): results of a qualitative study. *BMC Pulm Med.* 2015;15:155.
3. Overgaard D, Kaldan G, Marsaa K, Nielsen TL, Shaker SB, Egerod I. The lived experience with idiopathic pulmonary fibrosis: a qualitative study. *Eur Respir J.* 2016;47(5): 1472–1480.
4. Bonella F, Wijsenbeek M, Molina-Molina M, et al. European IPF Patient Charter: unmet needs and a call to action for healthcare policymakers. *Eur Respir J.* 2016;47(2):597–606.
5. Ahmadi Z, Wysham NG, Lundstrom S, Janson C, Currow DC, Ekstrom M. End-of-life care in oxygen-dependent ILD compared with lung cancer: a national population-based study. *Thorax.* 2016;71(6):510–516.
6. Garibaldi BT, Danoff SK. Symptom-based management of the idiopathic interstitial pneumonia. *Respirology.* 2016;21(8):1357–1365.
7. Continuous or nocturnal oxygen therapy in hypoxemic chronic obstructive lung disease: a clinical trial. Nocturnal Oxygen Therapy Trial Group. *Ann Intern Med.* 1980;93(3):391–398.
8. Bye PT, Anderson SD, Woolcock AJ, Young IH, Alison JA. Bicycle endurance performance of patients with interstitial lung disease breathing air and oxygen. *Am Rev Respir Dis.* 1982;126(6):1005–1012.
9. Parshall MB, Schwartzstein RM, Adams L, et al. An official American Thoracic Society statement: update on the mechanisms, assessment, and management of dyspnea. *Am J Respir Crit Care Med.* 2012;185(4):435–452.
10. Ryerson CJ, Abbritti M, Ley B, Elicker BM, Jones KD, Collard HR. Cough predicts prognosis in idiopathic pulmonary fibrosis. *Respirology.* 2011;16(6):969–975.
11. Key AL, Holt K, Hamilton A, Smith JA, Earis JE. Objective cough frequency in Idiopathic Pulmonary Fibrosis. *Cough.* 2010;6:4.
12. Hope-Gill BD, Hilldrup S, Davies C, Newton RP, Harrison NK. A study of the cough reflex in idiopathic pulmonary fibrosis. *Am J Respir Crit Care Med.* 2003;168(8):995–1002.
13. Horton MR, Santopietro V, Mathew L, et al. Thalidomide for the treatment of cough in idiopathic pulmonary fibrosis: a randomized trial. *Ann Intern Med.* 2012;157(6):398–406.
14. Harrison NK. Cough, sarcoidosis and idiopathic pulmonary fibrosis: raw nerves and bad vibrations. *Cough.* 2013;9(1):9.
15. Ryan NM, Birring SS, Gibson PG. Gabapentin for refractory chronic cough: a randomised, double-blind, placebo-controlled trial. *Lancet.* 2012;380(9853):1583–1589.
16. Wise PM, Breslin PA, Dalton P. Sweet taste and menthol increase cough reflex thresholds. *Pulm Pharmacol Ther.* 2012;25(3):236–241.
17. Millea PJ. N-acetylcysteine: multiple clinical applications. *Am Fam Physician.* 2009;80(3):265–269.
18. Bhagat S, Agarwal M, Roy V. Serratiopeptidase: a systematic review of the existing evidence. *Int J Surg.* 2013;11(3):209–217.
19. Behr J, Bendstrup E, Crestani B, et al. Safety and tolerability of acetylcysteine and pirfenidone combination therapy in idiopathic pulmonary fibrosis: a randomised, double-blind, placebo-controlled, phase 2 trial. *Lancet Respir Med.* 2016;4(6):445–453.
20. Oldham JM, Ma SF, Martinez FJ, et al. TOLLIP, MUC5B, and the response to N-acetylcysteine among Individuals with Idiopathic Pulmonary Fibrosis. *Am J Respir Crit Care Med.* 2015;192(12):1475–1482.
21. Sasaki S, Kawanami R, Motizuki Y, et al. Serrapeptase-induced lung injury manifesting as acute eosiniphilic pneumonia. *Nihon Kokyuki Gakkai Zasshi.* 2000;38(7): 540–544.
22. Hirahara K, Saitoh T, Terada I, et al. A case of pneumonitis due to serrapeptase. *Nihon Kyobu Shikkan Gakkai Zasshi.* 1989;27(10):1231–1236.
23. Kai N, Shirai R, Hirata N, et al. A case of eosinophilic pneumonia due to Nicolase (serrapeptase) after recovery from acute eosinophilic pneumonia. *Nihon Kokyuki Gakkai Zasshi.* 2009;47(3):254–258.
24. Dohmen KMK, Irie K, Shirahama M, et al. Granulomatous hepatitis induced by saridon and serrapeptase. *Hepatol Res.* 1998;11(2):133–137.
25. Badillo R, Francis D. Diagnosis and treatment of gastroesophageal reflux disease. *World J Gastrointest Pharmacol Ther.* 2014;5(3):105–112.
26. DeVault KR, Castell DO, American College of G. Updated guidelines for the diagnosis and treatment of gastroesophageal reflux disease. *Am J Gastroenterol.* 2005;100(1):190–200.
27. Johnston BT, Troshinsky MB, Castell JA, Castell DO. Comparison of barium radiology with esophageal pH monitoring in the diagnosis of gastroesophageal reflux disease. *Am J Gastroenterol.* 1996;91(6):1181–1185.

28. DeVault K, McMahon BP, Celebi A, et al. Defining esophageal landmarks, gastroesophageal reflux disease, and Barrett's esophagus. *Ann N Y Acad Sci*. 2013;1300: 278–295.

29. Raghu G, Freudenberger TD, Yang S, et al. High prevalence of abnormal acid gastro-oesophageal reflux in idiopathic pulmonary fibrosis. *Eur Respir J*. 2006;27(1): 136–142.

30. Tobin RW, Pope 2nd CE, Pellegrini CA, Emond MJ, Sillery J, Raghu G. Increased prevalence of gastroesophageal reflux in patients with idiopathic pulmonary fibrosis. *Am J Respir Crit Care Med*. 1998;158(6):1804–1808.

31. Dent J, El-Serag HB, Wallander MA, Johansson S. Epidemiology of gastro-oesophageal reflux disease: a systematic review. *Gut*. 2005;54(5):710–717.

32. Robinson NB, DiMango E. Prevalence of gastroesophageal reflux in cystic fibrosis and implications for lung disease. *Ann Am Thorac Soc*. 2014;11(6):964–968.

33. Havemann BD, Henderson CA, El-Serag HB. The association between gastro-oesophageal reflux disease and asthma: a systematic review. *Gut*. 2007;56(12):1654–1664.

34. Mokhlesi B, Morris AL, Huang CF, Curcio AJ, Barrett TA, Kamp DW. Increased prevalence of gastroesophageal reflux symptoms in patients with COPD. *Chest*. 2001;119(4):1043–1048.

35. Mays EE, Dubois JJ, Hamilton GB. Pulmonary fibrosis associated with tracheobronchial aspiration. A study of the frequency of hiatal hernia and gastroesophageal reflux in interstitial pulmonary fibrosis of obscure etiology. *Chest*. 1976;69(4):512–515.

36. Blondeau K, Mertens V, Vanaudenaerde BA, et al. Gastro-oesophageal reflux and gastric aspiration in lung transplant patients with or without chronic rejection. *Eur Respir J*. 2008;31(4):707–713.

37. Perng DW, Chang KT, Su KC, et al. Exposure of airway epithelium to bile acids associated with gastroesophageal reflux symptoms: a relation to transforming growth factor-beta1 production and fibroblast proliferation. *Chest*. 2007;132(5):1548–1556.

38. D'Ovidio F, Mura M, Tsang M, et al. Bile acid aspiration and the development of bronchiolitis obliterans after lung transplantation. *J Thorac Cardiovasc Surg*. 2005;129(5):1144–1152.

39. Raghu G, Yang ST, Spada C, Hayes J, Pellegrini CA. Sole treatment of acid gastroesophageal reflux in idiopathic pulmonary fibrosis: a case series. *Chest*. 2006;129(3): 794–800.

40. Ghebremariam YT, Cooke JP, Gerhart W, et al. Pleiotropic effect of the proton pump inhibitor esomeprazole leading to suppression of lung inflammation and fibrosis. *J Transl Med*. 2015;13:249.

41. Ghebremariam YT, Cooke JP, Khan F, et al. Proton pump inhibitors and vascular function: a prospective cross-over pilot study. *Vasc Med*. 2015;20(4):309–316.

42. Lee JS, Ryu JH, Elicker BM, et al. Gastroesophageal reflux therapy is associated with longer survival in patients with idiopathic pulmonary fibrosis. *Am J Respir Crit Care Med*. 2011;184(12):1390–1394.

43. Raghu G, Rochwerg B, Zhang Y, et al. An official ATS/ERS/JRS/ALAT Clinical Practice Guideline: treatment of Idiopathic Pulmonary Fibrosis. An Update of the 2011 Clinical Practice Guideline. *Am J Respir Crit Care Med*. 2015;192(2):e3–19.

44. Kedika RR, Souza RF, Spechler SJ. Potential anti-inflammatory effects of proton pump inhibitors: a review and discussion of the clinical implications. *Dig Dis Sci*. 2009;54(11):2312–2317.

45. Takagi T, Naito Y, Okada H, et al. Lansoprazole, a proton pump inhibitor, mediates anti-inflammatory effect in gastric mucosal cells through the induction of heme oxygenase-1 via activation of NF-E2-related factor 2 and oxidation of kelch-like ECH-associating protein 1. *J Pharmacol Exp Ther*. 2009;331(1):255–264.

46. Kreuter M, Wuyts W, Renzoni E, et al. Antacid therapy and disease outcomes in idiopathic pulmonary fibrosis: a pooled analysis. *Lancet Respir Med*. 2016;4(5): 381–389.

47. Linden PA, Gilbert RJ, Yeap BY, et al. Laparoscopic fundoplication in patients with end-stage lung disease awaiting transplantation. *J Thorac Cardiovasc Surg*. 2006;131(2):438–446.

48. University of California SF. *Treatment of IPF With Laparoscopic Anti-Reflux Surgery (WRAP-IPF)*; 2016. ClinicalTrials. gov Identifier: NCT01982968.

49. Ryerson CJ, Arean PA, Berkeley J, et al. Depression is a common and chronic comorbidity in patients with interstitial lung disease. *Respirology*. 2012;17(3):525–532.

50. Ryerson CJ, Berkeley J, Carrieri-Kohlman VL, Pantilat SZ, Landefeld CS, Collard HR. Depression and functional status are strongly associated with dyspnea in interstitial lung disease. *Chest*. 2011;139(3):609–616.

51. Holland AE, Fiore Jr JF, Bell EC, et al. Dyspnoea and comorbidity contribute to anxiety and depression in interstitial lung disease. *Respirology*. 2014;19(8): 1215–1221.

52. De Vries J, Kessels BL, Drent M. Quality of life of idiopathic pulmonary fibrosis patients. *Eur Respir J*. 2001;17(5): 954–961.

53. Akhtar AA, Ali MA, Smith RP. Depression in patients with idiopathic pulmonary fibrosis. *Chron Respir Dis*. 2013;10(3):127–133.

54. Lee JS, McLaughlin S, Collard HR. Comprehensive care of the patient with idiopathic pulmonary fibrosis. *Curr Opin Pulm Med*. 2011;17(5):348–354.

55. Lamers F, Jonkers CC, Bosma H, Chavannes NH, Knottnerus JA, van Eijk JT. Improving quality of life in depressed COPD patients: effectiveness of a minimal psychological intervention. *COPD*. 2010;7(5):315–322.

56. Kunik ME, Veazey C, Cully JA, et al. COPD education and cognitive behavioral therapy group treatment for clinically significant symptoms of depression and anxiety in COPD patients: a randomized controlled trial. *Psychol Med*. 2008;38(3):385–396.

57. Usmani ZA, Carson KV, Cheng JN, Esterman AJ, Smith BJ. Pharmacological interventions for the treatment of anxiety disorders in chronic obstructive pulmonary disease. *Cochrane Database Syst Rev*. 2011;(11):CD008483.

58. Rayner L, Price A, Evans A, Valsraj K, Higginson IJ, Hotopf M. Antidepressants for depression in physically ill people. *Cochrane Database Syst Rev.* 2010;(3):CD007503.

59. Rayner L, Price A, Evans A, Valsraj K, Hotopf M, Higginson IJ. Antidepressants for the treatment of depression in palliative care: systematic review and meta-analysis. *Palliat Med.* 2011;25(1):36–51.

60. Swigris JJ, Stewart AL, Gould MK, Wilson SR. Patients' perspectives on how idiopathic pulmonary fibrosis affects the quality of their lives. *Health Qual Life Outcomes.* 2005;3:61.

61. Mermigkis C, Bouloukaki I, Antoniou K, et al. Obstructive sleep apnea should be treated in patients with idiopathic pulmonary fibrosis. *Sleep Breath.* 2015;19(1):385–391.

62. Mermigkis C, Bouloukaki I, Antoniou KM, et al. CPAP therapy in patients with idiopathic pulmonary fibrosis and obstructive sleep apnea: does it offer a better quality of life and sleep? *Sleep Breath.* 2013;17(4):1137–1143.

63. Karmakar MK, Ho AM. Postthoracotomy pain syndrome. *Thorac Surg Clin.* 2004;14(3):345–352.

64. Solaini L, Prusciano F, Bagioni P, di Francesco F, Solaini L, Poddie DB. Video-assisted thoracic surgery (VATS) of the lung: analysis of intraoperative and postoperative complications over 15 years and review of the literature. *Surg Endosc.* 2008;22(2):298–310.

65. Patel NM, Lederer DJ, Borczuk AC, Kawut SM. Pulmonary hypertension in idiopathic pulmonary fibrosis. *Chest.* 2007;132(3):998–1006.

66. Song JW, Song JK, Kim DS. Echocardiography and brain natriuretic peptide as prognostic indicators in idiopathic pulmonary fibrosis. *Respir Med.* 2009;103(2):180–186.

67. Mejia M, Carrillo G, Rojas-Serrano J, et al. Idiopathic pulmonary fibrosis and emphysema: decreased survival associated with severe pulmonary arterial hypertension. *Chest.* 2009;136(1):10–15.

68. Idiopathic Pulmonary Fibrosis Clinical Research N, Zisman DA, Schwarz M, et al. A controlled trial of sildenafil in advanced idiopathic pulmonary fibrosis. *N Engl J Med.* 2010;363(7):620–628.

69. Raghu G, Behr J, Brown KK, et al. Treatment of idiopathic pulmonary fibrosis with ambrisentan: a parallel, randomized trial. *Ann Intern Med.* 2013;158(9):641–649.

70. Timms RM, Khaja FU, Williams GW. Hemodynamic response to oxygen therapy in chronic obstructive pulmonary disease. *Ann Intern Med.* 1985;102(1):29–36.

71. Nathan SD, Basavaraj A, Reichner C, et al. Prevalence and impact of coronary artery disease in idiopathic pulmonary fibrosis. *Respir Med.* 2010;104(7):1035–1041.

72. Nathan SD, Weir N, Shlobin OA, et al. The value of computed tomography scanning for the detection of coronary artery disease in patients with idiopathic pulmonary fibrosis. *Respirology.* 2011;16(3):481–486.

73. Fulton BG, Ryerson CJ. Managing comorbidities in idiopathic pulmonary fibrosis. *Int J Gen Med.* 2015;8:309–318.

74. Hubbard R, Venn A, Lewis S, Britton J. Lung cancer and cryptogenic fibrosing alveolitis. A population-based cohort study. *Am J Respir Crit Care Med.* 2000;161(1):5–8.

75. George TJ, Arnaoutakis GJ, Shah AS. Lung transplant in idiopathic pulmonary fibrosis. *Arch Surg.* 2011;146(10):1204–1209.

76. Yusen RD, Christie JD, Edwards LB, et al. The Registry of the International Society for Heart and Lung Transplantation: Thirtieth Adult Lung and Heart-Lung Transplant Report-2013; focus theme: age. *J Heart Lung Transplant.* 2013;32(10):965–978.

77. Yusen RD, Edwards LB, Kucheryavaya AY, et al. The Registry of the International Society for Heart and Lung Transplantation: Thirty-second Official Adult Lung and Heart-Lung Transplantation Report-2015; focus theme: early graft failure. *J Heart Lung Transplant.* 2015;34(10):1264–1277.

78. Christie JD, Edwards LB, Kucheryavaya AY, et al. The Registry of the International Society for Heart and Lung Transplantation: 29th adult lung and heart-lung transplant report-2012. *J Heart Lung Transplant.* 2012;31(10):1073–1086.

79. Paris W, Diercks M, Bright J, et al. Return to work after lung transplantation. *J Heart Lung Transplant.* 1998;17(4):430–436.

80. Suhling H, Knuth C, Haverich A, Lingner H, Welte T, Gottlieb J. Employment after lung transplantation–a single-center cross-sectional study. *Dtsch Arztebl Int.* 2015;112(13):213–219.

81. Lanuza DM, Lefaiver C, Mc Cabe M, Farcas GA, Garrity Jr E. Prospective study of functional status and quality of life before and after lung transplantation. *Chest.* 2000;118(1):115–122.

82. Myaskovsky L, Dew MA, McNulty ML, et al. Trajectories of change in quality of life in 12-month survivors of lung or heart transplant. *Am J Transplant.* 2006;6(8):1939–1947.

83. Singer JP, Singer LG. Quality of life in lung transplantation. *Semin Respir Crit Care Med.* 2013;34(3):421–430.

84. Martin JE, Zavala EY. The expanding role of the transplant pharmacist in the multidisciplinary practice of transplantation. *Clin Transplant.* 2004;18(suppl 12):50–54.

85. Weill D, Benden C, Corris PA, et al. A consensus document for the selection of lung transplant candidates: 2014–an update from the Pulmonary Transplantation Council of the International Society for Heart and Lung Transplantation. *J Heart Lung Transplant.* 2015;34(1):1–15.

86. Kenn K, Sczepanski B. Pulmonary rehabilitation before and after lung transplantation. *Pneumologie.* 2011;65(7):419–427.

87. Mathur S, Hornblower E, Levy RD. Exercise training before and after lung transplantation. *Phys Sportsmed.* 2009;37(3):78–87.

# CHAPTER 6

# Idiopathic Pulmonary Fibrosis: Diagnosis and Epidemiology

AMY L. OLSON • ZULMA X. YUNT • JEFFREY J. SWIGRIS

**KEY POINTS**

- Over the last several decades, results from several studies have advanced understanding of idiopathic pulmonary fibrosis (IPF): how it is diagnosed, its basic epidemiologic profile, and occupational or environmental exposures that may increase the risk for developing the disease.
- These results have reshaped how IPF is diagnosed, especially by highlighting the accuracy with which a characteristic HRCT identifies a UIP pattern of lung injury: patients with such an HRCT need not have a surgical lung biopsy for IPF to be diagnosed confidently.
- Making a diagnosis of IPF is complex, and whether a surgical lung biopsy is indicated or not, diagnostic accuracy is improved with multidisciplinary discussions in centers that specialize in the care of patients with this disease.

Idiopathic pulmonary fibrosis (IPF) is defined as a chronic fibrosing interstitial pneumonia of unknown cause with a histologic pattern of usual interstitial pneumonia (UIP) on surgical lung biopsy. IPF is a lung-limited process that tends to occur in older adults. It is the most common of the idiopathic interstitial pneumonias (IIPs), among which it has the worst prognosis, with median survival estimates ranging from 3 to 5 years after diagnosis.[1–3]

In 2000, the American Thoracic Society (ATS) and European Respiratory Society (ERS) published the first consensus statement providing guidelines on the diagnosis and treatment of IPF.[1] This statement presented, for the first time, diagnostic criteria for IPF and recommendations for treatment. Over the past decade, results from several studies have reshaped the thinking on IPF, and as a result, the guidelines have been recently revised using an evidence-based approach.[2] Meanwhile, several epidemiologic studies have yielded data that identify potential risk factors and that better define the societal burden of IPF. This chapter summarizes the approach to diagnosing IPF and reviews epidemiologic data on IPF.

## DIAGNOSIS OF IDIOPATHIC PULMONARY FIBROSIS

In recent years, emerging data have helped to refine the diagnostic criteria for IPF. The first collaborative effort, in 2000, among the ATS, ERS, and American College of Chest Physicians resulted in an international consensus statement for the diagnosis of IPF.[1] That statement, formulated on expert opinion and interpretation of available research at the time, held that a definitive diagnosis of IPF required a surgical lung biopsy showing a UIP pattern of lung injury and the following three criteria: (1) exclusion of other known causes of interstitial lung disease (ILD), including drug toxicities, environmental exposures, and collagen vascular diseases; (2) abnormal pulmonary function tests or impaired gas exchange; and (3) imaging consistent with this diagnosis. In the absence of a surgical lung biopsy, a diagnosis of probable IPF required all of the following four major criteria: (1) exclusion of other causes of ILD; (2) abnormal pulmonary function tests or impaired gas exchange; (3) bibasilar reticular abnormalities with minimal ground-glass opacities on high-resolution computed tomography (HRCT); and (4) transbronchial lung biopsy or bronchoalveolar lavage specimens without features to support an alternative diagnosis along with at least three of four minor criteria (age >50 years, the insidious onset of dyspnea, a duration of symptoms greater than 3 months, and bibasilar, inspiratory crackles).

Since that time, additional evidence has shown the value of HRCT in diagnosing IPF: when an experienced

## BOX 6.1
### Criteria for a Definite, Possible, and Inconsistent Usual Interstitial Pneumonia (UIP) Pattern on High-Resolution Computed Tomography Scan

**Definite UIP Pattern**
Subpleural, basal predominance
Reticular abnormality
Honeycombing without traction bronchiectasis
Absence of features (listed below) as inconsistent with UIP pattern

**Possible UIP Pattern**
Same as the criteria for a definite UIP pattern, although honeycombing is not present with or without traction bronchiectasis

**Inconsistent With UIP Pattern**
Upper-lung or midlung predominance
Peribronchovascular predominance
Extensive ground-glass abnormality (defined as the extent of the ground-glass abnormality is greater than the extent of the reticular abnormality)
Profuse micronodules
Discrete cysts
Diffuse mosaic attenuation or air-trapping (bilateral, in three or more lobes)
Consolidation in bronchopulmonary segments or lobes

Adapted from American Thoracic Society; European Respiratory Society. American Thoracic Society/European Respiratory Society International Multidisciplinary Consensus Classification of the Idiopathic Interstitial Pneumonias. This joint statement of the American Thoracic Society (ATS), and the European Respiratory Society (ERS) was adopted by the ATS board of directors, June 2001 and by the ERS Executive Committee, June 2001. *Am J Respir Crit Care Med.* 2001;165:277–304, with permission.

## BOX 6.2
### Criteria for a Definite, Probable, Possible, and Inconsistent Usual Interstitial Pneumonia (UIP) Pattern Based on Surgical Lung Biopsy

**Definite UIP Pattern**
Evidence of marked fibrosis/architectural distortion with or without honeycombing in a predominantly subpleural/paraseptal distribution
Fibrosis in a patchy distribution
Fibroblastic foci
Absence of features against a diagnosis of UIP (see below)

**Probable UIP Pattern**
Evidence of marked fibrosis/architectural distortion with or without honeycombing in a predominantly subpleural/paraseptal distribution
Absence of either patchy fibrosis or fibroblastic foci, but not both
Absence of features against a diagnosis of UIP (see below)
OR
Honeycomb changes only

**Possible UIP Pattern**
Patchy or diffuse involvement of lung parenchyma by fibrosis, with or without interstitial inflammation
Absence of other criteria for a definite UIP pattern
Absence of features against a diagnosis of UIP (see below)

**Inconsistent UIP Pattern**
Hyaline membranes (unless associated with an acute exacerbation of IPF)
Organizing pneumonia or granulomas (unless mild or occasional, respectively, but may otherwise suggest hypersensitivity pneumonitis)
Marked interstitial inflammation away from honeycombing
Predominant airway-centered disease
Other features suggesting an alternative diagnosis

Adapted from American Thoracic Society; European Respiratory Society. American Thoracic Society/European Respiratory Society International Multidisciplinary Consensus Classification of the Idiopathic Interstitial Pneumonias. This joint statement of the American Thoracic Society (ATS), and the European Respiratory Society (ERS) was adopted by the ATS board of directors, June 2001 and by the ERS Executive Committee, June 2001. *Am J Respir Crit Care Med.* 2001;165:277–304, with permission.

radiologist can say with high confidence that the pattern on HRCT is consistent with a histologic UIP pattern, UIP is the histologic pattern identified in more than 90% of cases.[4–7] Based on these and other data supporting the accuracy of HRCT, a surgical lung biopsy is no longer required for a definitive diagnosis of IPF in cases with a radiologic UIP pattern and a compatible clinical presentation,[3] and the characteristic HRCT pattern of a UIP pattern of lung injury has been defined (Box 6.1). Given a characteristic HRCT pattern, the diagnosis of IPF still requires exclusion of other known causes of ILD, including domestic, occupational, or environmental exposures, connective tissue diseases, and drug toxicities.

For diagnosing IPF, the sensitivity of HRCT is significantly lower than its positive predictive value[4–9]; thus, when the characteristic HRCT pattern is absent, a surgical lung biopsy showing a UIP pattern is still required to make a definitive diagnosis of IPF.[3] Histologic criteria have been devised to allow pathologists

to categorize findings in surgical lung biopsy specimens as definite, possible, probable, or not UIP (Box 6.2). In addition, the recently published evidence-based guidelines provide a framework for interpreting permutations of HRCT and histologic data (Table 6.1).

## Challenges in Diagnosing Idiopathic Pulmonary Fibrosis

A threat to making a confident diagnosis of IPF arises when, as is the case in 12.5–26% of patients who have a multilobe surgical lung biopsy, a UIP pattern is found

**TABLE 6.1**

**Criteria for a Definite, Probable, and Possible Diagnosis of Idiopathic Pulmonary Fibrosis (IPF) Based on Both High-Resolution Computed Tomography (HRCT) Pattern and Surgical Lung Biopsy Findings**

| HRCT Pattern | Surgical Lung Biopsy Pattern | Diagnosis of IPF |
|---|---|---|
| UIP | UIP | IPF |
| | Probable UIP | IPF |
| | Possible UIP | IPF |
| | Nonclassifiable fibrosis | IPF |
| | Not UIP | Not IPF |
| Possible UIP | UIP | IPF |
| | Probable UIP | IPF |
| | Possible UIP | Probable IPF |
| | Nonclassifiable fibrosis | Probable IPF |
| | Not UIP | Not IPF |
| Inconsistent with UIP | UIP | Possible IPF |
| | Probable UIP | Not IPF |
| | Possible UIP | Not IPF |
| | Nonclassifiable fibrosis | Not IPF |
| | Not UIP | Not IPF |

UIP, usual interstitial pneumonia.
Data from American Thoracic Society; European Respiratory Society. American Thoracic Society/European Respiratory Society International Multidisciplinary Consensus Classification of the Idiopathic Interstitial Pneumonias. This joint statement of the American Thoracic Society (ATS), and the European Respiratory Society (ERS) was adopted by the ATS board of directors, June 2001 and by the ERS Executive Committee, June 2001. *Am J Respir Crit Care Med.* 2001;165:277–304.

in samples from one lobe, but a different pattern is found in samples from another lobe (a scenario termed discordant UIP).[10,11] However, survival in patients with discordant UIP is similar to patients with concordant UIP (i.e., surgical lung biopsy samples from all lobes having UIP patterns).[10,12] Thus, if a surgical lung biopsy is performed, multiple lobes should be sampled, and a diagnosis of definite IPF can be made when a UIP pattern is identified in any.

Further complicating a confident diagnosis of IPF includes a recent study that utilized imaging and pathology from a prior multicenter study of IPF with a focus on discordance between imaging and a histologic diagnosis of UIP.[13] Of the 241 HRCT from IPF cases that were reviewed, 75 cases (31.1%) had HRCT findings that were inconsistent with IPF based on criteria noted earlier (Box

6.1). Of these inconsistent imaging cases, 94.7% were found to have either definite or probable UIP pattern on pathologic review—and were termed discordant cases. Discordant cases were then compared to concordant cases (imaging with a UIP pattern and pathology with either a definite or a probable UIP pattern). Discordant cases were younger and had less of a smoking history, smaller lung volumes, and slightly higher $FEV_1/FVC$ ratio than those in the concordant group. In addition, no significant difference in survival was found. Among the discordant cases, the inconsistent CT findings were most often the result of a diffuse mosaic pattern/air-trapping (71.8%), followed by a diffuse cradiocaudal distribution (39.4%), diffuse axial distribution (26.8%), predominance of signs in the upper zone or midzone of the lungs (23.9%), extensive ground-glass abnormalities (22.5%), and peribronchovascular predominance (12.7%). Thus, these findings further complicate the diagnosis, indicate that the term "inconsistent with IPF" is misleading, and stress the importance of surgical lung biopsy in those patients without a definite UIP—and even inconsistent with UIP—pattern on imaging.

As noted, making a diagnosis of IPF can be difficult, but the accuracy and confidence of an IPF diagnosis increase with multidisciplinary discussions among clinicians, radiologists, and pathologists. In a study of 58 consecutive cases of suspected IIP, Flaherty and colleagues[14] sequentially gave expert clinicians, radiologists, and pathologists more and more information about a case of ILD and then allowed them to discuss their impressions as a group. As more information was divulged and cross-disciplinary discussions took place, the level of agreement about the diagnosis (and the degree of certainty in that diagnosis) improved. Not surprisingly, centers with expertise in IPF are more accurate at diagnosing IPF than community-based, referral practices.[5] For unclear reasons, early referral to such a center seems to improve survival in patients with IPF.[15]

## EPIDEMIOLOGY OF IDIOPATHIC PULMONARY FIBROSIS

### Background

Epidemiology is defined as "the study of the distribution and determinants of health-related states or events (including disease)," and the goal of epidemiologists is to apply findings to control diseases or health issues.[16–18] Specific objectives include determining the extent and effects of disease: by defining its prevalence, incidence, and mortality; by identifying its risk factors or causes; and by examining its natural history and prognosis. This information then allows for the evaluation of preventive and therapeutic interventions and builds a foundation for policies and regulatory decisions to be made that alleviate the burden of disease.[18]

The relative rarity of IPF has challenged investigators with an interest in its epidemiology and, before 1990, discouraged large-scale epidemiologic studies from being performed.[19] Although Leibow and Carrington first defined a UIP pattern in 1969,[20] IPF was not given a diagnostic code in the International Classification of Diseases (ICD) until the ninth revision (ICD-9) at the end of the 1970s.[21] This coding system gave investigators an opportunity to use ICD-coded mortality data to study the burden of IPF at the population level. Johnston and colleagues[22] did so and published their results of mortality (discussed later) in 1990.

## Mortality and Mortality Trends Over Time

Disease-specific mortality is calculated by determining the number of deaths per year resulting from a specific cause, divided by the number of persons alive in the midyear population. In a disease that is lethal, and when survival is short, as occurs in IPF, mortality serves as a surrogate for the incidence of disease.[18]

Death certificate and census data are vital statistics recorded in several countries, and these data have provided investigators with the means to study mortality and mortality trends over time. Little is known about the validity of death certificate ICD coding in IPF, so results from studies using death certificate data should be interpreted with some caution. Investigators in the United Kingdom found that in 23 decedents with a diagnosis of IPF (ICD-9 code 516.3) recorded on a death certificate, 19 (83%) had premortem clinical information confirming either definite or possible IPF.[22] Conversely, among 45 patients with a premortem diagnosis of IPF (ICD-9 code 516.3), IPF was recorded on the death certificate only about 50% of the time. Before the ICD-10 coding system (which combines IPF and postinflammatory pulmonary fibrosis [PIPF]),[23] diagnostic transfer (or coding IPF as PIPF on the death certificate) was also reported to occur commonly. Of 20 decedents coded with PIPF (ICD-9 code 515) on the death certificate, nearly 50% had IPF (ICD-9 code 516.3) diagnosed before death. These data suggest IPF is likely underrecorded as the cause of death, and a significant proportion of decedents coded as dying from PIPF died of IPF. Although these findings are based on a small number of decedents from the United Kingdom, Coultas and Hughes[24] identified similar issues in mortality data from New Mexico.

Because the ICD-10 coding system combined PIPF and IPF into one diagnostic code (J84.1),[23] researchers

calculating mortality with data after 1998 are likely including some decedents with progressive, fibrosing ILD that is not IPF. Investigators who have used this diagnostic code (J84.1) and who have systematically excluded cases with known-cause pulmonary fibrosis (PF) have termed this entity general PF.[25,26] Other investigators have not excluded concurrent conditions that may result in PF and have termed this entity IPF clinical syndrome (IPF-CS).[27] Regardless of the precise diagnosis (i.e., IPF vs. other progressive, fibrotic ILD) for decedents in such studies, trends in mortality reveal that PF is a daunting public health problem.[25-27]

Johnston and colleagues[22] were the first to calculate IPF (previously termed cryptogenic fibrosing alveolitis in the United Kingdom) mortality in a large-scale epidemiologic study. They found that in England and Wales, from 1979 to 1988, deaths from IPF (ICD-9 code, 516.3) more than doubled. IPF-associated mortality was more common in men (odds ratio [OR] = 2.24; 95% confidence interval [CI] = 2.11–2.38) and increased progressively with age: the risk of IPF in those aged 75 years or more was eight times the risk for those aged 45–54 years. Greater mortality was found in the central, industrialized areas of England and Wales, suggesting that environmental/occupational exposures could be a risk factor for IPF.

Hubbard and colleagues[28] extended on the work of Johnston and colleagues by investigating available mortality data for both IPF (ICD-9 code 516.3) and PIPF (ICD-9 code 515) from England, Wales, Scotland, Germany, Australia, New Zealand, Canada, and the United States from 1979 to 1992. They found that mortality from IPF was the highest in England and Wales and rates were increasing not only in these countries but also in Scotland, Australia, and Canada. Mortality from IPF was stable in New Zealand and Germany and had decreased over time in the United States. Mortality from PIPF was the highest in the United States and increased over the study period in the United States, the United Kingdom, Canada, and Australia, with stable mortality again noted in New Zealand and Germany. The increase in mortality from PF could not be explained by diagnostic transfer (e.g., a change in coding practices from PIPF to IPF, or PIPF to IPF over time), although systematic diagnostic transfer (always coding IPF as PIPF, because of different terminology and coding rules)[25] may have explained the higher mortality of PIPF in the United States.

Mannino and colleagues[25] examined PF mortality data in the United States from 1979 to 1991. To capture all decedents with IPF, given the coding issues noted earlier, these investigators defined PF by combing

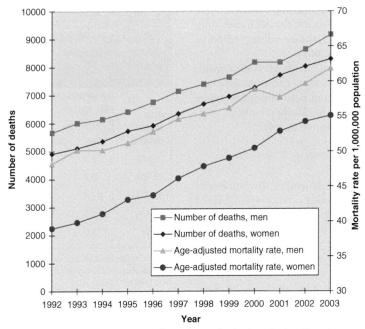

FIG. 6.1 Number of deaths per year and age-adjusted mortality in decedents with pulmonary fibrosis (PF) per 1,000,000 population from 1992 to 2003 in the United States. Mortality is standardized to the 2000 US census population. (From Olson AL, Swigris JJ, Lezotte DC, et al. Mortality from pulmonary fibrosis increased in the United States from 1992 to 2003. *Am J Respir Crit Care Med*. 2007;176:278; with permission.)

ICD-9 diagnostic codes 515 (PIPF) and 516.3 (IPF) and eliminated cases with concurrent diagnostic codes for conditions with known associations with PF, including radiation fibrosis, collagen vascular diseases, or asbestosis. Over that 13-year period, age-adjusted mortality from PF increased 4.7% in men (from 48.6 per million to 50.9 per million) and increased 27.1% in women (from 21.4 per million to 27.2 per million). PF-associated mortality increased with increasing age. States with the highest PF-associated mortality were in the west and southeast, and those with the lowest rates were in the midwest and northeast.

Data from the 1990s to early 2000 show a further increase, and acceleration, in PF-associated mortality. Using US mortality data from 1992 to 2003 and applying methods similar to those of Mannino and colleagues, Olson and colleagues[26] analyzed more than 28 million death records and found that the age-adjusted and standardized (to the year 2000) mortality increased 29.4% in men (from 49.7 deaths per million to 64.3 deaths per million) and 38.1% in women (from 42.3 deaths per million to 58.4 deaths per million) (Fig. 6.1). Rates increased with increasing age. Compared with the previous decade, mortality over this period increased at a significantly faster pace in both

men and women. From 1992 to 2003, rates rose more steeply in women than in men. Mortality was greater among white non-Hispanics than black non-Hispanics or Hispanics, suggesting that race and ethnicity may also play a role in the susceptibility to IPF.

Similar trends were reported in the United Kingdom: age-adjusted and sex-adjusted mortality from IPF-CS (ICD-9 code 515 or 516.3, or ICD-10 code J84.1) had reached 51 per million person-years by 2008 (an increase of 5% per year since the late 1960s).[27]

Hutchinson and colleagues recently determined IPF mortality rates from 10 countries over the period of 1999–2012.[29] To compare mortality rate among these countries, ICD-10 code J84 (other ILDs) was used given that not all countries had data available for more specific subcodes of J84.1 (IPF) and J84.9 (interstitial pulmonary disease, unspecified). Overall, age-standardized mortality rates ranged between 4.68 and 13.36 per 100,000 population (for the latest years of available data, ranging from 2010 to 2012) with lower rates identified in Sweden, Spain, and New Zealand; slightly higher rates noted in Australia, Canada, and the USA; and the highest rates found in England and Wales, Japan, Scotland, and Northern Ireland. Overall, there was a 2–3% annual increase in mortality over time; using the broad ICD-10 code J84, the overall rate ratio was 1.03 (95% CI, 1.02–1.04; $P<.001$), and using the narrow ICD-10 code J84.1, the overall rate ratio was 1.02 (95% CI, 1.01–1.03; $P<.001$).

These studies suggest that, although once considered an orphan disease, PF is more common than several common malignancies and is an important public health concern, particularly in elderly people, as mortality rates—in general—continue to rise.[26–29]

## Prevalence and Incidence, and Trends Over Time

The prevalence of disease is defined as the number of persons with disease at a specific point in time divided by the total population at that time, and incidence is defined as the number of persons with newly diagnosed disease divided by the number of persons at risk for developing that disease over that period of time. Prevalence is a proportion; incidence is a rate. In disease processes in which the incidence and the duration of the disease are stable, the prevalence should reflect the incidence multiplied by the duration of the disease.[30]

Before 1994, little was known about the incidence or prevalence of ILD in general or IPF in particular.[31,33] Coultas and colleagues[34] performed one of the first large-scale epidemiologic investigations to determine the prevalence and incidence of IPF. Using several, broad case-finding methods, they established a population-based registry of ILD in Bernalillo County, New Mexico. From 1988 to 1993, they found that IPF was the most common ILD in this region, accounting for 22.5% of prevalent cases and 31.2% of incident cases. The prevalence and incidence of IPF were higher in men (20.2 cases per 100,000 persons and 13.2 cases per 100,000 person-years, respectively) than women (10.7 per 100,000 persons and 7.4 per 100,000 person-years, respectively). Both the prevalence and incidence of IPF increased dramatically with age (Table 6.2). Limitations to this study included that these data came from only one county in New Mexico, so it was not known whether these were applicable to the United States as a whole.

More than a decade later, Raghu and colleagues[35] determined the prevalence and incidence of IPF using a large health-care claims database from a US health plan that covered ~3 million persons in 20 states. Using data from 1996 to 2000, they determined the prevalence and incidence of IPF using both a narrow and broad definition of IPF. The broad definition of IPF included any person 18 years of age or older, with one or more medical claims with a diagnosis of IPF (ICD-9

| TABLE 6.2 |
| :-- |
| The Prevalence and Incidence of Idiopathic Pulmonary Fibrosis (IPF) by Age Strata and Gender in Bernalillo County, New Mexico, From 1988 to 1993 |

| Age Strata (years) | IPF (PREVALENCE, PER 100,000 PERSONS) | | IPF (INCIDENCE, PER 100,000 PERSONS/ YEAR) | |
| :-- | :-- | :-- | :-- | :-- |
| | Men | Women | Men | Women |
| 35–44 | 2.7 | – | 4.0 | – |
| 45–54 | 8.7 | 8.1 | 2.2 | 4.0 |
| 55–64 | 28.4 | 5.0 | 14.2 | 10.0 |
| 65–74 | 104.6 | 72.3 | 48.6 | 21.1 |
| ≥75 | 174.7 | 73.2 | 101.9 | 57.0 |

Data from Coultas DB, Zumwalt RE, Black WC, et al. The epidemiology of interstitial lung diseases. *Am J Respir Crit Care Med.* 1994;150:967–72.

of 516.3), and without any other medical claims for a diagnosis of another ILD on or after the date of the last medical claim with this diagnostic code for IPF. The narrow definition of IPF included those criteria plus at least one claim for either a procedure code for surgical or transbronchial lung biopsy or a computed tomography scan of the thorax. They found that the overall prevalence of IPF was 14.0 or 42.7 per 100,000 persons, depending on whether the narrow or broad case definitions were used. These investigators found that the incidence of IPF was 6.8 or 16.3 per 100,000 person-years, depending on whether the narrow or broad case definitions were used. Similar to Coultas and colleagues, they also found that both the prevalence and incidence increased with age (Table 6.3). Compared with Coultas and colleagues, Raghu and colleagues calculated prevalence and incidence estimates that were greater, suggesting the burden of disease had increased over time (see Tables 6.2 and 6.3).

Studies performed outside the United States also suggest that the incidence of IPF has increased over time. Using a general practice database in the United Kingdom, Gribbin and colleagues[36] examined persons with a diagnosis of IPF from 1991 to 2003. During this period, the overall incidence of IPF was 4.6 per 100,000 person-years (numbers slightly lower than reported by either Coultas and colleagues or Raghu and colleagues). However, this study suggested that the burden of IPF had increased over time: the incidence had more than doubled, a finding not explained by an aging population.

**TABLE 6.3**

The Prevalence and Incidence of Idiopathic Pulmonary Fibrosis (IPF) by Age Strata and Gender From a Health Care Claims Processing System of a Large US Health Plan From 1996 to 2000 Using the Broad Case Definition (see text)

| Age Strata (years) | IPF (PREVALENCE, PER 100,000 PERSONS) | | IPF (INCIDENCE, PER 100,000 PERSONS/YEAR) | |
| --- | --- | --- | --- | --- |
| | Men | Women | Men | Women |
| 35–44 | 4.9 | 12.7 | 1.1 | 5.4 |
| 45–54 | 22.3 | 22.6 | 11.4 | 10.9 |
| 55–64 | 62.8 | 50.9 | 35.1 | 22.6 |
| 65–74 | 148.5 | 106.7 | 49.1 | 36.0 |
| ≥75 | 276.9 | 192.1 | 97.6 | 62.2 |

Data from Raghu G, Weycker D, Edelsberg J, et al. Incidence and prevalence of idiopathic pulmonary fibrosis. *Am J Respir Crit Care Med*. 2006;174:810–16.

Similar to the case with mortality, it is unclear if these studies that reported increases in incidence represent a true increase in disease occurrence or simply improved recognition of the disease. Case ascertainment may have increased over this period because of a growing use of HRCT in the evaluation of ILD. Increased public and community practice awareness of IPF may also account for these trends: during the 1990s, the first large, multicenter, therapeutic trial for IPF was conceptualized and began enrolling patients.[37]

Navaratnam and colleagues[27] reexamined the trends in incidence of PF in the United Kingdom through 2008. Using computerized primary care records in the United Kingdom, they found that the incidence of IPF-CS (defined from 1965 to 1978 as ICD, eighth edition code 517, from 1979 to 1999 as ICD-9 code 516.3 and 515, and from 2000 onward as ICD-10 code J84.1) increased at a rate of ~5% per year.

A recent systematic review regarding the global incidence of IPF, which summarized 34 studies of IPF incidence providing data from 21 countries, found that most studies showed an increase in incidence over time. Further, when using data from 2000 onward, Hutchinson and colleagues estimated an incidence of three to nine cases per 100,000 per year for Europe and North America and reported that incidence rates were lower in East Asia and South America.[38]

Additional data have been conflicting. One study from the United States suggested a different trend. Fernandez-Perez and colleagues[39] analyzed data

from Olmsted County, Minnesota, to determine incidence and prevalence of IPF from 1997 to 2005. They screened 596 patients in a population-based registry for PF. Overall, the age-adjusted and sex-adjusted incidence was 8.8/100,000 person-years based on a narrow-case definition of IPF (UIP pattern on surgical lung biopsy or characteristic HRCT) and 17.4/100,000 person-years based on a broad case definition (UIP pattern on surgical lung biopsy or either definite or possible characteristic HRCT). The incidence was higher in men than in women, and the incidence increased with advancing age in men and until the age of 80 years in women. Unlike any of the other investigators whose studies were described earlier, Fernandez-Perez and colleagues observed that the incidence significantly ($P < .001$) decreased over the study period (although peaks in incidence were noted in 1998 and 2001). In 2005, the age-adjusted and sex-adjusted prevalence of IPF was 27.9/100,000 and 63/100,000 (using the narrow and broad definition, respectively). However, given the aging population, these investigators project that the annual number of newly diagnosed cases of IPF in the US population by 2050 may reach 21,000. It is impossible to speculate whether these trends, observed in this one county, reflect the most current trends at a national or international level.

To further investigate trends at the national level, Raghu and colleagues recently examined US Medicare beneficiaries aged 65 years and more to determine the incidence and prevalence of IPF from 2001 to 2011.[40] These investigators found that the incidence of IPF remained stable over this period of time with an overall estimate of 93.7 cases per 100,000 person-years at risk (where the denominator is derived from the Medicare population) (95% CI, 91.9–95.4), while the annual cumulative prevalence increased steadily from 202.2 cases per 100,000 people in 2001 to 494.5 cases per 100,000 people in 2011. Given a stable incidence of IPF, but a steady increase in prevalence, the investigators hypothesized that at least part of the increase in prevalence was due to increasing survival time. Survival time was lower in patients diagnosed in 2007 (4.0 years; 95% CI, 3.8–4.5) compared to patients diagnosed in more recent years (3.3 years; 95% CI, 3.0–3.8).

**Risk Factors**

Although IPF is defined as an idiopathic disease, epidemiologic studies have identified several risk factors (including environmental and occupational exposures) associated with the diagnosis. These studies tend to be case-control studies and are subject to bias: recall bias occurs when persons with disease recall exposures differently from those without the disease, and diagnosis misclassification bias occurs when the number of individuals incorrectly diagnosed with IPF is not equally distributed between those with and those without the risk factor.[41] In addition, in case-control studies, the accurate assessment of dose and duration of exposure is challenging; thus, identifying a dose-response effect of the risk factor is frequently impossible.[42] Although case reports also suggest associations between IPF and several different exposures, the following discussion of exposures is limited to those in which the exposure was identified in two or more independent studies or via a metaanalysis. Clinical factors, including gastroesophageal reflux disease, diabetes, and infectious agents, have been implicated as risk factors for IPF, but are beyond the scope of this review.[3]

### Cigarette smoking

Several case-control studies have yielded data on the association between IPF and smoking. Baumgartner and colleagues[43] identified 248 IPF cases from 16 referral centers in the United States and matched these cases to 491 control individuals on sex, age, and geography. A smoking history was more common in those with IPF (72%) than controls (63%) (OR = 1.6; 95% CI = 1.1–2.4). Three other case-control studies from the United Kingdom and Japan found a similar association.[44-46] Scott and colleagues[32] found no association between IPF and smoking in a case-control study of 40 patients with IPF from Nottingham, United Kingdom, and 106 matched controls. Of all the studies on the topic, this one included the fewest cases. In a metaanalysis of these five studies, patients with IPF were significantly more likely than controls to report a smoking history (OR = 1.58; 95% CI = 1.27–1.97).[42]

In an attempt to identify a dose-response relationship between smoking and IPF, Baumgartner and colleagues[43] observed that, when compared with individuals who had a 20–pack-year or fewer smoking history, those with a 21–pack-year to 40–pack-year history had a greater odds of developing IPF (OR = 2.26; 95% CI = 1.3–3.8); however, for those with a history greater than 40 pack-years, there was no further increase in the risk of developing IPF (OR = 1.12; 95% CI = 0.7–1.9). After adjusting for age, sex, and region of residency, Miyake and colleagues[46] found an association between IPF and smoking in those with a 20–pack-year to 39.9–pack-year history (OR = 3.23; 95% CI = 1.01–10.84),

but not for those with either a fewer or greater pack-year history.

### Environmental and Occupational Exposures
Because other environmental exposures (including asbestosis, silicosis, and coal workers' pneumoconiosis) are known to cause fibrotic lung disease,[47–49] IPF is more likely to occur in men than in women (and men are more likely than women to work in jobs in which such exposures occur),[2] and IPF-associated mortality is higher in highly industrialized regions of some countries,[22] it has been hypothesized that environmental or occupational exposures may also be associated with IPF.

**Metal dust.** In several case-control studies and a metaanalysis, investigators have examined the association between a variety of environmental or occupational exposures and the risk of IPF. Each of the initial five studies yielded data that suggested an association between metal dust exposure and IPF (OR from the metaanalysis = 2.44, 95% CI = 1.74–3.40).[32,42,44–46,50] In two of these studies, a dose-response relationship was found.[44,50] In further support of this association, elemental microanalyses of hilar and mediastinal lymph nodes in patients with IPF have shown increased nickel,[51] silicon,[52] and aluminum[52] levels compared with controls.

In contrast, Gustafson and colleagues[53] recently found no association between metal dust exposure and IPF (OR = 0.9; 95% CI = 0.51–1.59) among 140 patients with IPF and 757 matched controls in Sweden; they did not assess for a dose-response relationship.

Hubbard and colleagues[54] assembled an historical cohort from the pension-fund archives of employees who had worked for Rolls-Royce plc in the United Kingdom to determine the risk of IPF in those exposed to metal dust. Among members of this cohort, there were 20,526 total deaths, and 55 were IPF associated. The number of IPF-associated deaths in this cohort was significantly greater than expected based on national mortality (proportional mortality ratio = 1.39; 95% CI = 1.07–1.82). Among the 22 decedents with available archive data, a dose-response relationship between metal exposure and IPF was identified (OR per 10 years of exposure = 1.71; 95% CI = 1.09–2.68).

Using US death certificate data from 1999 to 2003 and available industry/occupation codes for a proportion of decedents with PF (ICD-10 code J84.1), Pinheiro and colleagues[55] found an increase in the proportionate mortality (PM) for those decedents whose industry was recorded as metal mining (PM = 2.4; 95% CI = 1.3–4.0) and those whose industry was recorded as fabricated structural metal products (PM = 1.9; 95% CI = 1.1–3.1).

**Wood dust.** In the studies mentioned earlier and other case-controlled studies, researchers have examined the association between wood dust exposure and IPF.[32,42,44,46,50,56] Of the initial five studies, in only one did investigators observe a significantly increased risk of IPF in patients exposed to wood dust (OR = 1.71; 95% CI = 1.01–1.92).[44] However, when all of these studies were included in a metaanalysis, an increased risk of IPF was found in patients with exposure to wood dusts (OR = 1.94; 95% CI = 1.34–2.81).[42] In another study from Sweden, not included in the metaanalysis, there was no association between any wood dust and IPF among the entire study sample (OR = 1.2; 95% CI = 0.65–2.23); however, there was an increased risk of IPF in men exposed to birch dust (OR = 2.7, 95% CI = 1.30–5.65) or hardwood dust (OR = 2.7; 95% CI = 1.14–6.52). No association between IPF and fur or fir dust was identified. This finding suggests that in addition to gender, specific types of dust may play a role in the pathogenesis of IPF.[53]

**Sand, stone, and silica.** Three of four case-control studies have found an increased risk of IPF in patients with exposures to sand, stone, or silica, with a summary OR of 1.97 (95% CI = 1.09–3.55).[32,42,44,50,56]

**Farming and livestock.** Agriculture/farming-related and livestock-related exposures have been found to be associated with IPF. In two case-control studies, one from the United States and one from Japan, workers in the agriculture or farming sectors were found to have an increased risk of IPF (metaanalysis OR = 1.65, 95% CI = 1.20–2.26).[42,45,50] The study noted earlier from the United States and another study from the United Kingdom both found that exposure to livestock was associated with an increased risk of IPF (metaanalysis OR = 2.17, 95% CI = 1.28–3.68).[32,42,50] Furthermore, Baumgartner and colleagues[50] identified a dose–response relationship between livestock exposure and IPF. After adjusting for age and smoking history, they found no increased risk for IPF among patients exposed for less than 5 years (OR = 2.1; 95% CI = 0.7–6.1), but a significantly increased risk for IPF among those with 5 or more years of exposure (OR = 3.3; 95% CI = 1.3–8.3).

## SUMMARY

Over the last several decades, results from several studies have advanced understanding of IPF: how it is diagnosed, its basic epidemiologic profile, and occupational or environmental exposures that may increase the risk for developing the disease. These results have reshaped how IPF is diagnosed, especially by highlighting the accuracy with which a characteristic HRCT identifies a UIP pattern of lung injury: patients with such an HRCT need not have a surgical lung biopsy for IPF to be diagnosed confidently. However, making a diagnosis of IPF is complex, and whether a surgical lung biopsy is indicated or not, diagnostic accuracy is improved with multidisciplinary discussions in centers that specialize in the care of patients with this disease. Over the same period, the burden of IPF seems to have increased, with some incidence and mortality estimates placing IPF on par with certain relatively common malignancies. Although through case-control and cohort studies investigators have identified risk factors for IPF, these studies do not prove causality, and further research is needed not only to better understand the underlying pathobiology of this complex disease but also to find effective therapies for it.

## REFERENCES

1. American Thoracic Society. Idiopathic pulmonary fibrosis: diagnosis and treatment. International consensus statement. American Thoracic Society (ATS), and the European Respiratory Society (ERS). *Am J Respir Crit Care Med.* 2000;161:646–664.
2. American Thoracic Society, European Respiratory Society. American Thoracic Society/European Respiratory Society International Multidisciplinary Consensus Classification of the Idiopathic Interstitial Pneumonias. This joint statement of the American Thoracic Society (ATS), and the European Respiratory Society (ERS) was adopted by the ATS board of directors, June 2001 and by the ERS Executive Committee, June 2001. *Am J Respir Crit Care Med.* 2001;165:277–304.
3. Raghu G, Collard HR, Egan JJ, et al. An official ATS/ERS/JRS/ALAT statement: idiopathic pulmonary fibrosis: evidence-based guidelines for diagnosis and management. *Am J Respir Crit Care Med.* 2011;183:788–824.
4. Raghu G, Mageto YN, Lockhart D, et al. The accuracy of the clinical diagnosis of new-onset idiopathic pulmonary fibrosis and other interstitial lung disease: a prospective study. *Chest.* 1999;116:1168–1174.
5. Hunninghake GW, Zimmerman MB, Schwartz DA, et al. Utility of a lung biopsy for the diagnosis of idiopathic pulmonary fibrosis. *Am J Respir Crit Care Med.* 2001;164:193–196.

6. Swensen SJ, Aughenbaugh GL, Meyers JL. Diffuse lung disease: diagnostic accuracy of CT in patients undergoing surgical biopsy of the lung. *Radiology.* 1997;205:229–234.

7. Hunninghake GW, Lynch DA, Galvin JR, et al. Radiologic findings are strongly associated with a pathologic diagnosis of usual interstitial pneumonia. *Chest.* 2003;124: 1215–1223.

8. MacDonald SL, Rubens MB, Hansell DM, et al. Nonspecific interstitial pneumonia and usual interstitial pneumonia: comparative appearances at and diagnostic accuracy of thin-section CT. *Radiology.* 2001;221:600–605.

9. Johkoh T, Muller NL, Cartier Y, et al. Idiopathic interstitial pneumonias: diagnostic accuracy of thin-section CT in 129 patients. *Radiology.* 1999;211:555–560.

10. Monaghan H, Wells AU, Colby TV, et al. Prognostic implications of histologic patterns in multiple surgical lung biopsies from patients with idiopathic interstitial pneumonias. *Chest.* 2004;125:522–526.

11. Flaherty KR, Travis WD, Colby TV, et al. Histopathologic variability in usual and nonspecific interstitial pneumonias. *Am J Respir Crit Care Med.* 2001;164:1722–1727.

12. Flaherty KR, Thwaite EL, Kazerooni EA, et al. Radiological versus histological diagnosis in UIP and NSIP: survival implications. *Thorax.* 2003;58:143–148.

13. Yagihashi K, Huckleberry J, Colby TV, et al. Radiologic-pathologic discordance in biopsy-proven usual interstitial pneumonia. *Eur Respir J.* 2016;47:1189–1197.

14. Flaherty KR, King TE, Raghu G, et al. Idiopathic interstitial pneumonia: what is the effect of a multidisciplinary approach to diagnosis? *Am J Respir Crit Care Med.* 2004;170:904–910.

15. Lamas DJ, Kawut SM, Bagiella E, et al. Delayed access and survival in idiopathic pulmonary fibrosis: a cohort study. *Am J Respir Crit Care Med.* 2011;184(7):842–847.

16. World Health Organization. *Epidemiology.* Available at: http://www.who.int/topics/epidemiology/en/.

17. Last JM. *A Dictionary of Epidemiology.* 2nd ed. New York: Oxford University Press; 1998.

18. Gordis L. The epidemiologic approach to disease and intervention. In: Gordis L, ed. *Epidemiology.* 3rd ed. Philadelphia: Elsevier Saunders; 2004:1–14.

19. Coultas DB, Hubbard R. Epidemiology of idiopathic pulmonary fibrosis. In: Lynch JP, ed. *Idiopathic Pulmonary Fibrosis.* New York: Marcel Dekker; 2004:1–30.

20. Leibow AA, Carrington DB. The interstitial pneumonias. In: Simon M, Potchen EJ, LeMay M, eds. *Frontiers of Pulmonary Radiology.* New York: Grune & Stratton; 1969: 102–141.

21. World Health Organization. *International classification of diseases 1975.* 9th revision. Geneva, Switzerland: WHO; 1977.

22. Johnston I, Britton J, Kinnear W, et al. Rising mortality from cryptogenic fibrosing alveolitis. *BMJ.* 1990;301:1017–1021.

23. World Health Organization. *ICD-10: International Classification of Diseases and Related Health Problems.* 10th revision. Geneva, Switzerland: WHO; 2003.

24. Coultas DB, Hughes MP. Accuracy or mortality data for interstitial lung disease in New Mexico, USA. *Thorax.* 1996;51:717–720.

25. Mannino DM, Etzel RA, Parrish RG. Pulmonary fibrosis deaths in the United States, 1979-1991. *Am J Respir Crit Care Med.* 1996;153:1548–1552.

26. Olson AL, Swigris JJ, Lezotte DC, et al. Mortality from pulmonary fibrosis increased in the United States from 1992 to 2003. *Am J Respir Crit Care Med.* 2007;176:277–284.

27. Navaratnam V, Fleming KM, West J, et al. The rising incidence of idiopathic pulmonary fibrosis in the UK. *Thorax.* 2011;66:462–467.

28. Hubbard R, Johnston I, Coultas DB, et al. Mortality rates from cryptogenic fibrosing alveolitis in seven countries. *Thorax.* 1996;51:711–716.

29. Hutchinson JP, McKeever TM, Fogarty AW, et al. Increasing global mortality from idiopathic pulmonary fibrosis in the twenty-first century. *Ann Am Thorac Soc.* 2014;11:1176–1185.

30. Gordis L. Measuring the occurrence of disease: I. Morbidity. In: Gordis L, ed. *Epidemiology.* 3rd ed. Philadelphia: Elsevier Saunders; 2004:32–47.

31. Crystal RG, Bitterman PB, Rennard SI, et al. Interstitial lung diseases of unknown causes. Disorders characterized by chronic inflammation of the lower respiratory tract. *N Engl J Med.* 1984;310:154–166. 235–44.

32. Scott J, Johnston I, Britton J. What causes cryptogenic fibrosing alveolitis? A case-control study of environmental exposure to dust. *BMJ.* 1990;301:1015–1017.

33. U.S. Department of Health and Human Services. Vital and Health Statistics. *National Hospital Discharge Survey: Annual Summary, 1988.* Hyattsville, MD: DHHS; 1991:91–1101. No (PHS).

34. Coultas DB, Zumwalt RE, Black WC, et al. The epidemiology of interstitial lung diseases. *Am J Respir Crit Care Med.* 1994;150:967–972.

35. Raghu G, Weycker D, Edelsberg J, et al. Incidence and prevalence of idiopathic pulmonary fibrosis. *Am J Respir Crit Care Med.* 2006;174:810–816.

36. Gribbin J, Hubbard RB, Le Jeune I, et al. Incidence and mortality of idiopathic pulmonary fibrosis and sarcoidosis in the UK. *Thorax.* 2006;61:980–985.

37. Raghu G, Brown KK, Bradford WZ, et al. A placebo controlled trial of interferon gamma-1b in patients with idiopathic pulmonary fibrosis. *N Engl J Med.* 2004;350:125–133.

38. Hutchinson J, Fogarty A, Hubbard R, McKeever T. Global incidence and mortality of idiopathic pulmonary fibrosis: a systematic review. *Eur Respir J.* 2015;46:795–806.

39. Fernández-Pérez ER, Daniels CE, Schroeder DR, et al. Incidence, prevalence, and clinical course of idiopathic pulmonary fibrosis. *Chest.* 2010;137:129–137.

40. Raghu G, Chen SY, Yeh WS, et al. Idiopathic pulmonary fibrosis in US Medicare beneficiaries aged 65 and older: incidence, prevalence, and survival, 2001-2011. *Lancet Respir Med.* 2014;2:566–572.

41. Gordis L. Case-control and cross-sectional studies. In: Gordis L, ed. *Epidemiology*. 3rd ed. Philadelphia: Elsevier Saunders; 2004:159–176.

42. Taskar VS, Coultas DB. Is idiopathic pulmonary fibrosis an environmental disease? *Proc Am Thorac Soc*. 2006;3: 293–298.

43. Baumgartner KB, Samet JM, Stidley CA, et al. Cigarette smoking: a risk factor for idiopathic pulmonary fibrosis. *Am J Respir Crit Care Med*. 1997;155:242–248.

44. Hubbard R, Lewis S, Richards K, et al. Occupational exposure to metal or wood dust and aetiology of cryptogenic fibrosing alveolitis. *Lancet*. 1996;347:284–289.

45. Iwai K, Mori T, Yamada N, et al. Idiopathic pulmonary fibrosis epidemiologic approaches to occupational exposure. *Am J Respir Crit Care Med*. 1994;150:670–675.

46. Miyaka Y, Sasaki S, Yokoyama T, et al. Occupational and environmental factors and idiopathic pulmonary fibrosis in Japan. *Ann Occup Hyg*. 2005;49:259–265.

47. Weissman DN, Banks DE. Silicosis. In: Schwarz MI, King TE, eds. *Interstitial Lung Disease*. 4th ed. Ontario, Canada: BC Decker; 2003:387–401.

48. Banks DE. Coal workers' pneumoconiosis. In: Schwarz MI, King TE, eds. *Interstitial Lung Disease*. 4th ed. Ontario, Canada: BC Decker; 2003:402–417.

49. Steele M, Peterson MW, Schwarz DA. Asbestosis and asbestos-induced pleural fibrosis. In: Schwarz MI, King TE, eds. *Interstitial Lung Disease*. 4th ed. Ontario, Canada: BC Decker; 2003:418–434.

50. Baumgarter KB, Samet JM, Coutas DB, et al. Occupational and environmental risk factors for idiopathic pulmonary fibrosis: a multicenter case-control study. *Am J Epidemiol*. 2000;152:307–315.

51. Hashimoto H, Tajima H, Mizoguchi I, et al. Elemental analysis of hilar and mediastinal lymph nodes in idiopathic pulmonary fibrosis. *Nihon Kyobu Shikkan Gakkai Zasshi*. 1992;30:2061–2068. [in Japanese].

52. Kitamura H, Ichinose S, Hosoya T, et al. Inhalation of inorganic particles as a risk factor for idiopathic pulmonary fibrosis–elemental microanalysis of pulmonary lymph nodes obtained at autopsy cases. *Pathol Res Pract*. 2007;203:575–585.

53. Gustafson T, Dahlman-Höglund A, Nilsson K, et al. Occupational exposure and severe pulmonary fibrosis. *Respir Med*. 2007;110:2207–2212.

54. Hubbard R, Cooper M, Antaoniak M, et al. Risk of cryptogenic fibrosing alveolitis in metal workers. *Lancet*. 2000;355:466–467.

55. Pinheiro GA, Antao VC, Wood JM, et al. Occupational risks for idiopathic pulmonary fibrosis mortality in the United States. *Int J Occup Environ Health*. 2008;14: 117–123.

56. Mullen J, Hodgson MJ, DeGraff CA, et al. Case-control study of idiopathic pulmonary fibrosis and environmental exposures. *J Occup Environ Med*. 1998;40:363–367.

# CHAPTER 7

# Approach to the Diagnosis of Interstitial Lung Disease

JÜRGEN BEHR

---

**KEY POINTS**

- A comprehensive patient history taking is of crucial importance for the diagnosis of interstitial lung diseases (ILDs).
- Dyspnea with exertion or at rest is the predominant symptom in most ILDs.
- There are no specific laboratory tests that allow for the diagnosis of an ILD, but, in an appropriate clinical setting, laboratory test results may be strongly supportive of a specific diagnosis.

---

Interstitial lung diseases (ILDs) are a heterogeneous group of more than 150 disease entities that differ significantly with respect to prevention, therapy, and prognosis. The current classification scheme of ILDs is shown in Fig. 7.1.[1]

The diagnostic strategy in a patient with ILD is based on considerations regarding the dynamic time course (acute, subacute, chronic), the cause (known or unknown), and the context of the disease at presentation (presence of extrapulmonary/systemic disease manifestations). Fig. 7.2 summarizes the main disease categories that have to be differentiated during the diagnostic process.[1–3]

Once an interstitial disease process has been recognized in a patient, there are three crucial questions that have to be addressed in the diagnostic workup:

1. Is there a discernible cause for the disease?
2. If no cause is identifiable, is it idiopathic pulmonary fibrosis (IPF)?
3. If there is no cause of the disease and if it is not IPF, should surgical lung biopsy be recommended?

After a diagnosis has been established, the severity and dynamics of the disease have to be assessed and monitored, with or without therapy. Diagnosis and disease severity/dynamics are fundamental for treatment decisions and to predict prognosis. The diagnostic approach to ILD may have to be adapted to different clinical scenarios that eventually lead to presentation of a patient:

1. A patient presents with clinical symptoms (e.g., dry cough, dyspnea).
2. A patient is at risk of ILD because of known exposures (e.g., amiodarone, asbestos).
3. A patient is at risk of ILD because of family history.
4. A patient is asymptomatic but presents with chance finding on chest radiography or computed tomography.
5. A patient is asymptomatic but presents with chance finding on a pulmonary functioning test (e.g., restrictive pattern, reduced gas transfer).

This article deals with diagnostic approaches suitable for patients presenting with clinical symptoms of ILD in the first place.

## CLINICAL EVALUATION
### History Taking

A comprehensive history taking of a patient is of crucial importance for the diagnosis of ILD. There are four main questions to be answered: (1) When did respiratory symptoms start? (2) How did the disease develop over time to the present? (3) Are there or have there been any exposures to etiologic agents known to cause ILD? and (4) What is the severity of symptoms at presentation?[1]

The disease chronology can be subdivided into four categories: (1) acute, days up to a few weeks; (2) subacute, 4 to 12 weeks; (3) chronic, longer than 12 weeks; and (4) episodic, that is, symptomatic phases that are followed by asymptomatic phases. In addition, all available radiographs of the lung should be reviewed to characterize the nature and development of the radiologic pattern. Flitting opacities on chest imaging studies may drive the differential diagnosis to focus on eosinophilic pneumonia, hypersensitivity pneumonitis (HP), vasculitis, or organizing pneumonia.[1,3,4]

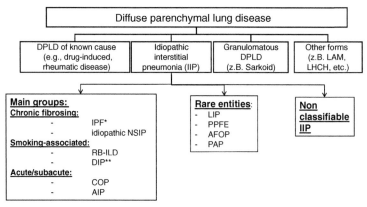

* Obligatory "usual interstitial pneumonia" (UIP) pattern;   ** occurs rarely in nonsmokers;

FIG. 7.1 New diffuse parenchymal lung disease (DPDL) classification, 2013. *AFOP*, acute fibrinoid organizing peumonia; *AIP*, acute interstitial pneumonia; *COP*, cryptogenic organizing pneumonia; *DIP*, desquamative interstitial pneumonia; *IPF*, idiopathic pulmonary fibrosis; *LAM*, lymphangioleiomyomatosis; *LCHC*, Langerhans cell histiocytosis; *LIP*, lymphoid interstitial pneumonia; *PAP*, pulmonary alveolar proteinosis; *PPFE*, pleuroparenchymal fibroelastosis; *RB-ILD*, respiratory bronchiolitis with interstitial lung disease. (From Travis et al. Am *J Respir Crit Care Med.* 2013;188[6]:733–48, with permission.)

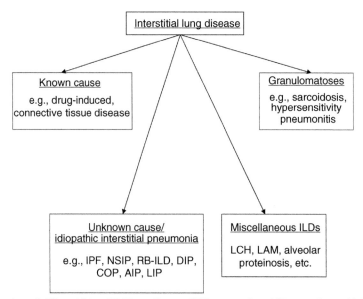

FIG. 7.2 Overview of different interstitial lung disease (ILD) categories. *AIP*, acute interstitial pneumonia; *COP*, cryptogenic organizing pneumonia; *DIP*, desquamative interstitial pneumonia; *IPF*, idiopathic pulmonary fibrosis; *LAM*, lymphangioleiomyomatosis; *LCH*, Langerhans cell histiocytosis; *LIP*, lymphoid interstitial pneumonia; *NSIP*, nonspecific interstitial pneumonia; *RB-ILD*, respiratory bronchiolitis and interstitial lung disease. (Data from American Thoracic Society/European Respiratory Society international multidisciplinary consensus classification of the idiopathic interstitial pneumonias. Am *J Respir Crit Care Med.* 2002;165:279.)

## ASSESSMENT OF SYMPTOMS

Dyspnea with exertion or at rest is the predominant symptom in most ILDs.[5,6] It is of importance to accurately assess the degree of exercise limitation and dyspnea in a reproducible manner by asking specific questions: after what distance, after how many steps, or after how many stairs or floors does dyspnea occur and for how long has the patient experienced this degree of dyspnea and how fast did it develop or when was the most recent change? The degree of dyspnea is linked to disease severity and prognosis.[5] It is also necessary to exclude nonrespiratory symptoms as a cause of the exercise limitation, for example, joint pains, muscle pains, or weakness.

Cough is the second most frequent symptom in patients with ILD and sometimes becomes really bothersome. Although a dry cough is common in IPF, cough is generally an airway symptom and therefore more indicative of airway-centered diseases such as sarcoidosis, HP, or organizing pneumonia. Increased secretions from ILD-associated bronchitis or bronchiectasis cause productive cough. Wheezing is another airway-associated symptom that is infrequent in ILD but may occur in certain entities such as Churg-Strauss syndrome, HP (e.g., pigeon breeder's lung), or airway-stenotic sarcoidosis.[7]

Pleural pain and effusion in the context of an ILD indicate connective tissue disease (e.g., systemic lupus erythematosus or rheumatoid arthritis) or drug-induced or asbestos-related disease. Differential diagnoses include complications such as infections or pulmonary embolism. Hemoptysis is always an alarming signal and may indicate manifestation of pulmonary hemorrhagic syndromes, for example, Goodpasture syndrome or granulomatosis with polyangiitis (GPA, previously called Wegener disease). Alternatively, infections, lung cancer, and pulmonary embolism have to be considered.[3] Gastroesophageal reflux is another common symptom in patients with ILD that is suspected of causing or at least exacerbating ILD. A history of acid reflux should, therefore, be taken in all patients with ILD.[8]

Extrapulmonary features of associated diseases may provide important hints to the correct diagnosis. Therefore joint pain and swelling (rheumatoid arthritis), cutaneous thickening, Raynaud phenomenon and dysphagia (systemic sclerosis), oculocutaneous albinism and colitis (Hermansky-Pudlak syndrome), chronic granulomatous sinusitis (GPA and Churg-Strauss syndrome), renal failure (Goodpasture syndrome), renal angiomyolipoma (lymphangioleiomyomatosis), and Crohn disease should be carefully asked about and sought for.[2,3,7]

## Next Step Is a Comprehensive Investigation of Possible Causes for Interstitial Lung Diseases

### Causative agents

A comprehensive history taking of all respiratory risk factors and exposures in the past and present is of utmost importance. Because history taking is a very complex and time-consuming task, it is often helpful to use a standardized questionnaire, such as that available from the American College of Chest Physicians.[9] The following items have to be checked: (1) smoking history, (2) hobbies, (3) travel, (4) occupations, and (5) drug history and treatments (e.g., radiation therapy).[3,10,11] Of special interest in this context is the family history as it becomes more and more clear that a considerable subset of patients and diseases do have hereditary traits.[2,3,12]

### Comorbid diseases

There are several diseases that mimic or that are associated with ILDs: (1) Infectious agents such as mycobacteria, cytomegalovirus, *Pneumocystis jiroveci*, and human immunodeficiency virus (HIV) and parasite infestations are able to cause an ILD-like condition. (2) Connective tissue diseases are frequently associated with ILDs. This is especially the case for systemic sclerosis and rheumatoid arthritis. (3) Vasculitides, for example, GPA, Churg-Strauss syndrome, and microscopic polyangiitis, are able to manifest in the lungs as ILD.[3,7]

## PHYSICAL EXAMINATION

On physical examination, inspection of the integument may reveal valuable findings: skin thickening and acral necrosis (scleroderma), oculocutaneous albinism (Hermansky-Pudlak syndrome), clubbing (up to 40% in all ILDs, up to 66% in IPF), livedo racemosa (systemic lupus erythematosus), cutaneous vasculitis (Churg-Strauss syndrome), and edematous-cyanotic skin (dermatomyositis, "disease lilac").[2,3,7] Palpation may reveal lymphadenopathy, hepatosplenomegaly pointing at sarcoidosis, HIV infection, or connective tissue disease.

On auscultation of the lungs, symmetric fine "Velcro-like" inspiratory crackles are found in more than 90% of patients with IPF and in about 60% of patients with connective tissue disease–associated ILD. Crackles are less frequent in HP and rare in sarcoidosis. Wheezing and inspiratory squeaks reflect bronchiolitis and/or bronchial obstruction and are associated with Churg-Strauss syndrome, HP, and rarely nonspecific interstitial pneumonia.[1-3] Cyanosis may be present and should be

**TABLE 7.1**

**Useful Laboratory Tests for Patients With Interstitial Lung Disease (ILD), Beyond Routine Laboratory Testing**

| Laboratory Test | Indication | Interpretation |
|---|---|---|
| ANA; rheumatoid factor; ANA differentiation, including Jo-1 or ScL-70 antibodies | Suspected CTD or idiopathic ILD for which CTD cannot be excluded | Low titers occur in up to 20% of patients with IPF, high titers suggest underlying CTD |
| Creatine kinase activity, myoglobin, aldolase | Suspected myositis | Elevated values support a diagnosis of dermatomyositis |
| Immunoglobulins | Suspicion of immunodeficiency | Decreased serum immunoglobulins suggest common variable immunodeficiency syndrome or LIP |
| c-ANCA, p-ANCA | Suspected vasculitis | c-ANCA suggestive of GPA (Wegener syndrome), microscopic polyangiitis; p-ANCA suggestive of CSS or MPA |
| Antiglomerular basement membrane antibody | Hemoptysis due to DAH, renal failure | Positive result is diagnostic of Goodpasture syndrome |
| Serum angiotensin-converting enzyme activity, serum-soluble interleukin-2 receptor | Sarcoidosis | Low sensitivity and specificity |
| Specific serum IgG antibodies | Exposure to antigens that cause HP | Valid only within an appropriate clinical context |

*ANA*, antinuclear antibody; *c-ANCA*, cytoplasmic antineutrophil cytoplasmic antibody (antiproteinase 3); *CSS*, Churg-Strauss syndrome; *CTD*, connective tissue disease; *DAH*, diffuse alveolar hemorrhage; *HP*, hypersensitivity pneumonitis; *GPA*, granulomatosis with polyangiitis; *IPF*, idiopathic pulmonary fibrosis; *LIP*, lymphocytic interstitial pneumonia; *MPA*, microscopic polyangiitis; *p-ANCA*, perinuclear antineutrophil cytoplasmic antibody (antimyeloperoxidase).

confirmed by pulse oximetry, which can be easily performed in clinics.[2,3,7]

## LABORATORY TESTING

There are no specific laboratory tests that allow for the diagnosis of an ILD, but, in an appropriate clinical setting, laboratory test results may be strongly supportive of a specific diagnosis. Routine laboratory testing should include a complete blood cell count; leukocyte differential; platelet count; erythrocyte sedimentation rate; determination of serum electrolyte levels, including calcium, serum urea nitrogen, and creatinine; liver function tests; and urinary sediment.[7] These laboratory values allow the exclusion or suggestion of an associated hematologic, liver, or kidney disease in a potential context of systemic disease (e.g., sarcoidosis, vasculitis, amyloidosis), malignancy (e.g., lymphoma), or infection (e.g., tuberculosis, HIV). To further evaluate the presence of connective tissue disease, systemic disease (e.g., sarcoidosis), or HP, additional measures may be appropriate as summarized in Table 7.1.

There have been multiple attempts to find biomarkers to monitor disease activity or to predict prognosis in different ILDs. Intraindividual changes of serum angiotensin-converting enzyme activity or of serum concentration of the soluble interleukin-2 receptor are to some extent helpful in monitoring disease activity in sarcoidosis.[13] The serum lactate dehydrogenase activity is to some extent predictive of prognosis in IPF. Limited data are available for serum levels of Krebs von der Lungen 6, a high-molecular-weight glycoprotein representing human MUC1 mucin, surfactant proteins A and D, matrix metalloproteinases, and CCL-18.[3,14] However, none of these biomarkers has been validated sufficiently to be recommended for the routine use in the monitoring and follow-up of patients with ILD.

## PULMONARY FUNCTION TESTING

Patients with ILD should undergo comprehensive pulmonary function testing, which includes arterial or capillary blood gas analysis at rest and eventually under exertion, spirometry, and body plethysmography, as well as measurement of the diffusion capacity using carbon monoxide as a tracer in the single-breath method (D$_{LCO}$).[1,3,4,15] In addition, measurement of compliance may be helpful in objectifying the elevated

**TABLE 7.2**
**Diagnostic Considerations Based on a Chest Radiograph**

| | |
|---|---|
| Low lung volumes | IPF; CTD-related ILD; chronic HP; asbestosis; chronic drug-induced fibrosis; chronic COP, CEP, or DIP |
| Preserved/increased lung volumes | RB-ILD, IPF plus emphysema, LCH, LAM, sarcoidosis, tuberous sclerosis, neurofibromatosis, bronchiolitis |
| Upper zone predominance | Sarcoidosis, silicosis, coal workers' pneumoconiosis, HP, LCH, berylliosis, CEP, Caplan syndrome, nodular rheumatoid arthritis |
| Lower zone predominance | IPF, CTD-associated ILD, asbestosis, DIP, chronic HP |
| Peripheral predominance | IPF, COP, CEP |
| Micronodular | Infection, sarcoidosis, HP, malignancy |
| Septa thickening | Malignancy, chronic left heart failure, infection, pulmonary venoocclusive disease |
| Honeycombing | IPF, asbestosis, CTD-associated ILD, chronic HP, sarcoidosis |
| Migratory opacities | Löffler disease, COP, HP, ABPA |
| Kerley-B lines | Chronic left-sided heart failure, lymphangitis carcinomatosa |
| Pleural disease | CTD-associated ILD, asbestosis, malignancy, radiation-induced ILD, sarcoidosis |
| Pneumothorax | LCH, LAM, tuberous sclerosis, neurofibromatosis |
| Mediastinal/hilar lymphadenopathy | Sarcoidosis, malignancy, silicosis, berylliosis, CTD-associated ILD, infection |
| Normal (about 10%) | HP, NSIP, CTD-associated ILD, RB-ILD, bronchiolitis, sarcoidosis |

*ABPA*, allergic bronchopulmonary aspergillosis; *CEP*, chronic eosinophilic pneumonia; *COP*, cryptogenic organizing pneumonia; *CTD*, connective tissue disease; *DIP*, desquamative interstitial pneumonia; *HP*, hypersensitivity pneumonitis; *ILD*, interstitial lung disease; *IPF*, idiopathic pulmonary fibrosis; *LAM*, lymphangioleiomyomatosis; *LCH*, Langerhans cell histiocytosis; *NSIP*, nonspecific interstitial pneumonia; *RB-ILD*, respiratory bronchiolitis and ILD.

stiffness of the lung.[15] Pulmonary function tests are in general not able to support a specific ILD diagnosis, but they are necessary to assess the respiratory limitations and to monitor the disease during follow-up.[2,3]

Lung function abnormalities generally reflect the effects of interstitial inflammation and scarring resulting in a restrictive ventilatory deficit and impaired gas exchange as well as reduced compliance. Airway obstruction and emphysema are not features of ILD; however, they may be present when bronchial asthma or chronic obstructive pulmonary disease coexists in the patient. Moreover, some diseases such as lymphangioleiomyomatosis, Langerhans cell histiocytosis, sarcoidosis, and HP may present with airway obstruction and/or hyperinflation as part of the underlying disease process or associated bronchiolitis.[3,7] A disproportionate decrease of the $D_{LCO}$ in comparison with the restrictive ventilatory deficit should prompt suspicion of emphysema or pulmonary hypertension (PH).[16]

During follow-up, changes in lung function parameters are widely used and helpful for disease monitoring.[2,3,15] Especially in IPF, a small decrease of only 5–10%

of forced vital capacity during an observation period of 6 months is already indicative of increased mortality.[17] Less well established are changes in $D_{LCO}$ and blood gases as prognostic predictors, but these parameters may well be used to support the clinical relevance of marginal changes in forced vital capacity. Calculated lung function indices may also be helpful to objectify the course and prognosis of the disease. The composite physiologic index (CPI) is such a calculated index that reflects the extent of fibrosis on high-resolution computed tomography (HRCT) and corrects for coexisting emphysema.[18] An increase in CPI indicates progression of fibrosis and is associated with increased mortality.[18–20]

## RADIOLOGIC ASSESSMENT

An abnormal chest radiograph is often the initial finding in patients with ILD. A diffuse reticulonodular pattern, ground-glass opacities, or both are the most common findings on a chest radiograph in patients with ILD. The pattern and distribution of radiologic appearances contribute to initial diagnostic considerations as summarized in Table 7.2.[1–3,7]

### TABLE 7.3
### Criteria Diagnostic for Idiopathic Pulmonary Fibrosis

| UIP Pattern (All Four Features) | Possible UIP Pattern (All Three Features) | Inconsistent With UIP Pattern (Any of the Seven Features) |
|---|---|---|
| • Subpleural basal predominance<br>• Reticular abnormality<br>• Honeycombing with or without traction bronchiectasis<br>• Absence of features listed as inconsistent with UIP pattern (see the third column) | • Subpleural basal predominance<br>• Reticular abnormality<br>• Absence of features listed as inconsistent with UIP pattern (see the third column) | • Upper-lung or midlung predominance<br>• Peribronchovascular predominance<br>• Extensive ground-glass abnormality (extent > reticular abnormality)<br>• Profuse micronodules (bilateral, predominantly upper lobes)<br>• Discrete cysts (multiple, bilateral, away from areas of honeycombing)<br>• Diffuse mosaic attenuation/air trapping (bilateral, in ≥ three lobes)<br>• Consolidation in bronchopulmonary segments/lobes |

UIP, usual interstitial pneumonia.
From Raghu G, Collard HR, Egan JJ, et al. An Official ATS/ERS/JRS/ALAT statement: idiopathic pulmonary fibrosis: evidence-based guidelines for diagnosis and management. *Am J Respir Crit Care Med*. 2011;183:794; with permission.

### TABLE 7.4
### High-Resolution Computed Tomography (HRCT) Findings Suggesting Specific Alternative Diagnoses Other Than Idiopathic Pulmonary Fibrosis (IPF)

| HRCT Features Atypical for IPF | Probable Diagnosis |
|---|---|
| Centrilobular nodules, air trapping, ground-glass opacities, relative sparing of bases | HP |
| Pleural effusion, pleural thickening, esophageal dilation | Collagen vascular disease |
| Pleural plaques, pleural thickening | Asbestosis |
| Focal abnormality | Localized scar |

HP, hypersensitivity pneumonitis.

### TABLE 7.5
### Diagnostic Considerations Based on High-Resolution Computed Tomography (HRCT) Patterns

| Specific Computed Tomographic Findings | Entity |
|---|---|
| Cysts | Langerhans cell histiocytosis<br>Lymphangioleiomyomatosis<br>Lymphoid interstitial pneumonia<br>Birt-Hogg-Dubé syndrome |
| Perilymphatic nodules | Sarcoidosis<br>Chronic beryllium disease<br>Lymphangitic carcinoma<br>Lymphoma |
| Centrilobular nodules | HP<br>Respiratory bronchiolitis |
| Tree-in-bud pattern | Infection<br>Aspiration<br>Other forms of bronchiolitis |
| Mosaic attenuation | HP<br>Obliterative bronchiolitis<br>Pulmonary thromboembolism |

HP, hypersensitivity pneumonitis.

For a more subtle diagnosis, HRCT is the key diagnostic procedure and is sufficient for diagnosis in a significant number of patients with IPF.[2] The criteria that aid in making a confident diagnosis of IPF are presented in Table 7.3.[3] HRCT findings suggestive of an alternative diagnosis other than IPF are shown in Tables 7.4 and 7.5.

Interpretation of chest radiographs and HRCTs should always include a complete review of all images available for a specific patient and should be done in direct communication between the pulmonologist and the radiologist to optimize the diagnostic yield.

## BRONCHOSCOPY

In patients with ILD, bronchoscopy can be performed to obtain materials for microbiological, cytologic, and histologic analyses. The applied techniques encompass bronchoalveolar lavage (BAL), transbronchial lung biopsy (TBLB), and transbronchial needle aspiration (TBNA) for cytologic or histologic (Wang needle) analyses. However, bronchoscopy is associated with some morbidity and even a very low rate of mortality and therefore is not an obligatory diagnostic procedure for all patients with ILD.[2,3] Moreover, to make bronchoscopy and BAL/TBLB a valuable tool in the workup of patients with ILD, each clinical site must establish routine methods for handling and analysis of the materials.[2] Best use of this BAL/TBLB requires that the clinician identify very clear questions that are to be addressed with the biologic materials obtained and that it is reasonable these questions can be answered with these materials before the procedure is performed. If these obligatory prerequisites are fulfilled, bronchoscopy and BAL with or without TBLB are valuable tools in the diagnostic workup of patients with ILD.[21]

With the use of BAL, TBLB, and/or TBNA (eventually endobronchial ultrasonography guided), a diagnosis of sarcoidosis, lymphangitis carcinomatosa, eosinophilic pneumonia, alveolar proteinosis, Langerhans cell histiocytosis, lymphoid interstitial pneumonia, and several bacterial, viral, and fungal infections can be confirmed, thus avoiding more invasive procedures such as mediastinoscopy, video-assisted thoracoscopic (VATS) biopsy, or open surgical lung biopsy. In several patients with probable or possible IPF, bronchoscopic techniques may be used to rule out alternative diagnoses, such as HP in selected patients,[21] especially if VATS biopsy seems too risky or has to be performed in elderly patients. However, especially in patients with IPF, bronchoscopy and BAL have the potential of triggering acute exacerbation of IPF, so the indication for bronchoscopic evaluation should be discussed critically in every individual patient.[2] Bronchoscopic transbronchial cryobiopsy has recently evolved to an interesting method that may add to the diagnostic confidence in the differential diagnosis of ILD, but it still needs further evaluation in clinical trials.[22]

## SURGICAL LUNG BIOPSY

Surgical lung biopsy, nowadays preferentially performed during VATS, is the most invasive diagnostic procedure used for diagnosis of ILD. It is associated with significant morbidity and mortality and should be reserved for those patients in whom the management and treatment could change depending on the result of biopsy.[2,3,23,24] In IPF, histologic analysis from a surgical lung biopsy is no longer the gold standard of diagnosis because it has become clear that because of sampling error and uniformity of disease pattern in patients with advanced disease, histologic examination

will not provide the diagnostic clue in many patients.[2] Consequently, in IPF, the multidisciplinary discussion (MDD) involving the pulmonologist, radiologist, and pathologist has become the gold standard for diagnosis. This also seems the appropriate approach to diagnosis for the vast majority of patients with ILD. Because IPF is one if not the most important differential diagnosis in most patients with ILD, an MDD seems to be the most promising approach to reach a confident diagnosis.[2,25]

## ASSESSMENT OF PULMONARY HYPERTENSION

PH is frequently associated with ILD. Among patients with advanced disease on the waiting list for lung transplantation, 40–80% have PH. In patients with less advanced disease, still 10% have significant PH. Moreover, PH in ILD is clinically relevant because it is associated with an excess exercise intolerance and mortality. Consequently, this condition is of clinical relevance for the general management of patients with ILD to diagnose PH, even though no targeted therapy is yet approved for this condition. In patients with ILD, the diagnosis of associated PH may avoid overtreatment with immunosuppressive agents and provide early indication for the initiation of long-term oxygen therapy or listing for lung transplantation. In addition, identification of PH may support the diagnosis of other treatable conditions, such as left-sided heart disease.[16,26]

To find PH in patients with ILD, clinical symptoms are rather unspecific. Lung function showing a disproportionate reduction in $D_{LCO}$ and very low oxygen partial pressures in arterial or capillary blood at rest and/or during mild exercise may indicate the presence of PH. Doppler echocardiography is suitable as a screening tool to support a clinical suspicion of PH, but about one-third of the patients will have a technically insufficient result. Brain natriuretic peptide may be used as a biomarker but is per se not sufficient to prove or exclude PH.[16,26–28] In patients with signs and symptoms of PH associated with ILD, in whom a therapeutic consequence is feasible, a right-sided heart catheterization should be performed to make a firm diagnosis of PH and to differentiate precapillary and postcapillary PH.[16] Right-sided heart catheterization may prompt the performance of left-sided heart catheterization and coronary angiography in addition to showing or ruling out treatable left-sided heart disease.

## DIAGNOSTIC ALGORITHM

A diagnostic algorithm for patients with ILD is shown in Fig. 7.3. After differentiating ILDs with known causes

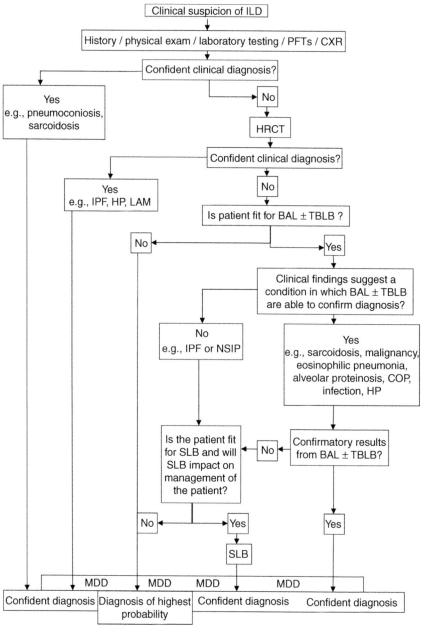

FIG. 7.3 Algorithm for the diagnosis of interstitial lung disease (ILD). *BAL*, bronchoalveolar lavage; *COP*, cryptogenic organizing pneumonia; *CXR*, chest radiography; *HP*, hypersensitivity pneumonitis; *HRCT*, high-resolution computed tomography; *LAM*, lymphangioleiomyomatosis; *MDD*, multidisciplinary discussion; *NSIP*, nonspecific interstitial pneumonia; *PFT*, pulmonary function testing; *SLB*, surgical lung biopsy; *TBLB*, transbronchial lung biopsy. (Data from Raghu G, Mageto YN, Lockhart D, et al. The accuracy of the clinical diagnosis of new-onset idiopathic pulmonary fibrosis and other interstitial lung disease: a prospective study. *Chest*. 1999;116:1168–1174; Bradley B, Branley HM, Egan JJ, et al. British Thoracic Society Interstitial Lung Disease Guideline Group, British Thoracic Society Standard of Care Committee; Thoracic Society of Australia; New Zealand Thoracic Society; Irish Thoracic Society. Interstitial lung disease guideline. *Thorax*. 2008;63[suppl 5]:v57.)

**TABLE 7.6**
**Characterization of Different Disease Patterns as a Guide to Treatment Approach and Monitoring Strategy**

| Pattern of Disease | Broad Treatment Approach | Monitoring Strategy |
|---|---|---|
| Self-limited inflammation | Remove cause/observe or treat (usually with steroid therapy) in short term | Short-term monitoring to confirm disease regression |
| Major inflammation with risk of progression to fibrosis | Antiinflammatory therapy (eventually high dose) for a response, then rationalize lower-dose therapy to maintain response | Monitor in short term to quantify the response to high-dose treatment. Monitor less frequently in long term to ensure that gains are preserved |
| Stable fibrosis | Observation alone (in treatment-naive patients, a treatment trial may be considered) | Long-term monitoring to ensure ongoing stability |
| Progressive fibrosis with stabilization realistic | Treat with steroid or immunosuppressive therapy, high dose if necessary to stabilize; consider antifibrotic drugs | Long-term monitoring to confirm absence of progression |
| Inexorably progressive fibrosis | Consider therapy to slow progression but avoid toxic agents | Long-term monitoring to quantify rapidity of progression with a view to transplant or for effective palliation |

Data from Wells AU. Diffuse parenchymal lung disease: an introduction. In: Warrell DA, Cox TM, Firth JD, eds. *Oxford textbook of medicine.* 5th ed. Vol. 2. Oxford, United Kingdom: Oxford University Press; 2010. 3365–3375.

from those with unknown causes, HRCT is the crucial diagnostic procedure that leads to a final diagnosis, for example, IPF, or that prompts further diagnostic steps, which eventually include bronchoscopic techniques such as BAL and TBLB or VATS lung biopsy. The evolution of the prognostic process may vary depending on the clinical presentation or setting, that is, symptomatic patients or asymptomatic patients with risk factors for ILD or chance findings of ILD. In all cases, an MDD involving pulmonologists, radiologists, and pathologists should be used to establish a confident diagnosis.[2]

## CLASSIFICATION OF DISEASE BEHAVIOR

In addition to a diagnosis based on nosology, it is of critical importance to also stratify a particular patient with ILD according to the disease behavior, which may have a more profound impact on management and therapy of an individual patient than the specific ILD diagnosis by itself. In Table 7.6, a classification scheme for the disease behavior is proposed that will guide the choice of treatment options. Obviously, there is an interaction between the underlying diagnosis and the prevalence of one or another pattern of disease behavior. Nonetheless, it seems very helpful to select the broad treatment approach in an individual patient by applying the patterns of disease behavior characterized in Table 7.6.

## REFERENCES

1. Travis, et al. *Am J Respir Crit Care Med.* 2013;188(6):733–748.
2. Raghu G, Collard HR, Egan JJ, et al. An official ATS/ERS/JRS/ALAT statement: idiopathic pulmonary fibrosis: evidence-based guidelines for diagnosis and management. *Am J Respir Crit Care Med.* 2011;183:788–824.
3. Bradley B, Branley HM, Egan JJ, et al. Interstitial lung disease guideline. *Thorax.* 2008;63(suppl 5):v1–v58.
4. Raghu G, Mageto YN, Lockhart D, et al. The accuracy of the clinical diagnosis of new-onset idiopathic pulmonary fibrosis and other interstitial lung disease: a prospective study. *Chest.* 1999;116:1168–1174.
5. King Jr TE, Tooze JA, Schwarz MI, et al. Predicting survival in idiopathic pulmonary fibrosis: scoring system and survival model. *Am J Respir Crit Care Med.* 2001;164:1171–1181.
6. Gribbin J, Hubbard RB, Le Jeune I, et al. Incidence and mortality of idiopathic pulmonary fibrosis and sarcoidosis in the UK. *Thorax.* 2006;61:980–985.
7. Yang S, Raghu G. Clinical evaluation. In: Costabel U, duBois RM, Egan MM, eds. *Diffuse Parenchymal Lung Disease.* Basel, Switzerland: Karger; 2007:22–28.
8. Raghu G, Freudenberger TD, Yang S, et al. High prevalence of abnormal acid gastro-oesophageal reflux in idiopathic pulmonary fibrosis. *Eur Respir J.* 2006;27:136–142.
9. Diffuse Lung Disease Questionnaire for Patients. Available at: www.chestnet.org/accp/patient-guides/interstitial-diffuse-lung-disease-questionnaire-accp-members.
10. Cooper Jr JA, White DA, Matthay RA. Drug-induced pulmonary disease. Part 1: cytotoxic drugs. *Am Rev Respir Dis.* 1986;133:321–340.

11. Cooper Jr JA, White DA, Matthay RA. Drug-induced pulmonary disease. Part 2: noncytotoxic drugs. *Am Rev Respir Dis.* 1986;133:488–505.

12. Steele MP, Speer MC, Loyd JE, et al. Clinical and pathologic features of familial interstitial pneumonia. *Am J Respir Crit Care Med.* 2005;172:1146–1152.

13. Costabel U, Hunninghake GW. ATS/ERS/WASOG statement on sarcoidosis. Sarcoidosis Statement Committee. American Thoracic Society. European Respiratory Society. World Association for Sarcoidosis and Other Granulomatous Disorders. *Eur Respir J.* 1999;14:735–737.

14. Prasse A, Probst C, Bargagli E, et al. Serum CC-chemokine ligand 18 concentration predicts outcome in idiopathic pulmonary fibrosis. *Am J Respir Crit Care Med.* 2009;179:717–723.

15. Behr J, Furst DE. Pulmonary function tests. *Rheumatology.* 2008;47(suppl 5):v65–v67.

16. Hoeper MM, Andreas S, Bastian A, et al. Pulmonary hypertension due to chronic lung disease. Recommendations of the Cologne Consensus Conference 2010. *Dtsch Med Wochenschr.* 2010;135(suppl 3):S115–S124. [in German].

17. Zappala CJ, Latsi PI, Nicholson AG, et al. Marginal decline in forced vital capacity is associated with a poor outcome in idiopathic pulmonary fibrosis. *Eur Respir J.* 2010;35:830–835.

18. Wells AU, Desai SR, Rubens MB, et al. Idiopathic pulmonary fibrosis: a composite physiologic index derived from disease extent observed by computed tomography. *Am J Respir Crit Care Med.* 2003;167:962–969.

19. Latsi PI, du Bois RM, Nicholson AG, et al. Fibrotic idiopathic interstitial pneumonia: the prognostic value of longitudinal functional trends. *Am J Respir Crit Care Med.* 2003;168:531–537.

20. Behr J, Demedts M, Buhl R, IFIGENIA study group, et al. Lung function in idiopathic pulmonary fibrosis—extended analyses of the IFIGENIA trial. *Respir Res.* 2009;10:101.

21. Ohshimo S, Bonella F, Cui A, et al. Significance of bronchoalveolar lavage for the diagnosis of idiopathic pulmonary fibrosis. *Am J Respir Crit Care Med.* 2009;179:1043–1047.

22. Tomassetti S, Wells AU, Costabel U, et al. Bronchoscopic lung cryobiopsy increases diagnostic confidence in the multidisciplinary diagnosis of idiopathic pulmonary fibrosis. *Am J Respir Crit Care Med.* 2016;193(7):745–752.

23. Chechani V, Landreneau RJ, Shaikh SS. Open lung biopsy for diffuse infiltrative lung disease. *Ann Thorac Surg.* 1992;54:296–300.

24. Kreider M, Hansen-Flaschen J, Ahmad N, et al. Complications of video-assisted thoracoscopic lung biopsy in patients with interstitial lung disease. *Ann Thorac Surg.* 2007;83(3):1140–1144.

25. Flaherty KR, King Jr TE, Raghu G, et al. Idiopathic interstitial pneumonia: what is the effect of a multidisciplinary approach to diagnosis? *Am J Respir Crit Care Med.* 2004;170:904–910.

26. Galiè N, Hoeper MM, Humbert M, et al. Guidelines for the diagnosis and treatment of pulmonary hypertension. The Task Force for the Diagnosis and Treatment of Pulmonary Hypertension of the European Society of Cardiology (ESC) and the European Respiratory Society (ERS), endorsed by the International Society of Heart and Lung Transplantation (ISHLT). *Eur Respir J.* 2009;34:1219–1263.

27. Leuchte HH, Neurohr C, Baumgartner R, et al. Brain natriuretic peptide and exercise capacity in lung fibrosis and pulmonary hypertension. *Am J Respir Crit Care Med.* 2004;170:360–365.

28. Leuchte HH, Baumgartner RA, Nounou ME, et al. Brain natriuretic peptide is a prognostic parameter in chronic lung disease. *Am J Respir Crit Care Med.* 2006;173:744–750.

# CHAPTER 8

# Palliative and End-of-Life Care in Idiopathic Pulmonary Fibrosis

KATHLEEN OARE LINDELL

---

**KEY POINTS**

- Idiopathic pulmonary fibrosis (IPF) is a fatal, progressive, scarring lung disease with a variable course.
- The goals of palliative care are to provide symptom management, prevent and relieve suffering, and support the best possible quality of life, regardless of stage of the disease or need for other therapies.
- Palliative care, integrated early, may reduce symptom burden in patients with idiopathic pulmonary fibrosis (IPF).

---

## INTERSTITIAL LUNG DISEASE

The interstitial lung diseases (ILDs) are a complex group of disorders, with idiopathic pulmonary fibrosis (IPF), hypersensitivity pneumonitis, connective tissue–associated lung disease, and sarcoidosis constituting the majority of cases seen in clinical practice.[1] These diseases are highly disabling and share the common characteristic of lung scarring and progressive loss of normal gas transfer.[2-4] Patients experience a loss of functional ability, resulting in dyspnea, dry cough, and fatigue as the disease advances. Death ultimately results from acute respiratory failure.[2] ILDs can be difficult to diagnose and treatment options are limited, posing a medical challenge.[1]

### Chronic Illness

All patients diagnosed with progressive ILD share problems common to those with a chronic illness. Chronic illness, a permanently altered health state, results from a nonreversible pathologic condition.[5] The consequence is a residual disability that cannot be corrected by a surgical procedure or cured by medical therapy.[6] The diagnosis of a chronic illness can produce an emotional response, sometimes in a manner disproportionate to the extent of physical disability and major life changes.[7] Major challenges include coping with progression of the disease and the associated disability, which vary across patients and diagnoses, and attempting to best maintain quality of life.

### Idiopathic Pulmonary Fibrosis

IPF is one of the most common, relentlessly progressive, and best-studied ILDs regarding symptom burden and perceived benefits and barriers to use of palliative care (PC). Therefore, the focus of this chapter will be on use of PC in IPF.

IPF is a progressive life-limiting lung disease that affects ~128,000 newly diagnosed individuals in the United States annually.[8] IPF, a disease of aging associated with intense medical and financial burden, is expected to grow in incidence within the US population.[9] The prognosis is poor.[10] Median survival from diagnosis is 3.8 years, with some patients succumbing to a rapid death within 6 months.[9,11] New therapies have recently become available. These medications slow the rate of deterioration of lung function, but have no proven impact on ultimate survival or quality of life.[12,13] Although transplantation is an effective surgical therapy,[14,15] less than 20% of patients ever receive a lung transplant.[11] The remaining 80% have few treatment options and are predicted to experience a progressive downhill course. Patients report great symptom burden and impaired quality of life.[16-19] As fibrosis advances and lung function deteriorates, patients experience a progressive increase in shortness of breath, cough, and fatigue. These symptoms are distressing to patients and family caregivers and present a challenge in maintaining quality of life as the disease relentlessly progresses.[16,20] Despite the fatal prognosis, patients and caregivers often fail to understand the poor prognosis.[20]

### Palliative Care—Goals and Timing

PC is a comprehensive treatment of the discomfort, symptoms, and stress of serious illness[21] and should be offered at the time of diagnosis of a serious illness[22] (Fig. 8.1).

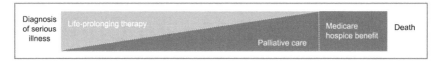

FIG. 8.1 Conceptual framework for the role of palliative care in the course of chronic illness. (Adapted from Dahlin C. *Clinical Practice Guidelines for Quality Palliative Care On behalf of the National Consensus Project for Quality Palliative Care Task Force. National Consensus Project for Quality Palliative Care.* 2009, with permission.)

PC involves management of symptoms, which is relevant even in patients with mild to moderate disease. Patients receive emotional and spiritual support focused on enabling them to live better with the consequences of an incurable illness.[23] PC can be a means to assist patients and families through the process of reflection, discussion, and communication of treatment preferences for end-of-life (EOL) care.[24] This process, termed advance care planning, is "a more deliberate, organized, and ongoing process of communication to help an individual identify, reflect upon, discuss, and articulate values, beliefs, goals, and priorities to guide personal care decisions up to and including EOL care."[25,26] The mantra "It is wise to hope for and expect the best, but it is also wise to prepare for the worst" is a way to introduce advance care planning to patients with IPF and their caregivers.[27]

PC can be delivered by an interdisciplinary team, referred to as specialty PC, or a member of the clinical care team, referred to as primary PC.[28] PC practitioners are trained in conducting discussions regarding EOL planning and, therefore, may be helpful in initiating and facilitating such discussions.[29] Often being confused with hospice (Table 8.1), PC has different goals. Because PC focuses on assisting patients/family caregivers to better manage symptoms associated with disease progression, primary and/or specialty PC should ideally occur early following diagnosis.[30] For patients with IPF, this is particularly important, as disease progression is difficult to predict.[18]

Consensus guidelines for implementation of PC have been developed through the work of several professional organizations. The National Consensus Project for Quality Palliative Care evolved from the work of four PC organizations: the American Academy of Hospice and Palliative Medicine; Center to Advance Palliative Care; Hospice and Palliative Nurses Association; and the National Hospice and Palliative Care Organization. The mission of the National Consensus Project for Quality Palliative Care was to create guidelines that improved the quality of PC in the United States.[29] Stakeholders from these organizations developed

### TABLE 8.1
### Differences Between Palliative Care and Hospice

| Palliative Care | Hospice |
| --- | --- |
| Provided in an inpatient facility or as an outpatient at the time of diagnosis of serious illness; may be short or long-term need | Provided in an inpatient facility or at the patient's home, to patients with a terminal prognosis who are medically certified at hospice onset to have ≤6 months to live |
| Services focus on minimizing symptom burden improving quality of life, providing emotional and spiritual support, and identifying end-of-life preferences | Services typically include care that focuses on pain and symptom control; counseling to help with psychologic, spiritual, and end-of-life issues; respite care, support for a family after the patient's death |
| Curative care continues | Care options are limited |

clinical practice guidelines that cover the eight domains identified as being crucial to the delivery of comprehensive PC[29] (Box 8.1). The goal is to promote quality PC, foster consistent and high standards in delivery of PC, and encourage continuity of care across settings.

Since introduction to the United States, PC has grown rapidly. Referral to PC has become an integral part of the care of patients with malignant disease and is commonly part of the care of critically ill patients because of high risk for mortality. In this setting, referral has the additional benefit of providing support to family caregivers who are asked to serve as surrogate decision-makers.

### Palliative Care Versus Hospice

In 1967, Dame Cicely Saunders (who trained as a nurse, a social worker, and a physician) founded the St. Christopher's Hospice in London, the first inpatient, home care, research, and teaching hospice.[31] The hospice movement came to the United States in the mid-1970s, when Dr. Florence Wald, a nursing pioneer, led an interdisciplinary team to create the first American hospice.[32] Hospice care became a Medicare benefit in the United States in the 1980s. While both PC and hospice share the same principles of providing comfort and support for patients, hospice is designated for patients with a life expectancy of 6 months or less certified by a physician. An important difference between hospice and PC relates to the use of life-prolonging therapy. This is not allowed as part of hospice, but is fully permitted as part of PC[29] (Table 8.1).

### Palliative Care in Patients With Malignant Disease

In patients with metastatic lung cancer, early and integrated PC, with a focus on communication regarding disease severity and treatment choices, has been found to improve quality of life, reduce symptom burden, and improve survival in comparison to usual care.[33] In one study comparing healthcare utilization and quality of care for patients with cancer who received early versus late PC, early PC was associated with less intensive medical care, improved quality outcomes, and cost savings at EOL.[34] Blackhall et al. measured timing of referral to outpatient PC and impact on EOL care in patients with advanced cancer and found that referral to outpatient patient care occurred in approximately half of patients with incurable cancer. Those patients referred had improved EOL care and reduced costs with fewer hospitalizations at the EOL and were less likely to die in hospital.[35]

Despite these positive findings, studies continue to indicate unmet needs. A 2016 survey conducted in the United States that enrolled a diverse sample of patients diagnosed with cancer in terms of ethnicity, income, education, geography, age, insurance, cancer type, and treatment stage revealed serious communication problems that compromised their EOL care. The findings of the survey entitled the CancerCare Patient Access and Engagement Report included (1) less than half of respondents said their care team knew their EOL wishes; (2) approximately one-third or less of the respondents said they felt adequately informed about other treatment options their care team considered, the responsibilities of their caregivers, and clinical trial opportunities; and (3) between 22% and 37% of respondents said that additional information about PC, living wills, or hospice care would have been helpful to them.[36]

### Palliative Care in Patients With Advanced Lung Disease

Despite higher symptom burden, worse quality of life, and more social isolation, patients with chronic lung disease have been found to receive PC less likely than patients with cancer.[37] In a study of 2400 deaths in patients with chronic illness, Beernaert and colleagues reported that patients with chronic obstructive pulmonary disease (COPD) (20%), heart failure (34%), and severe dementia (37%) were less likely to receive a PC referral than patients diagnosed with cancer (60%).[38] This and other studies reinforce the conclusions that discussion of PC by clinicians who manage the care of patients with advanced lung diseases, such as COPD, occurs less frequently than for other life-limiting conditions, such as cancer.[38–40] Brown and colleagues in an opinion editorial posed several reasons for fewer referrals. These included uncertainty in prognosis, lack of provider skill to engage in discussions about PC, fear of using opioids among patients with chronic lung disease, fear of diminishing hope, and perceived and implicit bias against patients with smoking-related lung disease.[41]

## PALLIATIVE CARE IN IDIOPATHIC PULMONARY FIBROSIS
### Supporting Research

Prior studies support that, as in other advanced lung diseases, referral to PC occurs infrequently and late in patients with IPF.[42–46] In a retrospective study, Lindell and colleagues identified the location of death and frequency of referral to PC for patients with IPF managed at a specialty lung center from 2001 to 2012. Of 277 IPF decedents whose location of death could be determined, over half died in the hospital (57%). Only 38 (13.7%) had a formal PC referral.[42] Most referrals (71%) occurred within 1 month of death, often after admission to the intensive care unit (ICU).[43] The most common reason for referral was "to discuss goals of care."[43] From a study of 45 patients with IPF, Bajwah and colleagues[46] reported the majority (76%) died in a hospital setting and a minority (38%) had PC team involvement, supporting limited referral.

To elicit perspectives of patients and family caregivers, Lindell conducted focus groups consisting of patients currently living with the disease, caregivers for patients living with the disease, and caregivers of a deceased family member.[47] Findings revealed overwhelming symptom burden, with cough being a particularly debilitating symptom, frustration with the need to use oxygen therapy, and worry about finances and the cost of medications. Participants also verbalized hesitance to engage in advance care planning, which was recognized as a need, but avoided because it was perceived as loss of hope. Caregivers of the patients living with the disease were vocal about "only wanting positive options," including research participation opportunities. Patients were not aware of the scope of support offered through PC, for example, reducing symptom burden. In addition, there was confusion with hospice.[47] Family members of decedents were more likely to receive a formal PC referral, suggesting clinician reluctance to suggest this option early in the disease course. This outcome, while logical, can be counterproductive as symptoms of IPF may escalate rapidly, resulting in acute respiratory failure and the need to make EOL care decisions at the time of critical illness.

Several additional qualitative studies have attempted to identify reasons for hesitancy in initiating referral to PC. Bajwah and colleagues reported findings from a survey of 124 general practitioners that attempted to elicit barriers to implementation. Respondents viewed PC services positively, but felt the support the care provided was sufficient and the referral was not indicated.[48] To gain further understanding, Bajwah and colleagues found in a qualitative study of 18 patients with fibrotic ILD and their informal caregivers and health professionals that patients experience substantial distress from the impact of their symptoms and psychosocial needs were often not being met. Health professionals had varied knowledge and confidence in managing these concerns and tended to underestimate patient concerns.[49]

Findings from this study prompted the authors to develop an educational plan using a case conference approach entitled *Hospital2Home*.[49] In a randomized control trial of 53 patients with advanced fibrotic lung disease, 26 of whom were randomized to receive the intervention, findings supported benefits. A PC specialist nurse delivered the intervention in patient homes. Prior to the conference, the nurse telephoned the patient and carer to identify current concerns and goals for the visit. Patients related physical, emotional, social, spiritual, and EOL concerns. A mutual action plan was developed with telephone follow-up at 2 weeks, 1 month, and 2 months, and as needed. Patients reported that the sessions improved their ability to manage their symptoms and quality of life, demonstrating this type of intervention can improve patient care.[50]

Sampson and colleagues conducted a qualitative study of IPF patients and their caregivers to explore their perspectives across the IPF spectrum and inform the development of clinical pathways and multidisciplinary service interventions. Because the nature of disease progression in IPF is uncertain, specialists in PC and ILD generated a disease typology to classify patients into four stages related to their disease progression. The intervention focused on using clinical visits to identify changes in health status and functional activity, patient understanding of symptoms, interventions to improve symptoms, coping strategies, and caregiver roles. Three important areas for improvement were identified: (1) including a focus on supportive interventions and symptom self-management in discussion during clinic visits, (2) recognition of importance of family caregivers, and (3) appreciation of differences in patients and caregivers regarding need for information and change in needs over time. Findings revealed that patients initially had a clear understanding of their prognosis, but were uncertain about how their disease would progress and be managed.[51] This study is important as it addresses ways to incorporate concepts of PC into the clinical care continuum.

## Caregiver Perspective

Decades of research have identified the stress experienced by caregivers of patients with high care needs.[52-55] Patient suffering, whether physical, psychosocial, or spiritual, has been found to have a major impact on family caregivers.[56] Family caregivers are essential to the well-being of patients with serious illness[57,58] In testing an interdisciplinary PC intervention in family caregivers in lung cancer, caregivers experienced improvement in social well-being and psychological distress and less caregiver burden after participating in interdisciplinary care meetings and receiving four educational sessions.[59]

Caregivers of patients with IPF are a unique and critical population in which to study approaches for improving the quality of PC because of their critical role in physical and emotional assistance. In testing a disease management intervention that included a session on advance care planning, Lindell[20] found the content reduced perceived stress among caregivers who participated in the study. Belkin and colleagues conducted a study capturing caregiver perspectives on the effects of IPF and reported that caregivers experienced hardships throughout the disease course, including dealing with their own emotional issues and the patient's physical limitations, which were increased by the need to use supplemental oxygen.[60]

### Critical Care Perspective

The Study to Understand Prognoses and Preferences for Outcomes and Risks of Treatment (SUPPORT) conducted in the early 1990s produced findings that prompted the discussion of the need for more proactive measures to improve quality of care for seriously ill and dying patients.[61] As a result, hospitals created PC service to provide specialty consult services to address symptom burden and quality of life. Team PC is now available in more than 70% of US hospitals with at least 50 beds.[62]

To evaluate impact, Roczen and colleagues conducted a review of 12 studies evaluating the effects of PC programs in ICUs from 2000 to 2013. Common findings included that PC interventions did not necessarily change hospital or ICU mortality, but length of stay was often significantly reduced, especially ICU length of stay.[63] Nevertheless, evidence continues to suggest that for patients with advanced lung disease, including those with IPF, referral is infrequent. From a study that examined medical record documentation of PC in patients admitted to 15 hospitals, Brown and colleagues[40] reported that, compared with patients with metastatic cancer, patients with ILD, including those with IPF, and COPD who died in an ICU were less likely to have documentation of a discussion of their prognosis or a "do not resuscitate" order at the time of their death. This is concerning because the onset of acute respiratory failure in patients with IPF is associated with extremely high mortality.[64–68]

### Lung Transplant Perspective

Lung transplantation remains the only treatment that has the potential to extend life for patients with IPF.[69] A significant percentage of patients hospitalized with advanced lung fibrosis or an acute exacerbation of their ILD will develop respiratory failure. In the absence of discussion of advance care planning, the consequence of this outcome may be admission to the ICU and mechanical ventilation. If so, mortality is extremely high and few patients survive to ICU discharge. Even fewer survive months and there are almost no survivors

at 12 months.[67,68] The need for ICU admission and mechanical ventilation typically precludes selection for transplant because of time constraints involved in the evaluation process, organ availability, and risk for complications during the ICU. Therefore, it is advisable to introduce the potential of evaluation for transplant early following diagnosis. A book, written by a transplant recipient and entitled *Partners for Life*,[70] provides a patient's perspective of this journey and can be of assistance in answering patients' questions.

PC is often not prescribed for lung transplant candidates. Barriers include fear that referral will signal abandonment by the transplant team and concern over opioid use.[71] Colman and colleagues did a retrospective case series reviewing outcomes of 64 lung transplant candidates comanaged by PC. There were no episodes of opioid toxicity or respiratory depression, and they concluded that PC could be an important means to reduce symptom burden in lung transplant candidates.[69]

## OVERCOMING BARRIERS

As noted in this chapter, there are a number of reasons for late PC referral, including the discomfort of many physicians, caregivers, and family members with this suggestion and fear that the discussion will diminish hope.[71,72] In addition, many equate PC, which can be provided at any point in the disease course, with hospice care. While concerns about adverse impact are not supported by evidence, perceptions on the part of clinicians, patients, and family caregivers can be extremely difficult to change. A potential means to address such concerns may involve using different terminology, such as substituting the term "supportive care" for PC. In patients with advanced cancer, the term "supportive care" was associated with better understanding, more favorable impressions, and higher future perceived need compared with the term PC.[73,74]

### Who Should Deliver Palliative Care?

Hospice and palliative medicine is now recognized as a medical subspecialty by the American Board of Medical Subspecialties, as well as in Canada, England, Ireland, Australia, and New Zealand. Many other European countries are in the process of developing PC certification. PC can be provided by an interdisciplinary team of specially trained physicians, nurses, social workers, chaplains, and other specialists with advanced training in PC; they work with the patient's other clinician(s) with the goal of providing an "extra layer" of support. In addition, concepts of PC can be delivered by the patient's primary clinician(s), coined as "primary

PC," in addition to PC specialists, coined as "secondary or subspecialty PC." Optimal PC for patients with chronic lung disease should incorporate both primary and subspecialty PC.[28] Challenges facing subspecialty PC include increasing demands on limited resources.[75] It is estimated that there is at present 1 PC physician for every 1200 patients with serious illness in the United States.[76] This shortage means that providing PC will fall to the patient's clinician(s).[77]

## How to Deliver Palliative Care

*What to say and do.* PC serves to address symptom management and advance care planning. Delivery of

PC must be done with great care and sensitivity. The video *The Human Connection of Palliative Care: What to Say and Do* from the Center to Advance Palliative Care describes the human connection of PC and identifies 10 steps for what to say and do.[78]

*Pharmacologic and nonpharmacologic strategies.* There is a lack of evidence-based literature on best practices in pharmacologic and nonpharmacologic management of symptoms experienced by patients with IPF. Empiric practice, therefore, is borrowed from strategies found effective in other types of lung diseases. Please refer to Table 8.2. A variety of therapies, including cough suppressants, thalidomide, and

## TABLE 8.2
## Symptom Management Chart

| Symptom | Evidence | Treatment Summary |
|---|---|---|
| Dyspnea | Although studies have not been done directly with idiopathic pulmonary fibrosis there have been several randomized controlled trials in COPD:<br>1. Abernethy AP et al. Randomised, double blind, placebo controlled crossover trial of sustained release morphine for the management of refractory dyspnoea. *BMJ*. 2003;327(7414):523–528.<br>2. Jennings AL et al. A systematic review of the use of opioids in the management of dyspnoea. *Thorax*. 2002;57(11):939–44.<br>3. Marciniuk DD et al. Managing dyspnea in patients with advanced chronic obstructive pulmonary disease: a Canadian Thoracic Society clinical practice guideline. *Can Respir J*. 2011;18(2):69–78.<br>4. Galbraith S et al. Does the use of a handheld fan improve chronic dyspnea? A randomized, controlled crossover trial. *J Pain Symptom Management*. 2010;(5):831.<br>5. Holland AE. Short term improvement in exercise capacity and symptoms following exercise training in interstitial lung disease. *Thorax*. 2008;63:549–54. | Abernethy: Benefits found with low-dose opiates<br>Jennings: Patients were started on a very-low-dose oral morphine and given a weekly set titration protocol; of the 32 patients enrolled, 20 ended the trial on long-acting doses of oral morphine, and of the remaining patients 9 continued to take immediate-release morphine. In addition, 43% of patients reported the morphine to be very helpful<br>Marciniuk: Pursed lip breathing has also been shown to be effective for dyspnea<br>Galbraith: Use of a handheld fan has been found to be effective at "reducing the sensation of breathlessness"<br>Holland: Pulmonary rehabilitation has been found to improve breathlessness and fatigue and is thought to improve emotional function |
| Anxiety/depression | 1. Kunik ME et al. COPD education and cognitive behavioral therapy group treatment for clinically significant symptoms of depression and anxiety in COPD patients: a randomized controlled trial. *Psychological Medicine*. 2008;38(3):385–396.<br>2. Ekstrom MP et al. Safety of benzodiazepines and opioids in very severe respiratory disease: national prospective study. *BMJ*. 2014;348:g445.<br>3. Sertraline for chronic obstructive pulmonary disease and comorbid anxiety and mood disorders. *Am J Psychiatry*. 1995;152(10):1531a–1531. | Kunik: Cognitive behavioral therapy is an excellent first step in managing anxiety and has been found to be effective as well as to improve quality of life<br>Ekstrom: Low-dose benzodiazepine therapy can be used; however, the clinician should be cautious as such agents have been associated with slightly increased mortality rates<br>*American Journal of Psychiatry*: Selective serotonin inhibitors have been thought to be effective in managing anxiety in COPD. A small pilot study was performed using sertraline, in which patients reported a better sense of well-being |

**TABLE 8.2**
**Symptom Management Chart—cont'd**

| Symptom | Evidence | Treatment Summary |
|---|---|---|
| Insomnia | 1. Roth T. Hypnotic use for insomnia management in chronic obstructive pulmonary disease. *Sleep Med.* 2009;10(1):19–25. | Roth: Benzodiazepine receptor agonists such as zolpidem are found to be effective |
| Cough | 1. Davis CL. ABC of palliative care: breathlessness, cough and other respiratory problems. *BMJ.* 1997;315:931–934.<br>2. Chung KF. Currently available cough suppressants for chronic cough. *Lung.* 2008. doi:10.007/SOO408-007-9030.<br>3. Horton MR. Thalidomide for the treatment of cough in idiopathic pulmonary fibrosis: a randomized trial. *Ann Intern Med.* 2012 Sep 18;157(6):398–406. doi:10.7326/0003-4819-157-6-201209180-00003. | Davis: Opioids are most effective when treating cough; cough suppressants, mucolytics, and nebulizer can also be used<br>Chung: Morphine extended-release has been reported to be helpful for refractory cough. In addition, there are case reports discussing the usefulness of amitriptyline, paroxetine, gabapentin, and carbamazepine for chronic cough<br>Horton: Thalidomide has been reported to be helpful in improving cough quality of life in IPF |

*COPD*, chronic obstructive pulmonary disease; *IPF*, idiopathic pulmonary fibrosis.

opioids, can be used to diminish dyspnea and cough. The effectiveness of these approaches varies, necessitating an approach tailored to the patient's response.[79] In addition, a variety of nonpharmacologic strategies including pursed lip breathing, use of a fan to relieve dyspnea, and cognitive behavioral therapy may be helpful.

Supplemental oxygen may be beneficial, but comes with its own burden[16] because of the equipment required and its impact on body image. Provision of PC could be extremely helpful in this situation, as it could serve as a means to address the benefits of oxygen regarding fatigue, quality of life, and greater potential to continue to engage in activities desired. As the prescription of oxygen increases, diligence should be paid to the delivery devices to ensure that the patient is able to receive the accurate dose of oxygen, and humidification should be added to the inspired oxygen to avoid excessive drying of the nasal mucosa.[28]

## FUTURE DIRECTIONS

In 2014, 40 years after the first hospice opened in the United States, Ferrell and Grant addressed the benefits of PC and advocated that PC is still needed from the time of initial diagnosis through long-term survivorship or EOL care in patients with cancer.[80] PC models of care include ambulatory-based PC clinics, home-based PC, inpatient PC units, and inpatient consultation services.[81] While all four exist along a continuum of service delivery, ambulatory- and home-based have the greatest potential to reduce the soaring costs of hospital-based care. All of these delivery systems have "the potential to improve quality of life, improve pain and symptom management, and deliver goal-directed care to patients with cancer and other serious illnesses."[81]

## SUMMARY/DISCUSSION

Patients with IPF represent a group of individuals with a chronic respiratory disease who are without disease-reversing treatment options and, in the absence of lung transplantation, inevitably face progressive decline and death. The goals of PC are to prevent and relieve suffering, support the best quality of life for patients facing serious illness and their families, and encourage discussions regarding EOL preferences. Studies have reported that even when patients and their caregivers understood the terminal nature of the disease, they did not appreciate that symptoms could escalate rapidly, resulting in death. Because the disease course of IPF is unpredictable, early introduction of PC should be considered as a standard of care to maximize benefits and improve quality of life (Box 8.2).

**BOX 8.2**
**Case Study**

A 63-year-old man was referred for specialty pulmonary evaluation for a potential diagnosis of idiopathic pulmonary fibrosis. He had a 1-year history of shortness of breath and cough with exertion, and his chest CT, pulmonary function test, and lab findings supported the diagnosis. The pulmonologist referred him for lung transplant evaluation. He completed the evaluation process and was deemed too well for transplant at that time. He participated in a clinical trial, and his symptoms remained stable over an 18-month period. During this time, he was examined every 3 to 4 months by his pulmonologist. His symptoms took a marked change, and he developed an increase in shortness of breath with rest, and his oxygen requirements increased to 6 LPM with rest and 15 LPM with exertion. He was seen in follow-up by his pulmonologist, who referred him back for lung transplant evaluation. Consequently he was seen and deemed to be "too sick" at this time and declined as a transplant candidate. The patient and his wife became very angry and he said, "I did everything you asked me to." Naturally this became a tense situation. Engagement of a specialty palliative care nurse practitioner (PC NP) involved assessment of his physical and psychological state and confirmed that this recent exacerbation caused a marked decline in his activities of daily living and a predicted mortality of less than 6 months. It also provided the ability for him and his wife to acclimate to this decline and vent their frustration. The PC NP was able to provide a prescription for an opioid and asked him to trial it to see if it would help with his dyspnea. Both the patient and wife were surprised and relieved with improvement in dyspnea. Despite this symptom relief, his disease continued to progress, and after a few visits, the PC NP was able to engage home hospice for this patient, and 1 month later, she received a call of thanks from his wife for a "beautiful death."

# REFERENCES

1. Wallis ASK. The diagnosis and management of interstitial lung diseases. *BMJ.* 2015:350.
2. Schwarz M, King TE. Interstitial Lung Disease. In: Cosgrove G, Schwarz MI, eds. *Approach to the Evaluation and Diagnosis of Interstitial Lung Disease.* 5th ed. Shelton, Connecticut: People's Medical Publishing House-USA; 2011.
3. Coultas DB, et al. The epidemiology of interstitial lung diseases. *Am J Respir Crit Care Med.* 1994;150(4):967–972.
4. Holland A, Fiore JF, Goh N, et al. Be honest and help me prepare for the future: what people with interstitial lung disease want from education in pulmonary rehabilitation. *Chron Respir Dis.* 2015;12(2):93–101.
5. Miller J. *Coping with Chronic Illness; Overcoming Powerlessness.* Philadelphia: FA Davis; 1992.
6. Newby NM. Chronic illness and the family life-cycle. *J Adv Nurs.* 1996;23(4):786–791.
7. Lewis KS. Emotional adjustment to a chronic illness. *Lippincotts Prim Care Pract.* 1998;2(1):38–51.
8. Raghu GCH, Egan JJ, Martinez FJ, et al. An official ATS/ERS/JRS/ALAT statement: idiopathic pulmonary fibrosis: evidence-based guidelines for diagnosis and management. *Am J Respir Crit Care Med.* 2011;183(6):788–824.
9. Raghu GCS, Yeh WS, Maroni B, Li Q, Lee YC3, Collard HR. Idiopathic pulmonary fibrosis in US Medicare beneficiaries aged 65 years and older: incidence, prevalence, and survival, 2001-11. *Lancet Respir Med.* 2014;2(7):566–572.
10. Vancheri C, Failla M, Crimi N, Raghu G. Idiopathic pulmonary fibrosis: a disease with similarities and links to cancer biology. *Eur Respir J.* 2010;35:496–504.
11. Richards TJ, et al. Peripheral blood proteins predict mortality in idiopathic pulmonary fibrosis. *Am J Respir Crit Care Med.* 2012;185(1):67–76.
12. King T, Bradford WZ, Castro-Bernardini S, et al. A phase 3 trial of pirfenidone in patients with idiopathic pulmonary fibrosis. *N Engl J Med.* 2014;370:2083–2092.
13. Richeldi L, du Bois RM, Raghu G, et al. Efficacy and Safety of Nintedanib in Idiopathic Pulmonary Fibrosis. *N Engl J Med.* 2014;370:2071–2082.
14. King Jr TE, Pardo A, Selman M. Idiopathic pulmonary fibrosis. *Lancet.* 2011;378(9807):1949–1961.
15. Martinez FJ, et al. The clinical course of patients with idiopathic pulmonary fibrosis. *Ann Intern Med.* 2005;142(12 Pt 1):963–967.
16. Belkin A, Albright K, Swigris JJ. Interstitial lung disease – original article: a qualitative study of informal caregivers' perspectives on the effects of idiopathic pulmonary fibrosis. *BMJ Open Respir Res.* 2014:1.
17. De Vries J, Kessels BL, Drent M. Quality of life of idiopathic pulmonary fibrosis patients. *Eur Respir J.* 2001;17(5):954–961.
18. Egan JJ. Follow-up and nonpharmacological management of the idiopathic pulmonary fibrosis patient. *Eur Respir Rev.* 2011;20(120):114–117.
19. Collard HR, Ward AJ, Lanes S, et al. Burden of illness in idiopathic pulmonary fibrosis. *Eur Respir Rev.* 2012;15:829–835.
20. Lindell KOOE, Song M, Zullo TJ, Gibson KF, Kaminski, Hoffman LA. Impact of a disease-management program on symptom burden and health-related quality of life in patients with idiopathic pulmonary fibrosis and their care partners. *Heart Lung.* 2010;39(4):302–313.
21. (NINR), N.I.o.N.R. *Palliative Care: The Relief You Need When You're Experiencing the Symptoms of Serious Illness;* 2012. Available from: https://www.ninr.nih.gov/newsandinformation/publications/palliative-care-brochure -.V13QwlfLGFA.
22. Dahlin C. *Clinical Practice Guidelines for Quality Palliative Care on behalf of the National Consensus Project for Quality Palliative Care Task Force. National Consensus Project for Quality Palliative Care.* 2nd ed. 2009.

23. Clark D. From margins to centre: a review of the history of palliative care in cancer. *Lancet Oncol.* 2007;8(5):430–438.
24. Dahlin C. It takes my breath away end-stage COPD. Part 2: pharmacologic and nonpharmacologic management of dyspnea and other symptoms. *Home Healthcare Nurse.* 2006;24(4):218–226.
25. Simpson C. Advance care planning in COPD: care versus "code status". *Chron Respir Dis.* 2012;9(3):193–204.
26. Sudore R, Schickedanz AD, Landefield CS, et al. Redefining the "planning" in advance care planning: preparing for end-of-life decision making. *Ann Intern Med.* 2010;153(4):256–261.
27. Hansen-Flaschen J. Advanced lung disease. Palliation and terminal care. *Clin Chest Med.* 1997;18(3):645–655.
28. Reinke L, Janssen D, Curtis JR. Palliative care issues in adults with nonmalignant pulmonary disease. In: Hollingsworth DM, ed. *Up to Date;* 2015.
29. Dahlin C. *Clinical Practice Guidelines for Quality Palliative Care On behalf of the National Consensus Project for Quality Palliative Care Task Force;* 2013. 3rd ed., Available from: http://www.nationalconsensusproject.org/NCP_Clinical_Practice_Guidelines_3rd_Edition.pdf.
30. Ferrell B, Connor SR, Cordes A, et al. The national agenda for quality palliative care: the national consensus project and the national quality forum. *J Pain Symptom Manage.* 2007;33(6):737–744.
31. Coyle N. Introduction to palliative care nursing. In: Ferrell B, Coyle N, Paice J, eds. *Oxford Textbook of Palliative Nursing.* New York, New York: Oxford University Press, Inc; 2015.
32. Wald F. Hospice care in the United States: a conversation with Florence S. Wald. *JAMA.* 1999;281:1683–1685.
33. Temel JS, et al. Early palliative care for patients with metastatic non-small-cell lung cancer. *N Engl J Med.* 2010;363(8):733–742.
34. Scibetta C, Kerr K, Mcguire J, Rabow MW. The costs of waiting implications of the timing of palliative care consultation among a cohort of decedents at a comprehensive care center. *J Palliative Med.* 2015;19(1).
35. Blackhall L, Read P, Stukenborg G, et al. CARE track for advanced cancer: impact and timing of an outpatient palliative care clinic. *J Palliative Med.* 2015;19(1).
36. *2016 CancerCare Patient Access and Engagement Report;* 2016. Available from: http://www.cancercare.org/accessengagementreport.
37. Bausewein C, Booth S, Gysels M, Kuhnbach R, Haberland B. Understanding breathlessness: cross-sectional comparison of symptom burden and palliative care needs in chronic obstructive pulmonary disease and cancer. *J Palliative Med.* 2010;13:1109–1118.
38. Beernaert K, et al. Referral to palliative care in COPD and other chronic diseases: a population-based study. *Respir Med.* 2013;107(11):1731–1739.
39. Rocker G, Simpson AC, Horton R. Palliative care in advanced lung disease: the challenge of integrating palliation into everyday care. *Chest.* 2015;148(3):801–809.
40. Brown CE, et al. Palliative care for patients dying in the intensive care unit with chronic lung disease compared with metastatic cancer. *Ann Am Thorac Soc.* 2016;13(5):684–689.
41. Brown C, Jecker NS, Curtis JR. Inadequate palliative care in chronic lung disease. *Ann Am Thorac Soc.* 2016;13(3):311–316.
42. Lindell K, Liang Z, Hoffman L, et al. Palliative care and location of death in decedents with idiopathic pulmonary fibrosis. *Chest.* 2015;147(2):423–429.
43. Liang Z, Hoffman LA, Nouraie M, et al. *Referral to Palliative Care Infrequent in Patients with Idiopathic Pulmonary Fibrosis Admitted to an Intensive Care Unit.* 2016;20(2).
44. Wijsenbeek M, Erasmus MC, Bendstrup E, Ross J, Wells A. Cultural difference in palliative care in patients with idiopathic pulmonary fibrosis. *Chest.* 2015;148(2):e57–e58.
45. Lindell K, Rosenzweig MQ, Pilewski JM, Hoffman LA, Gibson KF, Kaminski N. Invited correspondence to european experience of location of death for patients with idiopathic pulmonary fibrosis. *Chest.* 2015;148(2):e57–e58.
46. Bajwah S, et al. Specialist palliative care is more than drugs: a retrospective study of ILD patients. *Lung.* 2012;190(2):215–220.
47. Lindell K, Kavalieratos D, Gibson kf, Tycon L, Rosenzweig PQ. The palliative care needs of patients with idiopathic pulmonary fibrosis: a qualitative study of patients and family caregivers [in review]. 2016;46(1).
48. Bajwah SH, Higginson IJ. General practitioners' use and experiences of palliative care services: a survey in south east England. *BMC Palliative Care.* 2008;7(18).
49. Bajwah S, et al. The palliative care needs for fibrotic interstitial lung disease: a qualitative study of patients, informal caregivers and health professionals. *Palliative Med.* 2013;27(9):869–876.
50. Bajwah S, Ross JR, Wells AU, et al. Palliative care for patients with advanced fibrotic lung disease: a randomised controlled phase II and feasibility trial of a community case conference intervention. *Thorax.* 2015;70:830–839.
51. Sampson CGB, Harrison NK, Nelson A, Byrne A. The care needs of patients with idiopathic pulmonary fibrosis and their carers (CaNoPy): results of a qualitative study. *BMC Pulmonary Medicine.* 2015;15(155).
52. Schulz RBS, Cook TB, Martire LM, Tomlinson JM, Monin JK. Predictors and consequences of perceived lack of choice in becoming an informal caregiver. *Aging Mental Health.* 2012;16(6).
53. Herbert R, Schulz R, Copeland VC, Arnold RM. Preparing family caregivers for death and bereavement. Insights from caregivers of terminally ill patients. *J Pain Symptom Manage.* 2009;37(1):3–12.
54. Teno JM, et al. Patient-focused, family-centered end-of-life medical care: views of the guidelines and bereaved family members. *J Pain Symptom Manage.* 2001;22(3):738–751.
55. Siegel K, et al. Caregiver burden and unmet patient needs. *Cancer.* 1991;68(5):1131–1140.
56. Hebert RS, Arnold RM, Schulz R. Improving well-being in caregivers of terminally ill patients. Making the case for patient suffering as a focus for intervention research. *J Pain Symptom Manage.* 2007;34(5):539–546.

57. Lingler JH, et al. Conceptual challenges in the study of caregiver-care recipient relationships. *Nurs Res.* 2008;57(5):367–372.

58. Hebert RS, et al. Pilot testing of a question prompt sheet to encourage family caregivers of cancer patients and physicians to discuss end-of-life issues. *Am J Hosp Palliative Care.* 2009;26(1):24–32.

59. Sun V, Grant M, Koczywas M, et al. Effectiveness of an interdisciplinary palliative care intervention for family caregivers in lung cancer. *Cancer.* 2015:3737–3745.

60. Belkin ASJ. Pulmonary fibrosis – Original article: a qualitative study of informal caregivers' perspectives on the effects of idiopathic pulmonary fibrosis. *BMJ Open Respir Res.* 2014;1.

61. A controlled trial to improve care for seriously ill hospitalized patients: the study to understand prognoses and preferences for outcomes and risks of treatments (SUPPORT). *JAMA.* 1995;274(20):1591–1598.

62. Center to Advance Palliative Care. *Improving Palliative Care in the ICU.* 2016. Available from: https://www.capc.org/ipal/ipal/icu/.

63. Roczen M, White KR, Epstein EG. Palliative care and intensive care units. *J Hospice Palliative Nurs.* 2016;18(3):201–211.

64. Saydain G, et al. Outcome of patients with idiopathic pulmonary fibrosis admitted to the intensive care unit. *Am J Respir Crit Care Med.* 2002;166(6):839–842.

65. Mallick S. Outcome of patients with idiopathic pulmonary fibrosis (IPF) ventilated in intensive care unit. *Respir Med.* 2008;102(10):1355–1359.

66. Rush B, et al. The use of mechanical ventilation in patients with idiopathic pulmonary fibrosis in the United States: a nationwide retrospective cohort analysis. *Respir Med.* 2016;111:72–76.

67. Vianello A, Arcaro G, Battistella L, et al. Noninvasive ventilation in the event of acute respiratory failure in patients with idiopathic pulmonary fibrosis. *J Crit Care.* 2014;29(562–7).

68. Gaudry S, Vincent F, Rabbat A, et al. Invasive mechanical ventilation in patients with fibrosing interstitial pneumonia. *J Thorac Cardiovasc Surg.* 2014;147:47–53.

69. Colman R, Singer LG, Barua R, Downar J. Outcomes of lung transplant candidates referred for co-management by palliative care: a retrospective case series. *Palliative Med.* 2015;29(5):429–435.

70. Uhrig J. *Partners 4 Life: The Importance of Partners in Surviving an Organ Transplant.* IUniverse; 2014.

71. Colman RE, Curtis JR, Nelson JE, et al. Barriers to optimal palliative care of lung transplant candidates. *Chest.* 2013;143:736–743.

72. Dellon EP, Sawicki GS, Shores MD, Wolfe J, Hanson LC. Physician practices for communicating with patients with cystic fibrosis about the use of noninvasive and invasive mechanical ventilation. *Chest.* 2012;141:1010–1017.

73. Maciasz RM, Arnold RM, Chu E, et al. Does it matter what you call it? A randomized trial of language used to describe palliative care services. *Supportive Care Cancer.* 2013;21:3411–3419.

74. Zimmerman C, Swami N, Krzyzanowska M, et al. Perceptions of palliative care among patients with advanced cancer and their caregivers. *CMAJ.* 2016;188(10).

75. O'Connor NCDJ. Which patients need palliative care most? Challenges of rationing in medicine's newest specialty. *J Palliative Med.* 2016;19(7):1–2.

76. America's Care of Serious Illness: 2015. State-By-State Report Card on Access to Palliative Care in Our Nation's Hospitals. 2015 June 8, 2016; Available from: https://reportcard.capc.org.

77. Blinderman CD, Billings JA. Comfort care for patients dying in the hospital. *N Engl J Med.* 2015;373(26):2549–2561.

78. Meier DE. *The Human Connection of Palliative Care: What to Say and Do*; 2016. June 8, 2016; Available from: https://www.capc.org/providers/palliative-care-videos-podcasts/palliative-care-and-the-human-connection-ten--steps-for-what-to-say-and-do/.

79. Lee JS, McLaughlin S, Collard HR. Comprehensive care of the patient with idiopathic pulmonary fibrosis. *Curr Opin Pulm Med.* 2011;17(5):348–354.

80. Ferrell BGM. The future of palliative care. *Semin Oncol Nurs.* 2014;30(4):296–297.

81. Wiencer CCP. Palliative care delivery models. *Semin Oncol Nurs.* 2014;30(4):227–233.

# CHAPTER 9

# Lung Transplantation in Interstitial Lung Disease

LUCA PAOLETTI • TIMOTHY P.M. WHELAN

**KEY POINTS**

- For selected parenchymal lung disease (DPLD) patients who fail to respond to medical therapy and demonstrate declines in function that place them at increased risk for mortality, lung transplantation should be considered.
- Lung transplantation remains a complex medical intervention that requires a dedicated recipient and a medical team.
- Despite the challenges, lung transplantation affords appropriate patients a reasonable chance at increased survival and improved quality of life.
- Lung transplantation remains an appropriate therapeutic option for selected patients with DPLD.

There are over 120 distinct interstitial or diffuse parenchymal lung diseases (DPLDs). These diseases are often referred to as interstitial lung diseases; however, DPLD is a better term as the diseases affect the interstitium, pulmonary vasculature, small airways, and alveolar epithelial cells. DPLDs are typically associated with underlying autoimmune diseases, environmental/occupational exposures, medications, and radiation or are idiopathic in nature. A large percentage of these disorders (approximately 30–40%) are idiopathic. It is believed that previous prevalence estimates in the population have been grossly underestimated, and although DPLDs remain extremely rare in children, in adults the prevalence for parenchymal lung diseases is ~70 per 100,000 population.[1-4] Newer information indicates that the prevalence of the most common form of idiopathic interstitial pneumonia, idiopathic pulmonary fibrosis (IPF), is likely greater than previously expected. Clinical courses and prognoses across all types of DPLD are variable and dependent on the underlying subtype of lung disease. In addition, the literature consistently estimates the median survival for patients with newly diagnosed IPF is 2–5 years.[1,5-8] For IPF and the other DPLDs that progress despite best medical therapy, lung transplantation remains an appropriate treatment option for a select group of patients.

The first human lung transplantation was performed in 1963 at the University of Mississippi by Dr. James Hardy.[9] The patient succumbed 19 days later from preexisting renal disease, and on postmortem examination he was noted to have no evidence of acute rejection.[9] Multiple attempts between 1963 and 1981 ended in failure because of lack of adequate immunosuppressive therapy, which would allow allograft tolerance but would not result in multisystem organ failure from infection. The advent of cyclosporine A began a new era, and Reitz and Shumway performed the first successful heart and lung transplant at Stanford University in 1981.[10] Subsequently, in 1983, Cooper and the Toronto Lung Transplant Group successfully performed the first single lung transplant on a patient with IPF.[11] During the past 30 years, the number of transplants performed worldwide has increased from the single digits per year to over 3800 in 2013.[12] The major indications for lung transplantation include chronic obstructive pulmonary disease, IPF, and cystic fibrosis. Together these three diseases account for over 75% of all lung transplants performed.[12] Over the past decade, the proportion of transplants for IPF has consistently increased. This is most likely attributable to the change in organ allocation policies and implementation of the lung allocation score (LAS) in the United States. The LAS prioritizes organ placement; the calculation prioritizes based on risk of death while on the wait list. Prior to the LAS change, the percentage of transplant for IPF in the United States was ~20% between 2000 and 2004. Once the change occurred, over 35%[13] of the recipients between 2005 and 2012 had advanced lung disease due to IPF. This increase in the number of transplants differs with trends for idiopathic pulmonary arterial hypertension. With the advance of successful therapies for the treatment of pulmonary arterial hypertension, the number of transplants for this condition has significantly declined, now accounting for ~2% of all transplants in 2014 compared with ~13% of transplants performed in 1990.[14] This underscores the challenge that patients with IPF face: until 2014 there was a lack of beneficial therapy for this devastating disease.

## WHO SHOULD BE REFERRED AND BE LISTED FOR TRANSPLANT?

In 2015 the International Society for Heart and Lung Transplantation published an updated consensus report outlining appropriate guidelines for referral for transplantation and contraindications for transplantation.[12] The document also includes guidelines for actively placing a patient on a waiting list for transplant. The balance between providing a short-term survival benefit must be weighed against the reality that donor lungs are a limited resource. Therefore it is paramount that the appropriate transplant candidate be expected to have a reasonable opportunity to attain longer-term survival. Assessment for potential long-term survival must include an appraisal of potential recipients' comorbidities. The 2015 guideline statement outlines several absolute and relative contraindications to performing lung transplantation (Table 9.1). In addition to medical considerations, lung transplant recipients must actively participate in the management of a complex medical regimen. Adherence to this treatment is central to good outcomes. As a result, a social support system that enhances adherence is beneficial, if not vital.

Transplantation centers agree that the moment of referral should allow the potential recipient adequate time to consider this treatment option. The initial transplantation discussion should not occur as a last-ditch effort at improving a patient's outcome. In this or any document, there are limitations in defining the appropriate time for referral and transplantation. Consideration of referral to a transplant center should include the referring physician's assessment of the individual's quality of life as well as overall life expectancy without a transplant. In addition, the potential recipient's desire to learn more about this treatment option is a factor in considering referral. Early referral is crucial as it allows the potential recipient an opportunity to develop a relationship with the prospective transplant program. It also allows the patient an opportunity to learn about the entire process, from the surgery to the complex medical management one must adhere to after transplantation. The decision to actively list for transplant, alternatively, is based on organ allocation for a particular region, estimated risks and benefits based on the expertise of the individual transplant center, and the personal assessments of the transplant recipient.

### Choice of Procedure

There are three potential procedures for the interstitial lung disease recipient. These include heart and lung, single lung, and bilateral lung transplantation. Heart and lung transplantation was initially the procedure of choice during the 1980s, and many centers continued this practice into the 1990s. After successful lung transplantation and the realization that the dilated right ventricle can remodel with good outcomes, heart and lung transplantation numbers have significantly declined. In 2013, there were only 46 heart and lung transplants worldwide.[12] Currently, heart and lung transplantation is performed only on those patients with significant left ventricular dysfunction or non-operable congenital abnormalities. The decision to perform single lung versus bilateral lung transplant remains controversial today. The only absolute criterion for bilateral lung transplant is suppurative lung disease. This is due to concerns that the native lung will soil the transplanted allograft in a chronically immunosuppressed host and lead to poor outcomes. In addition to this absolute indication, it is now common practice to perform bilateral lung transplant for patients with idiopathic pulmonary hypertension. This population is at high risk of developing primary graft dysfunction (PGD) or early acute lung injury after transplantation. This risk is lower in patients who undergo bilateral lung transplantation.[15] For patients with very high pulmonary vascular resistance before transplant, the right ventricle becomes acutely unloaded with the reanastamosis of the normal allograft pulmonary vasculature. High cardiac output ensues with high flow rates that may increase the risk of endothelial injury and subsequent pulmonary edema. This impact is likely attenuated by double the vascular volume of a bilateral transplant. For patients with DPLD, it is less clear that individuals with secondary pulmonary hypertension receive an absolute benefit from bilateral lung transplantation. Several investigators have come to differing conclusions regarding the benefits of a particular procedure type in this population.[15,16] Because there are no randomized controlled trials evaluating single lung versus bilateral lung transplantation for pulmonary fibrosis, there are

**TABLE 9.1**
**Contraindications to Lung Transplantation**

| Absolute Contraindications | Comments |
|---|---|
| Malignancy within past 2 years | 2-year disease-free interval with low risk of recurrence is reasonable. However, because of the effects of chronic immunosuppression on malignancy, a 5-year disease-free interval is prudent |
| Untreatable dysfunction of other organs | Unless combined organ transplantation is performed |
| Uncorrected coronary artery disease | Coronary artery disease that is not amenable to revascularization by percutaneous transluminal coronary angioplasty |
| Uncorrectable bleeding problem | |
| Acute medical instability | Associated with increased perioperative mortality |
| Significant chest wall/spinal deformity | Prevents safe removal of native or donor lungs |
| Documented nonadherence to medical therapy | Includes the need for a consistent and reliable social support system. In addition, untreatable psychiatric conditions that would impair the ability of the recipient to remain adherent are included here |
| Substance abuse | Alcohol, tobacco, marijuana, illicit substances |
| Chronic infection with resistant organisms that are poorly controlled pretransplant | Increased risk of perioperative sepsis, empyema, wound healing, and infections |
| Obesity with BMI >35 kg/m$^2$ | Associated with poor short- and long-term outcomes |
| Severely limited functional status with poor rehabilitation potential | Decreased exercise tolerance is associated with worse outcomes |
| **Relative Contraindications** | **Comments** |
| Age >65 years | There is an increased risk of worse long-term survival with higher age likely related to increased comorbidities at transplant |
| Progressive or severe malnutrition | Impairs wound healing |
| Mechanical ventilation or extracorporeal life support (ECLS) | Carefully selected candidate without other acute or chronic organ dysfunction may be successfully transplanted, however |
| Noncurable chronic extrapulmonary infections | Chronic active hepatitis B, hepatitis C, and HIV patients should have transplant done only in experienced centers for those infections |
| Other chronic comorbidities that have not resulted in end-stage organ damage | All medical conditions should be optimized before consideration for listing for transplant, including chronic management of diabetes, hypertension, epilepsy, peptic ulcer disease, and gastroesophageal reflux before transplantation |

Absolute contraindications are determined by individual transplant programs and the balance of the risks and benefits is determined by the individual transplant center. Similarly, the presence of several relative contraindications may significantly increase the risk of poor transplant outcome and preclude listing for transplant.
Adapted from Yusen RD, Edwards LB, Kucheryavaya AY, et al. The Registry of the International Society for Heart and Lung Transplantation: thirty-second official adult lung and heart-lung transplantation report—2015; focus theme: early graft failure. *J Heart Lung Transplant.* 2015;34(10):1264–1277, with permission.

inherent selection biases that confound any retrospective cohort. There have been numerous studies in the past that suggest there may be a potential survival benefit in patients with IPF who have undergone a bilateral lung transplant even though there is an increased risk of complications early after transplant.[17–21] However, data also exist that show that there is no survival benefit for IPF patients who undergo bilateral vs. single lung transplantation.[18,22] Given the conflicting data, the debate on double vs. single lung transplant for patients with IPF will continue on with preference determined by each transplant center.

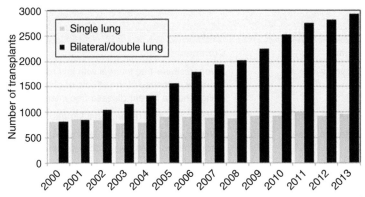

FIG. 9.1 Lung transplant volume: 75% of all transplants are now bilateral lung transplants. (Adapted from Yusen RD, Edwards LB, Kucheryavaya AY, et al. The Registry of the International Society for Heart and Lung Transplantation: thirty-second official adult lung and heart-lung transplantation report—2015; focus theme: early graft failure. *J Heart Lung Transplant.* 2015;34[10]:1264–1277, with permission.)

Regardless of the rationale for the choice of procedure, recent data indicate that bilateral lung transplantation is increasing in frequency (Fig. 9.1). In 2013, 75% of all transplant procedures were bilateral lung transplants.[12] During the same period, cystic fibrosis accounted for ~15% of transplants and idiopathic pulmonary hypertension for less than 3%, and the frequency of bilateral transplantation for patients with an underlying diagnosis of IPF is similarly increasing. One report evaluating wait list mortality demonstrated a higher risk for those IPF patients listed for bilateral lung transplant as their only option.[23] The impacts of current transplant procedure choice remain unclear on multiple variables, including its impact on the potential candidacy of a patient with DPLD, wait list mortality, and outcomes following lung transplant for all recipients.

## OUTCOMES AFTER TRANSPLANTATION FOR INTERSTITIAL LUNG DISEASE

The majority of information about outcomes after lung transplantation in DPLD comes from what is known about IPF recipients. Because the majority of DPLDs result in similar physiologic changes, with restrictive lung disease and high risk for the development of secondary pulmonary hypertension, some generalizations across the disease type are accurate. More specific disease considerations are discussed later.

Survival after lung transplantation has consistently improved by era from 1988 through June of 2013.[12] The most striking improvements in outcome

are during the perioperative period. These improvements are due to improved donor preservation, operative technique, and critical care management early after transplant. Currently, the median survival estimate for all recipients from 1994 through 2013 was 5.7 years.[12] The 90-day survival rate was 89%.[12] Although the impact has not been as great for long-term survival, this too is slowly improving. In the same era, unadjusted 10-year survival rates were 31%.[12] Survival for patients with an underlying diagnosis of DPLD is generally consistent with these reported outcomes. The largest cohort of interstitial lung disease transplanted remains IPF, and the median survival for this group is slightly above 4.5 years.[12] For those patients with sarcoidosis, median survival was 6.1 years.[12] These unadjusted survival rates need to be evaluated cautiously because additional recipient factors have an impact on survival after lung transplantation.

Early survival after transplantation is affected by numerous factors, including recipient- and donor-specific conditions before transplantation. However, PGD immediately following transplant is the top cause of early mortality. PGD is the consequence of ischemia-reperfusion injury with resultant development of reactive oxygen species. Ultimately, this leads to acute lung injury and capillary leak.[24] PGD is based on clinical findings early after transplantation (Table 9.2). Several studies have identified pulmonary fibrosis and pulmonary hypertension as having strong associations with the development of this complication.[25,26]

Furthermore, the severest form of PGD (grade 3 at 72 h after transplant) affects long-term survival

## TABLE 9.2
## Grading of Primary Graft Dysfunction Severity

| Grade | Pao$_2$/Fio$_2$ | Radiographic Infiltrates Consistent With Pulmonary Edema |
|-------|-----------------|----------------------------------------------------------|
| 0     | >300            | Absent                                                   |
| 1     | >300            | Present                                                  |
| 2     | 200–300         | Present                                                  |
| 3     | <200            | Present                                                  |

Adapted from Christie JD, Carby M, Bag R, et al. Report of the ISHLT working group on primary lung graft dysfunction part II: Definition. A consensus statement of the International Society for Heart and Lung Transplantation. *J Heart Lung Transplant.* 2005;24(10):1454–1459, with permission.

## TABLE 9.3
## Morbidity After Lung Transplantation

| Outcome | Within 1 year | Within 5 years |
|---------|---------------|----------------|
| Hypertension | 51.5% | 80.7% |
| Renal dysfunction | 22.5% | 53.3% |
| Creatinine <2.5 mg/dL | 15.7% | 35.3% |
| Creatinine >2.5 mg/dL | 5.0% | 14.3% |
| Chronic dialysis | 1.7% | 3.0% |
| Renal transplant | 0.1% | 0.8% |
| Hyperlipidemia | 26.2% | 57.9% |
| Diabetes mellitus | 23.0% | 39.5% |
| Bronchiolitis obliterans syndrome | 9.3% | 41.1% |

Data from Yusen RD, Edwards LB, Kucheryavaya AY, et al. The Registry of the International Society for Heart and Lung Transplantation: Thirty-second official adult lung and heart-lung transplantation report—2015; focus theme: early graft failure. *J Heart Lung Transplant.* 2015;34(10):1264–1277.

## TABLE 9.4
## Criteria for Grading Bronchiolitis Obliterans Syndrome

| Grade | Diagnostic Criteria |
|-------|---------------------|
| BOS 0 | FEV$_1$ >90% of baseline and FEF$_{25-75\%}$ >75% of baseline |
| BOS 0p | FEV$_1$ 81% to 90% of baseline and/or FEF$_{25-75\%}$ ≤75% of baseline |
| BOS 1 | FEV$_1$ 66% to 80% of baseline |
| BOS 2 | FEV$_1$ 51% to 65% of baseline |
| BOS 3 | FEV$_1$ 50% or less of baseline |

FEF$_{25-75\%}$—midexpiratory flow rate.
Baseline FEV$_1$ is based on the average of the two highest values obtained after transplants that are at least 3 weeks apart.
BOS grade is based on the subsequent average of two FEV$_1$ values that are obtained at least 3 weeks apart and compared with the baseline value.
*BOS,* bronchiolitis obliterans syndrome; *FEV$_1$,* forced expiratory volume in 1 s.
Data from Estenne M, Maurer JR, Boehler A, et al. Bronchiolitis obliterans syndrome 2001: an update of the diagnostic criteria. *J Heart Lung Transplant.* 2002;21(3):297–310.

and pulmonary function and increases the risk for development of bronchiolitis obliterans syndrome (BOS).[27] In addition to the recipient risk factors, there are donor factors that increase the risk of development of this complication. Currently, there are no recipient interventions to prevent its development. Further work into defining the best match for donor and recipient as well as the potential for conditioning of donor lungs may lead to improvements in the future.[28]

Patients are on lifelong immunosuppression and are typically treated with corticosteroids, a calcineurin inhibitor (tacrolimus or cyclosporine), and an antimetabolite (mycophenolate mofetil or azathioprine). Chronic immunosuppression places patients at risk for the development of comorbidities, including hypertension, diabetes, chronic kidney disease, and malignancy (Table 9.3). Notwithstanding the medical complexity, patients with DPLD who undergo lung transplantation garner a survival advantage from the procedure.[29,30] In addition, quality of life is significantly improved after transplantation in several studies.[31–34]

The main limitation to long-term survival after lung transplantation remains the development of BOS, or chronic rejection. BOS is defined by persistent airflow obstruction in comparison to a recipient's peak baseline values (Table 9.4). Complications that affect the allograft (acute rejection, anastomosis issues, disease recurrence) must first be ruled out in addition to documenting a decline in pulmonary function. There are several probable and possible risk factors that set up the lung transplant recipient for the development of chronic small airways disease, including recurrent acute rejection, viral infections, lymphocytic bronchiolitis, donor antigen specific reactivity, and aspiration of gastroesophageal refluxate. Ultimately, chronic obstruction increases the risk of infection and sets the stage for respiratory failure. The rate of BOS varies in different series but has an estimated prevalence of ~41% at 5 years.[12] Treatment interventions

for this syndrome are limited, but there are data that suggest the use of chronic azithromycin in these patients can
help slow down the progression of disease.[35–38]

## DISEASE-SPECIFIC CONSIDERATIONS
### Idiopathic Pulmonary Fibrosis

Over the past decade there has been an increase in disease awareness with IPF, while during the same period
there has been a shift in transplantation practices where
now programs are more willing to perform transplants
in older patients than in the past as these patients can
still garner a survival benefit. Based on these new practices it is felt that once a patient is diagnosed with IPF, he
or she should be referred to a transplant center (Box 9.1).
The appropriate time for listing for transplantation must

consider the potential survival benefit of the procedure
(Box 9.2). In the past decade there has been much work
to define risk factors associated with worse outcomes
in those with IPF before transplantation. Although the
overall prognosis is grim, the disease course remains
variable for individual patients. As a result, identifying
patients who are at particularly high risk is most appropriate when considering listing for lung transplantation.

Studies have focused on baseline characteristics as
well as the change in study values over time to identify
the group of patients at high risk for short-term mortality and, therefore, who are appropriate candidates for
lung transplantation. Most of these publications are
based on small series of retrospective data that have not
been prospectively validated. Nonetheless, several clinical indicators (Box 9.3) are worth discussion because
they likely portend a worse outcome and herald the
need for lung transplantation.

Computed tomography (CT) scan fibrosis scoring
has consistently correlated with risk for death. In several
studies, the extent of the fibrosis is an independent predictor of outcome.[39–43] The extent of honeycomb change
and reticulation is scored based on the percentage
involvement of the lung parenchyma. Although these
findings are consistent in the literature when interpreted
by a thoracic radiologist, the lack of consistently trained
radiologists limits its use in routine clinical practice.
Nonetheless, extensive reticulation and/or honeycombing should raise the suspicion for future poor outcome.

Unlike the CT scan fibrosis score, baseline pulmonary function tests alone seem less helpful than serial
measurements over time. The obvious advantage, however, is they are the easiest to measure. Martinez and
colleagues[45] demonstrated that IPF patients enrolled
in a clinical trial seemed at equal risk for subsequent decline regardless of their baseline pulmonary

function.[44] Subsequent evaluation has demonstrated that pulmonary function testing at baseline in conjunction with additional factors (gender, age, and physiology scores) is associated with risk for short- and mid-term mortality.[45] Furthermore, there are consistent data indicating that repeated measures of pulmonary function that demonstrate a decline in the forced vital capacity (FVC) are predictive of worse outcomes.[46,47] Several studies have used a 10% decline in FVC as a definition of significant decline to identify high-risk patients; however, a recent report suggests that smaller declines in FVC can also be clinically significant.[48] At this time, the absolute threshold for the decline in FVC to identify the highest-risk patient population remains unclear; however, any decline in FVC should warrant careful reevaluation for a change in a patient's clinical status.[46,49] Similarly, a drop in DLCO (diffusing capacity of the lungs for carbon monoxide) is important to identify as it is a sign that a patient is at higher risk of death.[46,49]

Assessment of a patient's exercise tolerance is also of independent value in determining prognosis of patients with IPF. Evidence of oxygen desaturation on a 6-min walk test has demonstrated an increased risk for poor outcome in several studies.[50–52] These studies consistently demonstrate an increased risk of death for those who desaturate below 89% during a 6-min walk test on room air. In addition, overall walk distance is independently associated with future outcome.[53,54] In two separate cohorts of IPF patients, one awaiting lung transplantation and another evaluated at a referral center, similar poor 6-min walk performance was associated with worse outcomes. One found a walk distance of less than 207 m associated with a fourfold increased risk of death over the subsequent 6 months. The other found that a walk distance of less than 212 m placed those individuals at high risk for mortality over the next 18 months. Consistent with the findings of pulmonary function testing, changes in exercise tolerance over time also seem predictive of outcome. Using data from a large randomized controlled trial, declines in 6-min walk distance of greater than 50 m over 24 weeks were associated with a fourfold increased risk of death during the next year.[50] These data indicate that poor exercise tolerance or falling exercise tolerance over time is indicative of a high-risk patient for mortality without transplantation.

To further complicate predicting the outcome of our patients with IPF, there is a subset of patients who develop acute respiratory deterioration that suggests a less predictable course. When the cause for the acute decline is unknown and there is evidence of new ground-glass opacity on CT imaging of the chest, this is termed an acute exacerbation of IPF.[55] Outcomes are variable; however, an exacerbation can be the defining event leading to frank respiratory failure. In a recent single institution study it was found that patients with fibrotic lung disease with and without IPF who suffered an acute respiratory worsening had a significantly high in-hospital mortality rate.[56] Outcomes following a well-defined acute exacerbation are poor with very high mortality as well as high risk for worse functional status and increased risk for subsequent complications.[57,58] The unpredictable nature of the acute exacerbation further supports early referral for those with IPF and no clear contraindication to transplantation.

The average IPF patient is diagnosed in the seventh decade. At this time, there is no absolute upper age limit for lung transplantation, although as patients age they are less likely to be candidates because of development of multiple relative contraindications.[59] Worldwide data demonstrate an increase in the number of lung transplants for those over age 65. In 2014, more than 25% of transplant patients were over the age of 65, indicating a clear trend toward offering transplant as a therapeutic option to older patients than in the past.[14] The International Society for Heart and Lung Transplantation Registry data indicate that those who are over age 65 suffer from worse long-term outcomes compared with those who are under age 50.[12] These data are difficult to interpret as they are inherently confounded and do not account for individual survival benefit. Furthermore, these data do not account for quality-of-life improvements. Nevertheless, available lung allografts remain a limited resource and transplant centers strive to identify candidates they believe will have an opportunity for long-term survival.

Until 2014, management of the patient with idiopathic pulmonary fibrosis (IPF) was limited. The primary interventions were supportive and targeted comorbidities to improve quality of life and functional status. With these interventions alone, retrospective analyses have consistently demonstrated a median survival of 3 to 5 years. Within the last several years, we have demonstrated that some common therapies for these patients are, in fact, harmful (azathioprine, prednisone, and N-acetylcysteine), and there are also two new proven antifibrotic therapies available. These changes to our practice will limit harmful interventions and provide disease-modifying therapy that will hopefully affect survival in the years to come. Both pirfenidone and nintedanib are conditionally recommended by the ATS/ERS/JRS/ALAT, recognizing that there remain gaps in our knowledge regarding these agents in populations without mild to moderate disease and regarding optimal duration of therapy.[60]

Pirfenidone is an oral antifibrotic agent with an unknown mechanism of action that has been shown to affect multiple pathways known to be important to the development of fibrosis in animal models.[61–64] Three large, placebo-controlled trials have evaluated its safety and efficacy in a population with mild to moderate IPF. Although the initial two studies had conflicting results regarding effect on FVC, the third trial demonstrated clear reduction in the decline of average FVC over 52 weeks. In addition, patients on pirfenidone were more likely to have progression-free survival compared with those receiving placebo (defined as a 10% decline in FVC, >50 m decline in 6-min walk test, or death). An additional analysis that used pooled data from all three trials demonstrated a mortality benefit for those on pirfenidone compared with placebo.[65]

Nintedanib is an oral medication that is an intracellular inhibitor of tyrosine kinases of multiple growth factor receptors, including fibroblast growth factor, vascular endothelial growth factor, and platelet-derived growth factor. As in the pirfenidone trials, it was studied in patients with mild to moderate disease due to IPF. Concurrent phase III double-blind placebo-controlled studies demonstrated that those on nintedanib had a slower decline in lung function at the end of 52 weeks compared with placebo. These trials also evaluated the effect of nintedanib on the development of an acute exacerbation over this same time frame. The trials had conflicting results with one study demonstrating a significant decrease in risk of AE for those on nintedanib, while the other study did not demonstrate a difference.[66]

Trials for both nintedanib and pirfenidone demonstrated that the medications will be well tolerated and for patients with well-defined IPF, use of these disease modifying agents is appropriate.

## Sarcoidosis

Sarcoidosis has a highly variable clinical course that is often extended over decades with the possibility of spontaneous remissions. Determining the right time for transplantation in these patients is very challenging, and characteristics associated with high risk for mortality come from limited data sources.[67–69] Sarcoidosis accounted for ~2.5% of all lung transplantations from 1995 to 2014.[12] Patients who are African-American, with high pulmonary hypertension, and requiring supplemental oxygen have a higher risk of death while on the United Network of Organ Sharing (UNOS) waiting list.[70] Posttransplant outcomes are consistent

with those of other indications, although there is an increased risk of early mortality.[71,72] This is most likely reflective of the increased rates of pulmonary hypertension.[70] However, despite that risk, the most recent data indicate a median survival of 6.1 years after transplant.[12] For patients who fail to response to conventional therapy for sarcoidosis and develop advanced lung disease, lung transplantation remains a viable therapeutic option.

Special considerations for those with sarcoidosis include its systemic nature. A thorough preoperative evaluation of these patients must be done to ensure that there is no other clinically significant end organ damage from sarcoidosis that could preclude lung transplantation. In addition, mycetomas are a common complication of cavitary lung disease and these can have an impact on transplant candidacy as well as pre- and postoperative management.[73] One unique feature of sarcoidosis after transplant is its common recurrence in the transplanted lung.[72,74–77] The reported prevalence of recurrent disease ranges from 20% to 80%. The granulomas are of recipient origin, and disease recurrence typically is of little clinical significance after transplantation. Because patients are living longer after transplant, it remains to be seen if there are any longer term complications from recurrence of disease.

## Scleroderma Lung Disease and Connective Tissue Disease–Associated Diffuse Parenchymal Lung Diseases

The number of lung transplants performed for underlying connective tissue disease remains low, accounting for 1.5% of all transplants up to June 2014.[12] Systemic sclerosis, rheumatoid arthritis, and undifferentiated connective tissue disease have all been associated with DPLD. The majority of data outlining outcomes after lung transplantation due to connective tissue disease are from patients with systemic sclerosis. With the advent of angiotensin-converting enzyme inhibitors, renal crisis is no longer the main cause of death, and this has been replaced with respiratory failure due to fibrosis and pulmonary hypertension.[78] Although the total number of transplants remains limited, several retrospective studies have demonstrated similar 1- and 3-year outcomes to those with pulmonary arterial hypertension.[79–83] These series are limited by their small size and lack of clear selection criteria, however, and further data are needed to define outcomes in this patient population. Also, in two recent papers it was suggestive that in highly selective patients with systemic sclerosis 5-year outcomes are similar to those with pulmonary fibrosis.[84,85] These were retrospective studies at single institutions; however, they have shown that systemic sclerosis should not be an absolute contraindication to lung transplantation, and for selected patients lung transplant can be a treatment option for end-stage lung disease.

As for patients with sarcoidosis, connective tissue diseases have systemic manifestations, and careful consideration of comorbidities that may hamper transplant outcome is imperative. One salient feature of systemic sclerosis is esophageal dysmotility. Several reports have associated chronic allograft dysfunction or BOS with gastroesophageal reflux.[86,87] Esophageal dysmotility may not only increase reflux episodes, but also preclude fundoplication that has been associated with improvements in lung function in selected patients.[88,89] Gastroparesis is a common complication after lung transplantation as well.[90] Combining esophageal dysmotility and gastroparesis can lead to significant aspiration events that lead to graft dysfunction and loss. Guidelines that specifically outline criteria for acceptable esophageal function in systemic sclerosis remain elusive. Individual transplant programs assess this feature of disease on a case-by-case basis, and it can vary from transplant center to transplant center.

Although further data and clarity are needed, lung transplantation remains a viable therapeutic option for select individuals with systemic sclerosis and CTD-DPLD.

## Lymphangioleiomyomatosis

Lymphangioleiomyomatosis (LAM) remains a rare indication for lung transplantation, accounting for 1% of all transplants performed between 1995 and 2014.[12] Initial reports suggested a far worse natural history for LAM than is currently known.[91] Despite this there is a subset of patients who decline over time and develop significant morbidity associated with the disease.[92] From a single center cohort, perioperative complications included significant blood loss with the removal of the explanted lungs and chylous effusions[93,94]; however, these findings did not preclude good outcomes.[95] An additional evaluation of the US transplant registry demonstrated outcomes with statistically significantly better 5-year survival (65%) compared with other indications for lung transplant.[96] In addition to mortality data, there is now information that demonstrates an improved quality of life for those who have undergone lung transplantation compared with those who have severe advanced disease due to LAM.[32]

A novel intervention for patients with LAM has been sirolimus. Sirolimus has been studied in a cohort of patients with moderate obstructive lung disease and was found to reduce the decline in forced expiratory volume in 1 s ($FEV_1$) over time.[97] This medication is being used in patients with LAM now; however, it should be avoided in all patients who are listed for transplantation. Sirolimus has a long half-life and has been associated with the development of bronchial wound dehiscence in clinical trials evaluating its safety and efficacy after lung transplantation.[98] This potentially fatal complication precludes the use of sirolimus in the perioperative periods of lung transplantation.

## Pulmonary Langerhans Cell Histiocytosis

Pulmonary Langerhans cell histiocytosis (PLCH) accounts for less than 0.5% of all lung transplants. Patients with this disorder typically have significant pulmonary hypertension. Lung transplant outcomes seem compatible with those for other patients with idiopathic pulmonary hypertension, although recurrence of disease does occur in the allograft at a high rate (20% in one series).[99] The greatest risk factor for disease recurrence was a past history of systemic disease. The recurrence of disease was not reported to have an impact on survival; however, conclusions regarding the impact of disease recurrence are limited because of the small numbers and short follow-up. PLCH has also been associated with malignancy in several reports. Vassallo and colleagues attempted to determine the risk for development of malignancy in their cohort, and a relationship could not be ruled in or ruled out.[100] These past reports suggest it is prudent to carefully prescreen potential lung transplant recipients for malignancy. Given the small numbers of transplants and the reported outcomes to date, lung transplantation remains an appropriate therapeutic option for patients with advanced disease due to PLCH.

## SUMMARY

For selected DPLD patients who fail to respond to medical therapy and demonstrate declines in function that place them at increased risk for mortality, lung transplantation should be considered. Lung transplantation remains a complex medical intervention that requires a dedicated recipient and medical team. Despite the challenges, lung transplantation affords appropriate patients a reasonable chance at increased survival and improved quality of life. Lung transplantation remains an appropriate therapeutic option for selected patients with DPLD.

# REFERENCES

1. Daniels CE, Lasky JA, Limper AH, et al. Imatinib treatment for idiopathic pulmonary fibrosis: randomized placebo-controlled trial results. *Am J Respir Crit Care Med*. 2010;181(6):604–610. http://dx.doi.org/10.1164/rccm.200906-0964OC.

2. Coultas DB, Zumwalt RE, Black WC, Sobonya RE. The epidemiology of interstitial lung diseases. *Am J Respir Crit Care Med*. 1994;150(4):967–972. http://dx.doi.org/10.1164/ajrccm.150.4.7921471.

3. Raghu G, Weycker D, Edelsberg J, Bradford WZ, Oster G. Incidence and prevalence of idiopathic pulmonary fibrosis. *Am J Respir Crit Care Med*. 2006;174(7):810–816. pii:200602-163OC.

4. 4th ed. Schwarz MIKT, King Jr TE, Schwarz MI, eds. *Interstitial Lung Disease*;2003. B.C. Decker; 2003:1.

5. Araki T, Katsura H, Sawabe M, Kida K. A clinical study of idiopathic pulmonary fibrosis based on autopsy studies in elderly patients. *Intern Med*. 2003;42(6):483–489.

6. Bjoraker JA, Ryu JH, Edwin MK, et al. Prognostic significance of histopathologic subsets in idiopathic pulmonary fibrosis. *Am J Respir Crit Care Med*. 1998;157(1):199–203. http://dx.doi.org/10.1164/ajrccm.157.1.9704130.

7. Nathan SD, Shlobin OA, Weir N, et al. Long-term course and prognosis of idiopathic pulmonary fibrosis in the new millennium. *Chest*. 2011;140(1):221–229. http://dx.doi.org/10.1378/chest.10-2572.

8. Sgalla G, Biffi A, Richeldi L. Idiopathic pulmonary fibrosis: diagnosis, epidemiology and natural history. *Respirology*. 2016;21(3):427–437. http://dx.doi.org/10.1111/resp.12683.

9. Hardy JD, Webb WR, Dalton Jr ML, Walker Jr GR. Lung homotransplantation in man. *JAMA*. 1963;186:1065–1074.

10. Reitz BA, Wallwork JL, Hunt SA, et al. Heart-lung transplantation: successful therapy for patients with pulmonary vascular disease. *N Engl J Med*. 1982;306(10):557–564. http://dx.doi.org/10.1056/NEJM198203113061001.

11. Unilateral lung transplantation for pulmonary fibrosis. Toronto Lung Transplant Group. *N Engl J Med*. 1986;314(18):1140–1145. http://dx.doi.org/10.1056/NEJM198605013141802.

12. Yusen RD, Edwards LB, Kucheryavaya AY, et al. The registry of the international society for heart and lung transplantation: thirty-second official adult lung and heart-lung transplantation report–2015; focus theme: early graft failure. *J Heart Lung Transplant*. 2015;34(10):1264–1277. http://dx.doi.org/10.1016/j.healun.2015.08.014.

13. Valapour M, Paulson K, Smith JM, et al. OPTN/SRTR 2011 annual data report: lung. *Am J Transplant*. 2013;13(suppl 1):149–177. http://dx.doi.org/10.1111/ajt.12024.

14. Valapour M, Skeans MA, Smith JM, et al. Lung. *Am J Transplant*. 2016;16(suppl 2):141–168. http://dx.doi.org/10.1111/ajt.13671.

15. Conte JV, Borja MJ, Patel CB, Yang SC, Jhaveri RM, Orens JB. Lung transplantation for primary and secondary pulmonary hypertension. *Ann Thorac Surg*. 2001;72(5):1673–1679. discussion 1679–1680. pii:S0003-4975(01)03081-8.

16. Whelan TP, Dunitz JM, Kelly RF, et al. Effect of preoperative pulmonary artery pressure on early survival after lung transplantation for idiopathic pulmonary fibrosis. *J Heart Lung Transplant*. 2005;24(9):1269–1274. pii:S1053-2498(04)00559-5.

17. Weiss ES, Allen JG, Merlo CA, Conte JV, Shah AS. Survival after single versus bilateral lung transplantation for high-risk patients with pulmonary fibrosis. *Ann Thorac Surg*. 2009;88(5):1616–1625. http://dx.doi.org/10.1016/j.athoracsur.2009.06.044. discussion 1625–1626.

18. Thabut G, Christie JD, Ravaud P, et al. Survival after bilateral versus single-lung transplantation for idiopathic pulmonary fibrosis. *Ann Intern Med*. 2009;151(11):767–774. http://dx.doi.org/10.7326/0003-4819-151-11-200912010-00004.

19. Force SD, Kilgo P, Neujahr DC, et al. Bilateral lung transplantation offers better long-term survival, compared with single-lung transplantation, for younger patients with idiopathic pulmonary fibrosis. *Ann Thorac Surg*. 2011;91(1):244–249. http://dx.doi.org/10.1016/j.athoracsur.2010.08.055.

20. Neurohr C, Huppmann P, Thum D, et al. Potential functional and survival benefit of double over single lung transplantation for selected patients with idiopathic pulmonary fibrosis. *Transpl Int*. 2010;23(9):887–896. http://dx.doi.org/10.1111/j.1432-2277.2010.01071.x.

21. Algar FJ, Espinosa D, Moreno P, et al. Results of lung transplantation in idiopathic pulmonary fibrosis patients. *Transplant Proc*. 2010;42(8):3211–3213. http://dx.doi.org/10.1016/j.transproceed.2010.05.046.

22. Chauhan D, Karanam AB, Merlo A, et al. Post-transplant survival in idiopathic pulmonary fibrosis patients concurrently listed for single and double lung transplantation. *J Heart Lung Transplant*. 2016;35(5):657–660. pii:S1053-2498(16)00025-5.

23. Nathan SD, Shlobin OA, Ahmad S, Burton NA, Barnett SD, Edwards E. Comparison of wait times and mortality for idiopathic pulmonary fibrosis patients listed for single or bilateral lung transplantation. *J Heart Lung Transplant*. 2010;29(10):1165–1171. http://dx.doi.org/10.1016/j.healun.2010.05.014.

24. de Perrot M, Liu M, Waddell TK, Keshavjee S. Ischemia-reperfusion-induced lung injury. *Am J Respir Crit Care Med*. 2003;167(4):490–511. http://dx.doi.org/10.1164/rccm.200207-670SO.

25. Lee JC, Christie JD, Keshavjee S. Primary graft dysfunction: definition, risk factors, short- and long-term outcomes. *Semin Respir Crit Care Med*. 2010;31(2):161–171. http://dx.doi.org/10.1055/s-0030-1249111.

26. Barr ML, Kawut SM, Whelan TP, et al. Report of the ISHLT working group on primary lung graft dysfunction part IV: recipient-related risk factors and markers. *J Heart Lung Transplant*. 2005;24(10):1468–1482. pii:S1053-2498(05)00136-1.

27. Whitson BA, Prekker ME, Herrington CS, et al. Primary graft dysfunction and long-term pulmonary function after lung transplantation. *J Heart Lung Transplant*. 2007;26(10):1004–1011. pii:S1053-2498(07)00531-1.

28. Cypel M, Yeung JC, Liu M, et al. Normothermic ex vivo lung perfusion in clinical lung transplantation. *N Engl J Med*. 2011;364(15):1431–1440. http://dx.doi.org/10.1056/NEJMoa1014597.

29. Thabut G, Mal H, Castier Y, et al. Survival benefit of lung transplantation for patients with idiopathic pulmonary fibrosis. *J Thorac Cardiovasc Surg*. 2003;126(2):469–475. pii:S0022522303006007.

30. Kotloff RM. Does lung transplantation confer a survival benefit? *Curr Opin Organ Transplant*. 2009;14(5):499–503. http://dx.doi.org/10.1097/MOT.0b013e32832fb9f8.

31. Kugler C, Fischer S, Gottlieb J, et al. Health-related quality of life in two hundred-eighty lung transplant recipients. *J Heart Lung Transplant*. 2005;24(12):2262–2268. pii:S1053-2498(05)00494-8.

32. Maurer JR, Ryu J, Beck G, et al. Lung transplantation in the management of patients with lymphangioleiomyomatosis: baseline data from the NHLBI LAM registry. *J Heart Lung Transplant*. 2007;26(12):1293–1299. pii:S1053-2498(07)00724-3.

33. Santana MJ, Feeny D, Jackson K, Weinkauf J, Lien D. Improvement in health-related quality of life after lung transplantation. *Can Respir J*. 2009;16(5):153–158.

34. Kugler C, Tegtbur U, Gottlieb J, et al. Health-related quality of life in long-term survivors after heart and lung transplantation: a prospective cohort study. *Transplantation*. 2010;90(4):451–457. http://dx.doi.org/10.1097/TP.0b013e3181e72863.

35. Gerhardt SG, McDyer JF, Girgis RE, Conte JV, Yang SC, Orens JB. Maintenance azithromycin therapy for bronchiolitis obliterans syndrome: results of a pilot study. *Am J Respir Crit Care Med*. 2003;168(1):121–125. http://dx.doi.org/10.1164/rccm.200212-1424BC.

36. Verleden GM, Dupont LJ. Azithromycin therapy for patients with bronchiolitis obliterans syndrome after lung transplantation. *Transplantation*. 2004;77(9):1465–1467. pii:00007890-200405150-00028.

37. Yates B, Murphy DM, Forrest IA, et al. Azithromycin reverses airflow obstruction in established bronchiolitis obliterans syndrome. *Am J Respir Crit Care Med*. 2005;172(6):772–775. pii:200411-1537OC.

38. Vos R, Vanaudenaerde BM, Verleden SE, et al. A randomised controlled trial of azithromycin to prevent chronic rejection after lung transplantation. *Eur Respir J*. 2011;37(1):164–172. http://dx.doi.org/10.1183/09031936.00068310.

39. Lynch DA, Godwin JD, Safrin S, et al. High-resolution computed tomography in idiopathic pulmonary fibrosis: diagnosis and prognosis. *Am J Respir Crit Care Med*. 2005;172(4):488–493. pii:200412-1756OC.

40. Mogulkoc N, Brutsche MH, Bishop PW, et al. Pulmonary function in idiopathic pulmonary fibrosis and referral for lung transplantation. *Am J Respir Crit Care Med*. 2001;164(1):103–108. http://dx.doi.org/10.1164/ajrccm.164.1.2007077.

41. Gay SE, Kazerooni EA, Toews GB, et al. Idiopathic pulmonary fibrosis: predicting response to therapy and survival. *Am J Respir Crit Care Med*. 1998;157(4 Pt 1):1063–1072. http://dx.doi.org/10.1164/ajrccm.157.4.9703022.

42. Mooney JJ, Elicker BM, Urbania TH, et al. Radiographic fibrosis score predicts survival in hypersensitivity pneumonitis. *Chest*. 2013;144(2):586–592. http://dx.doi.org/10.1378/chest.12-2623.

43. Best AC, Meng J, Lynch AM, et al. Idiopathic pulmonary fibrosis: physiologic tests, quantitative CT indexes, and CT visual scores as predictors of mortality. *Radiology*. 2008;246(3):935–940. http://dx.doi.org/10.1148/radiol.2463062200.

44. Martinez FJ, Safrin S, Weycker D, et al. The clinical course of patients with idiopathic pulmonary fibrosis. *Ann Intern Med*. 2005;142(12 Pt 1):963–967. pii:142/12_Part_1/963.

45. Ley B, Ryerson CJ, Vittinghoff E, et al. A multidimensional index and staging system for idiopathic pulmonary fibrosis. *Ann Intern Med*. 2012;156(10):684–691. http://dx.doi.org/10.7326/0003-4819-156-10-201205150-00004.

46. Latsi PI, du Bois RM, Nicholson AG, et al. Fibrotic idiopathic interstitial pneumonia: the prognostic value of longitudinal functional trends. *Am J Respir Crit Care Med*. 2003;168(5):531–537. http://dx.doi.org/10.1164/rccm.200210-1245OC.

47. Collard HR, King Jr TE, Bartelson BB, Vourlekis JS, Schwarz MI, Brown KK. Changes in clinical and physiologic variables predict survival in idiopathic pulmonary fibrosis. *Am J Respir Crit Care Med*. 2003;168(5):538–542. http://dx.doi.org/10.1164/rccm.200211-1311OC.

48. Zappala CJ, Latsi PI, Nicholson AG, et al. Marginal decline in forced vital capacity is associated with a poor outcome in idiopathic pulmonary fibrosis. *Eur Respir J*. 2010;35(4):830–836. http://dx.doi.org/10.1183/09031936.00155108.

49. Ryerson CJ, Vittinghoff E, Ley B, et al. Predicting survival across chronic interstitial lung disease: the ILD-GAP model. *Chest*. 2014;145(4):723–728. http://dx.doi.org/10.1378/chest.13-1474.

50. du Bois RM, Albera C, Bradford WZ, et al. 6-minute walk test distance is an independent predictor of mortality in patients with idiopathic pulmonary fibrosis. *Eur Respir J*. 2013;10(47):18. pii:09031936.00131813.

51. Hallstrand TS, Boitano LJ, Johnson WC, Spada CA, Hayes JG, Raghu G. The timed walk test as a measure of severity and survival in idiopathic pulmonary fibrosis. *Eur Respir J*. 2005;25(1):96–103. pii:25/1/96.

52. Lama VN, Flaherty KR, Toews GB, et al. Prognostic value of desaturation during a 6-minute walk test in idiopathic interstitial pneumonia. *Am J Respir Crit Care Med*. 2003;168(9):1084–1090. http://dx.doi.org/10.1164/rccm.200302-219OC.

53. Caminati A, Bianchi A, Cassandro R, Mirenda MR, Harari S. Walking distance on 6-MWT is a prognostic factor in idiopathic pulmonary fibrosis. *Respir Med*. 2009;103(1):117–123. http://dx.doi.org/10.1016/j.rmed.2008.07.022.

54. Lederer DJ, Arcasoy SM, Wilt JS, D'Ovidio F, Sonett JR, Kawut SM. Six-minute-walk distance predicts waiting list survival in idiopathic pulmonary fibrosis. *Am J Respir Crit Care Med*. 2006;174(6):659–664. pii:200604-520OC.

55. Collard HR, Moore BB, Flaherty KR, et al. Acute exacerbations of idiopathic pulmonary fibrosis. *Am J Respir Crit Care Med.* 2007;176(7):636–643. pii:200703-463PP.

56. Moua T, Westerly BD, Dulohery MM, Daniels CE, Ryu JH, Lim KG. Patients with fibrotic interstitial lung disease hospitalized for acute respiratory worsening: a large cohort analysis. *Chest.* 2016;149(5):1205–1214. pii:S0012-3692(16)00443-8.

57. Collard HR, Yow E, Richeldi L, Anstrom KJ, Glazer C, IPFnet investigators. Suspected acute exacerbation of idiopathic pulmonary fibrosis as an outcome measure in clinical trials. *Respir Res.* 2013;14:73. http://dx.doi.org/10.1186/1465-9921-14-73.

58. Papiris SA, Kagouridis K, Kolilekas L, et al. Survival in idiopathic pulmonary fibrosis acute exacerbations: the non-steroid approach. *BMC Pulm Med.* 2015;15:162. http://dx.doi.org/10.1186/s12890-015-0146-4.

59. Weill D, Benden C, Corris PA, et al. A consensus document for the selection of lung transplant candidates: 2014–an update from the pulmonary transplantation council of the international society for heart and lung transplantation. *J Heart Lung Transplant.* 2015;34(1):1–15. http://dx.doi.org/10.1016/j.healun.2014.06.014.

60. Raghu G, Rochwerg B, Zhang Y, et al. An official ATS/ERS/JRS/ALAT clinical practice guideline: treatment of idiopathic pulmonary fibrosis. an update of the 2011 clinical practice guideline. *Am J Respir Crit Care Med.* 2015;192(2):e3–e19. http://dx.doi.org/10.1164/rccm.201506-1063ST.

61. Nakazato H, Oku H, Yamane S, Tsuruta Y, Suzuki R. A novel anti-fibrotic agent pirfenidone suppresses tumor necrosis factor-alpha at the translational level. *Eur J Pharmacol.* 2002;446(1–3):177–185. pii:S0014299902017582.

62. Oku H, Shimizu T, Kawabata T, et al. Antifibrotic action of pirfenidone and prednisolone: different effects on pulmonary cytokines and growth factors in bleomycin-induced murine pulmonary fibrosis. *Eur J Pharmacol.* 2008;590(1–3):400–408. http://dx.doi.org/10.1016/j.ejphar.2008.06.046.

63. Iyer SN, Gurujeyalakshmi G, Giri SN. Effects of pirfenidone on procollagen gene expression at the transcriptional level in bleomycin hamster model of lung fibrosis. *J Pharmacol Exp Ther.* 1999;289(1):211–218.

64. Iyer SN, Gurujeyalakshmi G, Giri SN. Effects of pirfenidone on transforming growth factor-beta gene expression at the transcriptional level in bleomycin hamster model of lung fibrosis. *J Pharmacol Exp Ther.* 1999;291(1):367–373.

65. King Jr TE, Bradford WZ, Castro-Bernardini S, et al. A phase 3 trial of pirfenidone in patients with idiopathic pulmonary fibrosis. *N Engl J Med.* 2014;370(22):2083–2092. http://dx.doi.org/10.1056/NEJMoa1402582.

66. Richeldi L, du Bois RM, Raghu G, et al. Efficacy and safety of nintedanib in idiopathic pulmonary fibrosis. *N Engl J Med.* 2014;370(22):2071–2082. http://dx.doi.org/10.1056/NEJMoa1402584.

67. Arcasoy SM, Christie JD, Pochettino A, et al. Characteristics and outcomes of patients with sarcoidosis listed for lung transplantation. *Chest.* 2001;120(3):873–880. pii:S0012-3692(15)50170-0.

68. Shorr AF, Davies DB, Nathan SD. Outcomes for patients with sarcoidosis awaiting lung transplantation. *Chest.* 2002;122(1):233–238.

69. Shorr AF, Davies DB, Nathan SD. Predicting mortality in patients with sarcoidosis awaiting lung transplantation. *Chest.* 2003;124(3):922–928. pii:S0012-3692(15)37649-2.

70. Shlobin OA, Nathan SD. Management of end-stage sarcoidosis: pulmonary hypertension and lung transplantation. *Eur Respir J.* 2012;39(6):1520–1533. http://dx.doi.org/10.1183/09031936.00175511.

71. Shorr AF, Helman DL, Davies DB, Nathan SD. Sarcoidosis, race, and short-term outcomes following lung transplantation. *Chest.* 2004;125(3):990–996. pii:S0012-3692(15)31937-1.

72. Milman N, Burton C, Andersen CB, Carlsen J, Iversen M. Lung transplantation for end-stage pulmonary sarcoidosis: outcome in a series of seven consecutive patients. *Sarcoidosis Vasc Diffuse Lung Dis.* 2005;22(3):222–228.

73. Hadjiliadis D, Sporn TA, Perfect JR, Tapson VF, Davis RD, Palmer SM. Outcome of lung transplantation in patients with mycetomas. *Chest.* 2002;121(1):128–134. pii:S0012-3692(15)34650-X.

74. Milman N, Andersen CB, Burton CM, Iversen M. Recurrent sarcoid granulomas in a transplanted lung derive from recipient immune cells. *Eur Respir J.* 2005;26(3):549–552. pii:26/3/549.

75. Ionescu DN, Hunt JL, Lomago D, Yousem SA. Recurrent sarcoidosis in lung transplant allografts: granulomas are of recipient origin. *Diagn Mol Pathol.* 2005;14(3):140–145. pii:00019606-200509000-00004.

76. Johnson BA, Duncan SR, Ohori NP, et al. Recurrence of sarcoidosis in pulmonary allograft recipients. *Am Rev Respir Dis.* 1993;148(5):1373–1377. http://dx.doi.org/10.1164/ajrccm/148.5.1373.

77. Yeatman M, McNeil K, Smith JA, et al. Lung transplantation in patients with systemic diseases: an eleven-year experience at Papworth Hospital. *J Heart Lung Transplant.* 1996;15(2):144–149.

78. Steen VD, Medsger TA. Changes in causes of death in systemic sclerosis, 1972-2002. *Ann Rheum Dis.* 2007;66(7):940–944. pii:ard.2006.066068.

79. Khan IY, Singer LG, de Perrot M, et al. Survival after lung transplantation in systemic sclerosis. A systematic review. *Respir Med.* 2013;107(12):2081–2087. http://dx.doi.org/10.1016/j.rmed.2013.09.015.

80. Bernstein EJ, Peterson ER, Sell JL, et al. Survival of adults with systemic sclerosis following lung transplantation: a nationwide cohort study. *Arthritis Rheumatol.* 2015;67(5):1314–1322. http://dx.doi.org/10.1002/art.39021.

81. Saggar R, Khanna D, Furst DE, et al. Systemic sclerosis and bilateral lung transplantation: a single centre experience. *Eur Respir J.* 2010;36(4):893–900. http://dx.doi.org/10.1183/09031936.00139809.

82. Shitrit D, Amital A, Peled N, et al. Lung transplantation in patients with scleroderma: case series, review of the literature, and criteria for transplantation. *Clin Transplant.* 2009;23(2):178–183. http://dx.doi.org/10.1111/j.1399-0012.2009.00958.x.

83. Rosas V, Conte JV, Yang SC, et al. Lung transplantation and systemic sclerosis. *Ann Transplant.* 2000;5(3):38–43.

84. Crespo MM, Bermudez CA, Dew MA, et al. Lung transplant in patients with scleroderma compared with pulmonary fibrosis. Short- and long-term outcomes. *Ann Am Thorac Soc.* 2016;13(6):784–792. http://dx.doi.org/10.1513/AnnalsATS.201503-177OC.

85. Miele CH, Schwab K, Saggar R, et al. Lung transplant outcomes in systemic sclerosis with significant esophageal dysfunction. A comprehensive single-center experience. *Ann Am Thorac Soc.* 2016;13(6):793–802. http://dx.doi.org/10.1513/AnnalsATS.201512-806OC.

86. D'Ovidio F, Mura M, Tsang M, et al. Bile acid aspiration and the development of bronchiolitis obliterans after lung transplantation. *J Thorac Cardiovasc Surg.* 2005;129(5):1144–1152. pii:S002252230401685X.

87. Murthy SC, Nowicki ER, Mason DP, et al. Pretransplant gastroesophageal reflux compromises early outcomes after lung transplantation. *J Thorac Cardiovasc Surg.* 2011;142(1):47–52.e3. http://dx.doi.org/10.1016/j.jtcvs.2011.04.028.

88. Hartwig MG, Anderson DJ, Onaitis MW, et al. Fundoplication after lung transplantation prevents the allograft dysfunction associated with reflux. *Ann Thorac Surg.* 2011;92(2):462–468. http://dx.doi.org/10.1016/j.athoracsur.2011.04.035. discussion; 468–469.

89. Palmer SM, Miralles AP, Howell DN, Brazer SR, Tapson VF, Davis RD. Gastroesophageal reflux as a reversible cause of allograft dysfunction after lung transplantation. *Chest.* 2000;118(4):1214–1217. pii:S0012-3692(15)37731-X.

90. Berkowitz N, Schulman LL, McGregor C, Markowitz D. Gastroparesis after lung transplantation. Potential role in postoperative respiratory complications. *Chest.* 1995;108(6):1602–1607. pii:S0012-3692(15)45115-3.

91. Taylor JR, Ryu J, Colby TV, Raffin TA. Lymphangioleiomyomatosis. clinical course in 32 patients. *N Engl J Med.* 1990;323(18):1254–1260. http://dx.doi.org/10.1056/NEJM199011013231807.

92. Kitaichi M, Nishimura K, Itoh H, Izumi T. Pulmonary lymphangioleiomyomatosis: a report of 46 patients including a clinicopathologic study of prognostic factors. *Am J Respir Crit Care Med.* 1995;151(2 Pt 1):527–533. http://dx.doi.org/10.1164/ajrccm.151.2.7842216.

93. Pechet TT, Meyers BF, Guthrie TJ, et al. Lung transplantation for lymphangioleiomyomatosis. *J Heart Lung Transplant.* 2004;23(3):301–308. http://dx.doi.org/10.1016/S1053-2498(03)00195-5.

94. Taveira-DaSilva AM, Moss J. Management of lymphangioleiomyomatosis. *F1000Prime Rep.* 2014;6:116. http://dx.doi.org/10.12703/P6-116. eCollection 2014.

95. Boehler A, Speich R, Russi EW, Weder W. Lung transplantation for lymphangioleiomyomatosis. *N Engl J Med.* 1996;335(17):1275–1280. http://dx.doi.org/10.1056/NEJM199610243351704.

96. Kpodonu J, Massad MG, Chaer RA, et al. The US experience with lung transplantation for pulmonary lymphangioleiomyomatosis. *J Heart Lung Transplant.* 2005;24(9):1247–1253. pii:S1053-2498(04)00543-1.

97. McCormack FX, Inoue Y, Moss J, et al. Efficacy and safety of sirolimus in lymphangioleiomyomatosis. *N Engl J Med.* 2011;364(17):1595–1606. http://dx.doi.org/10.1056/NEJMoa1100391.

98. Groetzner J, Kur F, Spelsberg F, et al. Airway anastomosis complications in de novo lung transplantation with sirolimus-based immunosuppression. *J Heart Lung Transplant.* 2004;23(5):632–638. http://dx.doi.org/10.1016/S1053-2498(03)00309-7.

99. Dauriat G, Mal H, Thabut G, et al. Lung transplantation for pulmonary langerhans' cell histiocytosis: a multicenter analysis. *Transplantation.* 2006;81(5):746–750. http://dx.doi.org/10.1097/01.tp.0000200304.64613.af.

100. Vassallo R, Ryu JH, Schroeder DR, Decker PA, Limper AH. Clinical outcomes of pulmonary langerhans'-cell histiocytosis in adults. *N Engl J Med.* 2002;346(7):484–490. http://dx.doi.org/10.1056/NEJMoa012087.

101. Christie JD, Carby M, Bag R, et al. Report of the ISHLT working group on primary lung graft dysfunction part II: definition. A consensus statement of the international society for heart and lung transplantation. *J Heart Lung Transplant.* 2005;24(10):1454–1459. pii:S1053-2498(04)00652-7.

102. Estenne M, Maurer JR, Boehler A, et al. Bronchiolitis obliterans syndrome 2001: an update of the diagnostic criteria. *J Heart Lung Transplant.* 2002;21(3):297–310. pii:S1053249802003984.

# Idiopathic Pulmonary Fibrosis: Phenotypes and Comorbidities

ADITI SHAH • CHARLENE D. FELL

---

**KEY POINTS**

- Idiopathic pulmonary fibrosis (IPF) may have multiple phenotypes, including combined pulmonary fibrosis and emphysema, rapidly progressive IPF, and pulmonary hypertension and IPF, each with different rates of progression and clinical outcome.
- Common comorbidities in IPF patients include cardiovascular disease, venous thromboembolism, gastroesophageal reflux, sleep apnea, lung cancer, and depression.
- Identification and management of comorbidities in IPF may improve patient well-being and outcomes.

---

Idiopathic pulmonary fibrosis (IPF) is a progressive fatal disease of the lung with unknown etiology and limited treatment options. It was once thought to be a slowly progressive disease, but more recent evidence suggests that there may be different phenotypes of IPF with different rates of disease progression. Furthermore, patients with comorbid disease, such as emphysema or pulmonary hypertension (PH), do more poorly than those with IPF alone. Rapidly progressive IPF, combined emphysema and pulmonary fibrosis, and IPF with PH may represent new disease phenotypes. Patients are often very discouraged to receive a diagnosis of IPF given its poor prognosis and limited treatment options. However, much can be done to identify and alleviate symptoms from comorbidities, potentially improving the overall quality of life of IPF patients. This chapter updates the evidence to support the hypothesis that there is more than one phenotype for IPF and describes the common comorbidities seen in this disease.[1]

## ARE THERE DISTINCT PHENOTYPES IN IDIOPATHIC PULMONARY FIBROSIS?

A phenotype is the outward manifestation of a gene or genes, may involve more than one organ system, and is dynamic, changing over time or in response to the environment.[2] In contrast, genotypes are stable over the lifespan of an individual. Defining a phenotype concisely and accurately is crucial, as phenotypes are used to predict prognosis, select patients for enrollment into clinical trials, and provide the foundation for studies exploring the pathobiology of disease. Some authors have suggested that the lack of significant and reproducible results in recent therapeutic trials may be due to the inclusion of several different as yet to be characterized phenotypes in IPF.[3] Three distinct phenotypes of IPF have been proposed: combined emphysema and pulmonary fibrosis,[4] disproportionate PH and IPF,[5] and IPF, which is rapidly progressive.[3]

### Combined Pulmonary Fibrosis and Emphysema

Smoking increases the risk of developing IPF,[6] and many patients exhibit features of IPF and emphysema. The prevalence of emphysema in IPF patients was 30% in a retrospective study from Mexico[7] and 47% at the time of diagnosis and 55% during follow-up in a European cohort.[8] Early reports describe patients with a clinical presentation of severe dyspnea, pulmonary fibrosis, preserved lung volumes, and a markedly reduced transfer factor for carbon monoxide.[9,10] These patients had characteristic radiographic features including upper lobe–predominant centrilobular or periseptal emphysema and lower lobe–predominant pulmonary fibrosis (Fig. 10.1).[8,10] The syndrome of combined pulmonary fibrosis and emphysema (CPFE) was coined by Cottin and colleagues in 2005 to describe this subgroup of IPF patients.[8] It is important to note that the CPFE

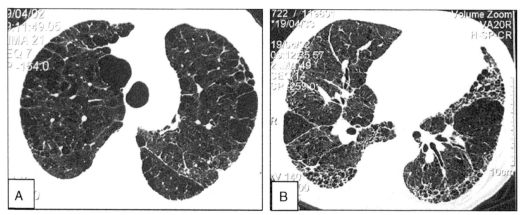

FIG. 10.1 High-resolution computed tomography images from a patient with combined pulmonary fibrosis and emphysema illustrating upper lobe emphysema (A) and lower lobe fibrosis with honeycomb change (B). (From Mejia M, Carrillo G, Rojas-Serrano J, et al. Idiopathic pulmonary fibrosis and emphysema: decreased survival associated with severe pulmonary arterial hypertension. *Chest*. 2009;136:10–15; with permission.)

phenotype is not limited to IPF; hypersensitivity pneumonitis, nonspecific interstitial pneumonia (NSIP), and other forms of fibrotic lung disease have also been described in CPFE.[1a]

The pathobiology of CPFE has not been established. Cigarette smoke is the most important trigger, but other environmental exposures, such as agrochemical compounds, may also contribute.[11] It is not known whether CPFE develops in individuals who inherit susceptibility to both chronic obstructive pulmonary disease (COPD) and IPF or if there is a distinct genetic basis for the syndrome.

Patients with CPFE have worse survival than those with IPF alone (25 vs. 34 months).[7] Prognosis of patients with concurrent pulmonary fibrosis and emphysema is even poorer if they develop PH.[8] When patients develop restriction (forced vital capacity [FVC] <50% predicted) in the setting of CPFE with PH, the prognosis is grim.[7]

Recent studies have attempted to determine models that could further help in the prognostication of patients with CPFE. Although the decline in FVC and diffusing capacity of the lungs for carbon monoxide ($D_{LCO}$) are important prognostic variables for IPF patients, they are not reliable indicators of disease in CPFE patients.[12] In a retrospective study conducted by Schmidt et al., decline in $FEV_1$ by 10% was a stronger predictor of mortality in CPFE patients than FVC, $D_{LCO}$, or composite physiologic index.[13] Kishaba et al. retrospectively examined ILD patients at their center; 93 had CPFE with either IPF or iNSIP as the fibrotic phenotype. The mean survival rate of these patients was 30.7 months. In this study, an overall ratio of %$FEV_1$ to %FVC of more than 1.2 and presence of finger clubbing were the best predictors of poor survival in patients with CPFE.[14]

Management of patients with CPFE should be directed to the underlying fibrotic lung disease, emphysema, and resulting aberrations in gas exchange. Smoking cessation is of paramount importance. Oral corticosteroids and immunosuppressive therapy are ineffective for the long-term management of CPFE patients,[8,9] but may be considered for management of acute exacerbations. Supplemental oxygen should be provided for hypoxemic patients. Anti-PH therapy has not been specifically evaluated in this population.

## Pulmonary Hypertension and Idiopathic Pulmonary Fibrosis

Multiple studies have examined PH in patients with IPF. PH is defined as a mean pulmonary arterial pressure (mPAP) ≥25 mm Hg at rest or ≥30 mm Hg with exercise.[15] Echocardiography is recommended as a screening test for identifying patients with PH.[15] In a study comparing echocardiographic and right-sided heart catheterization data for patients with advanced lung disease waiting for lung transplant, 48% of patients were misclassified with PH.[16] Thus echocardiographic data must be interpreted with caution, and right-sided heart catheterization is required to accurately confirm the presence and severity of PH in the IPF population.

Recent studies have investigated the utility of echocardiographic measurements of right ventricular structure and function to predict outcomes in

IPF-associated PH. A retrospective cohort study by Rivera-Lebron et al. reviewed 135 patients with IPF out of whom 29% had PH.[17] They reported an association between the ratio of right ventricle to left ventricle diameter greater than 1, TAPSE less than 1.6 cm, presence of moderate to severe right atrial or right ventricle dilation, and right ventricle dysfunction with increased risk of death.[17] Hence quantitative echocardiographic assessment of right ventricular structure and function can be clinically significant.[17] Other echocardiographic parameters such as right ventricular systolic pressure have limited accuracy in patients with advanced lung disease.[17-19]

Estimates of the prevalence of PH in IPF range between 31% and 85%[20-23] and are derived from data from patients awaiting lung transplantation. The incidence and severity of PH increase with time,[24] and thus the prevalence of PH in the general IPF population may be lower.

PH in IPF is associated with a higher mortality,[22] especially in patients with combined emphysema and pulmonary fibrosis.[15,16] Although mPAP ≥25 mm Hg is an accepted definition for PH, a recent analysis demonstrated that mPAP >17 mm Hg is the best discriminator of increased 5-year mortality for IPF patients.[25] Elevated pulmonary vascular resistance has also been associated with poor outcome in patients with IPF-PH.[17,18]

PH in IPF is the result of a number of proposed pathophysiologic mechanisms, including distortion and destruction of the vascular bed from fibrosis and chronic vasoconstriction due to hypoxemia.[5] PH usually develops in patients with severe IPF and is analogous to the development of PH in other chronic lung diseases, such as COPD. However, there exists a subset of IPF patients who develop PH at earlier stages of the disease.[22,26,27] These patients are hypothesized to represent a distinct phenotype of disproportionate PH in IPF.[5] Patients may have disproportionate PH in IPF due to episodic hypoxemia during sleep or exercise or may have an imbalance of angiogenesis and angiostasis in the lung.[5] Whether this represents a true novel phenotype remains to be explored, as do the underlying potential mechanisms of disproportional PH in IPF.

Recent advances in the understanding of the pathobiology of PH have resulted in the development of therapies that have greatly improved functional status and survival of select groups of patients with the disease.[28] Early trials of endothelin receptor antagonists in IPF provided promising results[29,30]; subsequent larger trials have failed to show a statistically significant

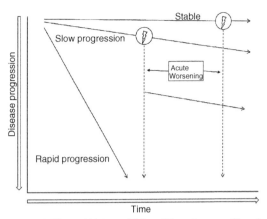

FIG. 10.2 Natural history of idiopathic pulmonary fibrosis. The majority of patients experience slow progression of the disease (slow progression), while some have more stable disease (stable). Patients with slow progression or stable disease may experience episodes of acute deterioration (lightning bolt; acute worsening). A subset of patients has rapidly progressive disease (rapid progression) and may encompass a distinct phenotype. (Adapted from Raghu G, Collard HR, Egan JJ, et al. An Official ATS/ERS/JRS/ALAT Statement: idiopathic pulmonary fibrosis: evidence-based guidelines for diagnosis and management. *Am J Respir Crit Care Med.* 2011;183:788; with permission.)

benefit.[31-33,9a] Other studies have been terminated early because of disease progression in IPF patients with PH treated with ambrisentan or riociguat.[8a,10a,11a] Based on a lack of evidence and potential for harm, treatment of PH in IPF is not recommended for the majority of patients.[34]

In patients with idiopathic PAH, there is evidence supporting the use of long-term anticoagulation for prevention of venous thromboembolism. However, currently there are no studies to support the use of long-term anticoagulation in IPF patients with PH.[35] Furthermore, a study that evaluated the use of warfarin in patients with progressive IPF was terminated early because of a trend toward higher mortality, hospitalization, and acute exacerbation of IPF in the warfarin group.[36]

## Rapidly Progressive Idiopathic Pulmonary Fibrosis

Patients with IPF may exhibit varying courses of their disease: some have slowly progressive disease, some experience acute exacerbations of IPF, and some experience a very rapid deterioration from the time of symptom onset (Fig. 10.2). Patients with rapid disease progression are hypothesized to represent a distinct phenotype of IPF. A study of 26 patients with rapidly progressive disease (<6 months of symptoms) and 88 patients with slowly progressive disease (>24 months of symptoms) found differential expression of genes between the groups, with the rapid progressors exhibiting upregulation of the several genes involved in cell motility, myofibroblast differentiation, coagulation, oxidative stress, and development, including the gene for the adenosine $A_{2B}$ receptor.[3] Another study showed elevated TLR9 gene expression in surgical lung biopsies of patients with rapidly progressive IPF compared with those with more stable disease.[37] A genomewide analysis in IPF patients identified gene expression from lung parenchyma of IPF patients that differentiated patients with rapid disease progression from those with stable disease.[38] These results suggest biologically plausible mechanisms underlying the difference between the proposed slowly and rapidly progressive phenotypes in IPF.

## Gastroesophageal Reflux Disease

Evidence that gastroesophageal reflux disease (GERD) is associated with IPF and recurrent silent aspiration of gastric acid is associated with acute exacerbations of IPF makes GERD an attractive hypothesis for the etiology of IPF.[39,40] Instillation of acid into the tracheobronchial tree produces pulmonary fibrosis in animal models,[41,42] and aspiration of gastric contents can cause pulmonary fibrosis in humans.[43]

The prevalence of GERD in IPF is estimated between 66% and 87%.[40,44,45] It should be noted that 33–53% of patients with documented acid reflux are asymptomatic.[40,44] In a study of patients with IPF being worked up for lung transplantation, symptoms of reflux were a poor predictor of acid reflux measured with esophageal pH monitoring with a sensitivity of 65% and specificity of 71%.[44] A small case series comparing bronchoalveolar lavage (BAL) pepsin levels found that patients with acute exacerbations of IPF had higher levels of BAL pepsin than stable IPF patients.[46] In a recent study, patients with asymmetric IPF were more likely to have GERD and have experienced acute exacerbations of IPF than patients with symmetric IPF.[39] The authors speculate that asymmetric IPF is caused by silent nocturnal aspiration and that acute exacerbations of IPF are also caused by silent aspiration.

There are limited data describing treatment outcomes for IPF patients with silent GERD. A small series of four IPF patients with silent GERD documented by 24-h pH measurements and treated with proton pump inhibitors (PPIs) and gastric fundoplication if required showed stabilization in lung function.[47] A retrospective study of IPF patients waiting for lung transplantation found that those who underwent Nissan fundoplication for severe symptomatic acid reflux had an improved posttransplant course compared with patients who did not undergo the procedure.[48]

Two recent post hoc studies show contrasting results. Lee et al. examined patients who were assigned to the placebo group of the three IPFnet randomized controlled trials. Out of 242 patients in placebo arms, 124 patients (51%) were taking PPI or H2 receptor blockers (H2B) at baseline. At 30 weeks the H2B/PPI group had smaller decrease in FVC (estimated difference between groups 0.07 L (95% CI 0.00, 0.14, P-value = .05) and fewer acute exacerbations compared with the group of patients not taking antacid therapy at baseline.[4a] Kreuter et al. analyzed patients who were randomly allocated to the placebo arms in three large clinical trials of pirfenidone.[49] Of the 624 patients included in the study cohort, 291 (47%) received antacid therapy (256 [88%] PPIs, 24 [8%] H2 blockers, and 11 [4%] both PPIs and H2 blockers) and 333 (53%) patients did not.[49] Antacid therapy users had similar disease progression at 1 year compared with no antacid therapy users (37·8% vs. 40·5%; P = .4002).[49] There were no significant differences in percent-change in FVC from baseline, 6-min walk distance, all-cause mortality and IPF-related mortality, and adverse events between the two groups.[49] However, there were more overall infections [107 (74%) vs. 101 (62%); P = .0174] and pulmonary infections [20 (14%) vs. 10 (6%); P = .0214] in patients with more advanced IPF treated with antacids than those who were not.[49] These observational and retrospective studies suggest that anti-GER therapy may improve lung function, but may be associated with an increased risk of pneumonia. Randomized controlled trials are needed. The most recent ATS/ERS/JRS/ALAT IPF guidelines provide a conditional recommendation for the use of antacid therapy for the treatment of IPF, with "very low confidence in effect estimates."[5a]

## Cardiovascular Disease and Venous Thromboembolic Disease

Several studies have demonstrated that IPF patients have a higher risk of developing acute vascular disease (cardiovascular disease and venous thromboembolic disease) than those with other lung diseases or the general population. In an uncontrolled autopsy study of IPF patients, nine patients (21%) died of cardiovascular events.[50] A cross-sectional study of 630 patients referred for lung transplantation at a tertiary hospital demonstrated that IPF patients have an increased risk of coronary artery disease identified at angiography than patients referred with other chronic lung disease (OR, 2.31; 95% CI, 1.11–4.82).[51] More recently, a large case-controlled study showed that patients with IPF are more likely to have a history of cardiovascular disease at the time of IPF diagnosis (OR, 1.53; 95% CI, 1.15–2.03) than controls and are more likely to have an acute coronary event during follow-up (RR, 3.14; 95% CI, 2.02–4.87).[52] IPF patients who were diagnosed with cardiovascular disease during follow-up for IPF had a greater mortality than those with preexisting cardiovascular disease at the time of IPF diagnosis (HR 4.7, 95% CI 2.0, 11.1; $P < .001$).[53] IPF patients have an increased risk of angina, atrial fibrillation, deep vein thrombosis, and stroke.[52]

Venous thromboembolic disease is also important in IPF patients. A large study of the Danish population examined whether thromboembolic disease is a risk factor for idiopathic interstitial pneumonia.[54] This study demonstrated that patients with deep venous thrombosis and pulmonary embolism have an increased risk of idiopathic interstitial pneumonia compared with controls (HR 1.3; 95% CI, 1.2–1.4; and HR 2.4; 95% CI, 2.3–2.6, respectively) with multivariate-adjusted analyses.[54] In a study of all decedents in the United States between 1988 and 2007, the risk of death from venous thromboembolic disease was greater for patients with pulmonary fibrosis compared with the general population (OR 1.35, 95% CI 1.29–1.38, $P < .0001$), patients with lung cancer (OR 1.45, 95% CI 1.39–1.48, $P < .0001$), or patients with COPD (OR 1.55, 95% CI 1.49–1.59, $P < .0001$).[55]

Current guidelines on the management of IPF do not discuss the identification and management of comorbid vascular disease in IPF patients. However, it is reasonable to screen patients for cardiovascular or thromboembolic disease if they clinically deteriorate. In particular, when assessing a patient with a possible acute exacerbation of IPF, one must rule out cardiovascular disease and pulmonary embolism as causes of the deterioration.[56]

## Lung Cancer

The risk of lung cancer for patients with IPF is high. When compared with that of the general population, the relative risk is 7.31 (95% CI, 4.47–11.93).[57] The prevalence of lung cancer among IPF patients followed in national registries ranges between 4.4% and 9.8%.[57–59] In a retrospective cohort study, the cumulative incidence of lung cancer among IPF patients was 3.3% at 1 year, 15.4% at 5 years, and 54.7% at 10 years.[60] The risk of developing lung cancer is greater for IPF patients who are male ever-smokers.[57,59,60] There are

three hypotheses to explain this relationship: pulmonary fibrosis causes lung cancer, lung cancer and/or its treatment causes pulmonary fibrosis, and/or common mediators cause lung cancer and pulmonary fibrosis.[61] Interestingly, in a study of molecular phenotypes of IPF, several genes that are upregulated in IPF (but not in normal lung tissue) are also upregulated in adenocarcinoma of the lung,[38] suggesting that the observed increased risk may be in part due to common biologic mechanisms.

Treatment of lung cancer in IPF is fraught with difficulties, including acute exacerbations of pulmonary fibrosis/acute lung injury associated with surgical resection of cancers,[62,63] radiation therapy,[64] and chemotherapy.[65] Existing guidelines do not specifically address this issue and the decision to proceed with treatment of cancer in IPF patients should be a carefully considered one.

## Depression

Quality of life in patients with pulmonary fibrosis is poor[66,67] and associated with dyspnea and impaired pulmonary function.[68–71] Dyspnea in IPF affects health-related quality of life differently in men and women: in men, dyspnea worsens physical quality of life domains, and in women, it worsens emotional domains.[72] Twenty three percent of patients with pulmonary fibrosis were found to have clinically significant depression in a recent study.[73] There is a strong correlation between depression and dyspnea in these patients; multivariate analysis suggests that depression is a major contributing factor in patients' perception of dyspnea and thus their quality of life.[73] Depression was found in 21% of a Danish cohort of IPF patients.[53] Treating depression may improve patients' dyspnea and quality of life; this hypothesis needs testing in clinical trials.

## Sleep Apnea and Idiopathic Pulmonary Fibrosis

Obstructive sleep apnea (OSA) affects 2–4% of the North American population.[74] Numerous studies show disruption of sleep architecture in ILD patients,[75] increased breathing frequency,[76,77] nocturnal cough,[76] and oxygen desaturation especially during rapid eye movement sleep.[77] The prevalence of OSA in IPF patients is estimated between 44% and 88%.[78,79]

Early recognition and treatment of OSA are important as untreated OSA is associated with high risk of adverse clinical outcomes including cardiovascular disease, type 2 diabetes mellitus, depression, PH, and cognitive impairment. Mortality and morbidity rates increase significantly when OSA occurs concurrently with other chronic lung diseases.[80] Several factors associated with OSA such as chronic gastroesophageal reflux, microaspiration, intermittent hypoxia, and intrathroacic mechanical strain may either contribute to the development of IPF or further promote its progression.[81] In addition, OSA may contribute to fatigue and poor sleep quality in affected patients.

Treatment of moderate to severe OSA in IPF patients results in overall improvement in the quality of life based on the Functional Outcome of Sleep Questionnaire, daily living activities, and sleep parameters.[82,83] Initiating CPAP therapy in the early stages of the disease may improve acclimation and compliance to CPAP.[83] However, in general, there is a paucity of literature looking at CPAP initiation in this patient population; future research is needed to investigate the potential role of OSA in progression and development of IPF.

## Diabetes Mellitus

A prospective Danish study of IPF patients noted that 17% of IPF patients had diabetes mellitus.[53] Survival of IPF patients with diabetes at the time of IPF diagnosis mellitus was significantly worse than for those without diabetes after adjusting for age, gender, and FVC (HR 2.47, 95% CI 1.04–5.88; $P = .041$).[53] The reason why IPF patients with diabetes mellitus have a higher risk of death than those without is not clear, and the relationship between diabetes mellitus and IPF warrants further investigation.

## SUMMARY

Patients with IPF face progressive dyspnea and disability, poor prognosis, and limited treatment options. Once thought to be a slowly progressive disease, IPF may have an accelerated variant phenotype. CPFE and disproportionate PH in IPF may also be distinct phenotypes; further investigation is needed to characterize these phenotypes and determine if there is a plausible biologic explanation for these entities. Identification and management of comorbidities may improve the overall quality of life and the well-being of these patients.

## REFERENCES

1. Fell CD. Idiopathic pulmonary fibrosis: phenotypes and comorbidities. *Clin Chest Med.* 2012;33:51–57.
2. Schulze TG, McMahon FJ. Defining the phenotype in human genetic studies: forward genetics and reverse phenotyping. *Hum Hered.* 2004;58:131.
3. Selman M, Carrillo G, Estrada A, et al. Accelerated variant of idiopathic pulmonary fibrosis: clinical behavior and gene expression pattern. *PLoS One.* 2007;2:e482.
4. Cottin V, Cordier JF. The syndrome of combined pulmonary fibrosis and emphysema. *Chest.* 2009;136:1.
5. Corte TJ, Wort SJ, Wells AU. Pulmonary hypertension in idiopathic pulmonary fibrosis: a review. *Sarcoidosis Vasc Diffuse Lung Dis.* 2009;26:7.
6. Baumgartner KB, Samet JM, Stidley CA, et al. Cigarette smoking: a risk factor for idiopathic pulmonary fibrosis. *Am J Respir Crit Care Med.* 1997;155:242.
7. Mejia M, Carrillo G, Rojas-Serrano J, et al. Idiopathic pulmonary fibrosis and emphysema: decreased survival associated with severe pulmonary arterial hypertension. *Chest.* 2009;136:10.
8. Cottin V, Nunes H, Brillet P, et al. Combined pulmonary fibrosis and emphysema: a distinct underrecognised entity. *Eur Res J.* 2005;26:586.
9. Doherty MJ, Pearson MG, O'Grady EA, et al. Cryptogenic fibrosing alveolitis with preserved lung volumes. *Thorax.* 1997;52:998.
10. Wiggins J, Strickland B, Turner-Warwick M. Combined cryptogenic fibrosing alveolitis and emphysema: the value of high resolution computed tomography in assessment. *Respir Med.* 1990;84:365.
11. Daniil Z, Koutsokera A, Gourgoulianis K. Combined pulmonary fibrosis and emphysema in patients exposed to agrochemical compounds. *Eur Respir J.* 2006;27:434.
12. Jankowich MD, Rounds SI. Combined pulmonary fibrosis and emphysema syndrome: a review. *Chest.* 2012;141(1):222–231.
13. Schmidt SL, Nambiar AM, Tayob N, et al. Pulmonary function measures predict mortality differently in IPF versus combined pulmonary fibrosis and emphysema. *Eur Respir J.* 2011;38(1):176–183.
14. Kishaba T, Shimaoka Y, Fukuyama H, et al. A cohort study of mortality predictors and characteristics of patients with combined pulmonary fibrosis and emphysema. *Respir Med.* 2012;2(3):1–5.
15. Barst RJ, McGoon M, Torbicki A, et al. Diagnosis and differential assessment of pulmonary arterial hypertension. *J Am Coll Cardiol.* 2004;43:40S.
16. Arcasoy SM, Christie JD, Ferrari VA, et al. Echocardiographic assessment of pulmonary hypertension in patients with advanced lung disease. *Am J Respir Crit Care Med.* 2003;167:735.
17. Rivera-Lebron BN, Forfia PR, et al. Echocardiographic and hemodynamic predictors of mortality in idiopathic pulmonary fibrosis. *Chest.* 2013;144(2):564–570.
18. Arcasoy SM, Christie JD, Ferrari VA, et al. Echocardiographic assessment of pulmonary hypertension in patients with advanced lung disease. *Am J Respir Crit Care Med.* 2003;167(5):735–740.
19. Nathan SD, Shlobin OA, Barnett SD, et al. Right ventricular systolic pressure by echocardiography as a predictor of pulmonary hypertension in idiopathic pulmonary fibrosis. *Respir Med.* 2008;102(9):1305–1310.

20. Shorr AF, Wainright JL, Cors CS, et al. Pulmonary hypertension in patients with pulmonary fibrosis awaiting lung transplant. *Eur Respir J.* 2007;30:715.

21. Agarwal R, Gupta D, Verma JS, et al. Noninvasive estimation of clinically asymptomatic pulmonary hypertension in idiopathic pulmonary fibrosis. *Indian J Chest Dis Allied Sci.* 2005;47:267.

22. Lettieri CJ, Nathan SD, Barnett SD, et al. Prevalence and outcomes of pulmonary arterial hypertension in advanced idiopathic pulmonary fibrosis. *Chest.* 2006;129:746.

23. Nadrous HF, Pellikka PA, Krowka MJ, et al. The impact of pulmonary hypertension on survival in patients with idiopathic pulmonary fibrosis. *Chest.* 2005;128:616S.

24. Nathan SD, Shlobin OA, Ahmad S, et al. Serial development of pulmonary hypertension in patients with idiopathic pulmonary fibrosis. *Respiration.* 2008;76:288.

25. Hamada K, Nagai S, Tanaka S, et al. Significance of pulmonary arterial pressure and diffusion capacity of the lung as prognosticator in patients with idiopathic pulmonary fibrosis. *Chest.* 2007;131:650.

26. Lederer DJ, Caplan-Shaw CE, O'Shea MK, et al. Racial and ethnic disparities in survival in lung transplant candidates with idiopathic pulmonary fibrosis. *Am J Transplant.* 2006;6:398.

27. Nathan SD, Shlobin OA, Ahmad S, et al. Pulmonary hypertension and pulmonary function testing in idiopathic pulmonary fibrosis. *Chest.* 2007;131:657.

28. Badesch DB, Abman SH, Simonneau G, et al. Medical therapy for pulmonary arterial hypertension: updated ACCP evidence-based clinical practice guidelines. *Chest.* 2007;131:1917.

29. Collard HR, Anstrom KJ, Schwarz MI, et al. Sildenafil improves walk distance in idiopathic pulmonary fibrosis*. *Chest.* 2007;131:897.

30. King Jr TE, Behr J, Brown KK, et al. BUILD-1: a randomized placebo-controlled trial of bosentan in idiopathic pulmonary fibrosis. *Am J Respir Crit Care Med.* 2008;177:75.

31. King Jr TE, Brown KK, Raghu G, et al. The BUILD-3 trial: a prospective, randomized, double-blind, placebo-controlled study of bosentan in idiopathic pulmonary fibrosis. *Am J Respir Crit Care Med.* 2010;181:A6838.

32. The Idiopathic Pulmonary Fibrosis Clinical Research Network. A controlled trial of sildenafil in advanced idiopathic pulmonary fibrosis. *N Engl J Med.* 2010;363:620.

33. Press release. *Actelion Reports Results of Exploratory Study with Macitentan in Patients with Idiopathic Pulmonary Fibrosis – Promising Long-Term Safety and Tolerability Profile – Efficacy Data Not Supportive of Phase III in IPF.* Actelion Pharmaceuticals Ltd; August 29, 2011.

34. Raghu G, Collard HR, Egan JJ, et al. An official ATS/ERS/JRS/ALAT statement: idiopathic pulmonary fibrosis: evidence-based guidelines for diagnosis and management. *Am J Respir Crit Care Med.* 2011;183:788.

35. Smith JS, Gorbett D, Mueller J, et al. Pulmonary hypertension idiopathic pulmonary fibrosis: a dastardly duo. *Am J Med Sci.* 2013;346(3):221–225.

36. Noth I, Anstrom KJ, Calvert SB, et al. A placebo-controlled randomized trial of warfarin in idiopathic pulmonary fibrosis. *Am J Respir Crit Care Med.* 2012;186:88–95.

37. Trujillo G, Meneghin A, Flaherty KR, et al. TLR9 differentiates rapid from slowly progressive forms of idiopathic pulmonary fibrosis. *Sci Transl Med.* 2010;2(57):57–82.

38. Boon K, Bailey NW, Yang J, et al. Molecular phenotypes distinguish patients with relatively stable from progressive idiopathic pulmonary fibrosis (IPF). *PLos One.* 2009;4(4):e5134.

39. Tcherakian C, Cottin V, Brillet PY, et al. Progression of idiopathic pulmonary fibrosis: lessons from asymmetrical disease. *Thorax.* 2011;66:226.

40. Raghu G, Freudenberger TD, Yang S, et al. High prevalence of abnormal acid gastro-oesophageal reflux in idiopathic pulmonary fibrosis. *Eur Respir J.* 2006;27:136.

41. Downs JB, Chapman Jr RL, Modell JH, et al. An evaluation of steroid therapy in aspiration pneumonitis. *Anesthesiology.* 1974;40:129.

42. Moran TJ. Experimental aspiration pneumonia. IV. Inflammatory and reparative changes produced by intratracheal injections of autologous gastric juice and hydrochloric acid. *Am Med Assoc Arch Pathol.* 1955;60:122.

43. Sladen A, Zanca P, Hadnott WH. Aspiration pneumonitis–the sequelae. *Chest.* 1971;59:448.

44. Sweet MP, Patti MG, Leard LE, et al. Gastroesophageal reflux in patients with idiopathic pulmonary fibrosis referred for lung transplantation. *J Thorac Cardiovasc Surg.* 2007;133:1078.

45. Han MK. High prevalence of abnormal acid gastro-oesophageal reflux in idiopathic pulmonary fibrosis. *Eur Respir J.* 2006;28:884.

46. Lee J, Song J, Wolters P, et al. Bronchoalveolar lavage pepsin levels in acute exacerbations of idiopathic pulmonary fibrosis. *Am J Respir Crit Care Med.* 2011:183.

47. Raghu G, Yang STY, Spada C, et al. Sole treatment of acid gastroesophageal reflux in idiopathic pulmonary fibrosis: a case series. *Chest.* 2006;129:794.

48. Linden PA, Gilbert RJ, Yeap BY, et al. Laparoscopic fundoplication in patients with end-stage lung disease awaiting transplantation. *J Thorac Cardiovasc Surg.* 2006;131:438.

49. Kreuter M, Wuyts W, Renzoni E, et al. Antacid therapy and disease outcomes in idiopathic pulmonary fibrosis: a pooled analysis. *Lancet Respir Med.* 2016;4(5):381–389.

50. Daniels CE, Yi ES, Ryu JH. Autopsy findings in 42 consecutive patients with idiopathic pulmonary fibrosis. *Eur Respir J.* 2008;32:170.

51. Kizer JR, Zisman DA, Blumenthal NP, et al. Association between pulmonary fibrosis and coronary artery disease. *Arch Intern Med.* 2004;164:551.

52. Hubbard RB, Smith C, Le Jeune I, et al. The association between idiopathic pulmonary fibrosis and vascular disease: a population-based study. *Am J Respir Crit Care Med.* 2008;178:1257.

53. Hyldgaard C, Hilberg O, Bendstrup E. How does comorbidity influence survival in idiopathic pulmonary fibrosis? *Resp Med.* 2014;108:647–653.

54. Sode BF, Dahl M, Nielsen SF, et al. Venous thromboembolism and risk of idiopathic interstitial pneumonia: a nationwide study. *Am J Respir Crit Care Med.* 2010;181:1085.

55. Olson A, Sprunger D, Huie T, et al. The prevalence of venous thromboembolism (vte) in pulmonary fibrosis (PF). *Am J Respir Crit Care Med.* 2011;183:A5305.

56. Collard HR, Moore BB, Flaherty KR, et al. Acute exacerbations of idiopathic pulmonary fibrosis. *Am J Respir Crit Care Med.* 2007;176:636.

57. Hubbard R, Venn A, Lewis S, et al. Lung cancer and cryptogenic fibrosing alveolitis. A population-based cohort study. *Am J Respir Crit Care Med.* 2000;161:5.

58. Turner-Warwick M, Burrows B, Johnson A. Cryptogenic fibrosing alveolitis: clinical features and their influence on survival. *Thorax.* 1980;35:171.

59. Harris JM, Johnston IDA, Rudd R, et al. Cryptogenic fibrosing alveolitis and lung cancer: the BTS study. *Thorax.* 2009;65:70.

60. Ozawa Y, Suda T, Naito T, et al. Cumulative incidence of and predictive factors for lung cancer in IPF. *Respirology.* 2009;14:723.

61. Daniels CE, Jett JR. Does interstitial lung disease predispose to lung cancer? *Curr Opin Pulm Med.* 2005;11:431.

62. Kushibe K, Kawaguchi T, Takahama M, et al. Operative indications for lung cancer with idiopathic pulmonary fibrosis. *Thorac Cardiovasc Surg.* 2007;55:505.

63. Shintani Y, Ohta M, Iwasaki T, et al. Predictive factors for postoperative acute exacerbation of interstitial pneumonia combined with lung cancer. *Gen Thorac Cardiovasc Surg.* 2010;58:182.

64. Takeda A, Enomoto T, Sanuki N, et al. Acute exacerbation of subclinical idiopathic pulmonary fibrosis triggered by hypofractionated stereotactic body radiotherapy in a patient with primary lung cancer and slightly focal honeycombing. *Radiat Med.* 2008;26:504.

65. Isobe K, Hata Y, Sakamoto S, et al. Clinical characteristics of acute respiratory deterioration in pulmonary fibrosis associated with lung cancer following anti-cancer therapy. *Respirology.* 2010;15:88.

66. De Vries J, Kessels BL, Drent M. Quality of life of idiopathic pulmonary fibrosis patients. *Eur Respir J.* 2001;17:954.

67. Swigris JJ, Kuschner WG, Jacobs SS, et al. Health-related quality of life in patients with idiopathic pulmonary fibrosis: a systematic review. *Thorax.* 2005;60:588.

68. Martinez T, Pereira C, dos Santos M, et al. Evaluation of the short-form 36-item questionnaire to measure health-related quality of life in patients with idiopathic pulmonary fibrosis. *Chest.* 2000;117:1627.

69. Chang JA, Curtis JR, Patrick DL, et al. Assessment of health-related quality of life in patients with interstitial lung disease. *Chest.* 1999;116:1175.

70. Baddini Martinez JA, Martinez TY, Lovetro Galhardo FP, et al. Dyspnea scales as a measure of health-related quality of life in patients with idiopathic pulmonary fibrosis. *Med Sci Monit.* 2002;8:R405.

71. Tzanakis N, Samiou M, Lambiri I, et al. Evaluation of health-related quality-of-life and dyspnea scales in patients with idiopathic pulmonary fibrosis. Correlation with pulmonary function tests. *Eur J Intern Med.* 2005;16:105.

72. Han MK, Swigris J, Liu L, et al. Gender influences health-related quality of life in IPF. *Respir Med.* 2010;104:724.

73. Ryerson CJ, Berkeley J, Carrieri-Kohlman VL, et al. Depression and functional status are strongly associated with dyspnea in interstitial lung disease. *Chest.* 2011;139:609.

74. Epstein LJ, Kristo D, Strollo Jr PJ, et al. Clinical guidelines for the evaluation, management and long-term care of obstructive sleep apnea in adults. *J Clin Sleep Med.* 2009;5(3):263–276.

75. Miliolia G, Bosib M, Potettib V, et al. Sleep and respiratory sleep disorders in idiopathic pulmonary fibrosis. *Sleep Med Rev.* 2015;26:57–63.

76. Mermigkis C, Stagaki E, Amfilochiou A, et al. Sleep quality and associated daytime consequences in patients with idiopathic pulmonary fibrosis. *Med Princ Pract.* 2009;18:10–15.

77. Bye P, Issa F, Berthon-Jones M, et al. Studies of oxygenation during sleep in patients with interstitial lung disease. *Am Rev Respir Dis.* 1984;129:27–32.

78. Lancaster LH, Mason WR, Parnell JA, et al. Obstructive sleep apnea is common in idiopathic pulmonary fibrosis. *Chest.* 2009;136(3):772–778.

79. Mermigkis C, Stagaki E, Tryfon S, et al. How common is sleep-disordered breathing in patients with idiopathic pulmonary fibrosis? *Sleep Breathing.* 2010;14(4):387–390.

80. Rasche K, Orth M. Sleep and breathing in idiopathic pulmonary fibrosis. *J Physiol Pharmacol.* 2009;5:13–14.

81. Schiza S, Merigkis C, Margaritopoulos GA, et al. Idiopathic pulmonary fibrosis and sleep disorders: no longer strangers in the night. *Eur Respir Rev.* 2015;24(136):327–339.

82. Mermigkis C, Bouloukaki I, Antoniou K, et al. Obstructive sleep apnea should be treated in patients with idiopathic pulmonary fibrosis. *Sleep Breath.* 2015;19:385–391.

83. Mermigkis C, Bouloukaki I, Katerina M, et al. CPAP therapy in patients with idiopathic pulmonary fibrosis and obstructive sleep apnea: does it offer a better quality of life and sleep? *Sleep Breathing.* 2013;17(4):1137–1143.

## Additional References

1a. Jankowich MD, Rounds SI. Combined pulmonary fibrosis and emphysema syndrome: a review. *Chest.* 2012;141(1):222–231.

2a. Cottin V, Cordier JF. Combined pulmonary fibrosis and emphysema in connective tissue disease. *Curr Opin Pulm Med.* 2012;18(5):418–427.

3a. Ryerson C, Hartman T, et al. Clinical features and outcomes in combined pulmonary fibrosis and emphysema in idiopathic pulmonary fibrosis. *Chest*. 2013;144(1):234–240.

4a. Lee JS, Collard HR, et al. Anti-acid treatment and disease progression in idiopathic pulmonary fibrosis: an analysis of data from three randomised controlled trials. *Lancet Respir Med*. 2013;1(5):369.

5a. Raghu G, Rochwerg B, et al. An Official ATS/ERS/JRS/ALAT Clinical Practice Guideline: treatment of idiopathic pulmonary fibrosis an update of the 2011 Clinical Practice Guideline. *Am J Respir Crit Care Med*. 2015;192(2):e3–e19.

6a. Kim WY, Mok Y, et al. Association between idiopathic pulmonary fibrosis and coronary artery disease: a case-control study and cohort analysis. *Sarcoidosis Vasc Diffuse Lung Dis*. 2015;31(4):289–296.

7a. Hubbard RB, Smith C, et al. The association between idiopathic pulmonary fibrosis and vascular disease: a population-based study. *Am J Respir Crit Care Med*. 2008;178(12):1257–1261.

8a. Raghu G, Behr J, et al. Treatment of idiopathic pulmonary fibrosis with ambrisentan: a parallel, randomized trial. *Ann Intern Med*. 2013;158(9):641–649.

9a. Raghu G, Million-Rousseau R, et al. Macitentan for the treatment of idiopathic pulmonary fibrosis: the randomized controlled MUSCI trial. *Eur Respir J*. 2013;42(6):1622–1632.

10a. Steven N, King C. Treatment of pulmonary hypertension in idiopathic pulmonary fibrosis: shortfall in efficacy or trial design? *Drug Des Dev Ther*. 2014;8:875–885.

11a. http://www.press.bayer.com/baynews/baynews.nsf/id/Bayer-Terminates-Phase-II-Study-Riociguat-Patients-Pulmonary-Hypertension-Associated-Idiopathic?OpenDocument&sessionID=1474254072.

# CHAPTER 11

# Acute Exacerbations in Patients With Idiopathic Pulmonary Fibrosis

DONG SOON KIM

---

**KEY POINTS**

- Acute exacerbation (AEx) of idiopathic pulmonary fibrosis (IPF) is an important event exerting a critical impact on the prognosis of the patients with IPF, but the real nature, etiology, the pathobiology, and therapy are not yet clear.
- Previously, it was defined as an idiopathic acute worsening of respiratory condition in the patients with IPF, but recently an international working group proposed a new definition, which removes "idiopathic" and thus excludes the necessity of invasive procedures for the diagnosis.
- It is hoped that this new definition and diagnostic criteria will improve the feasibility of future research to find effective treatment.

---

Acute exacerbation (AEx) of idiopathic pulmonary fibrosis (IPF) is now a well-known phenomenon during the course of IPF and has a critical impact on the natural course and prognosis.[1,2] However, the real nature of AEx and the exact pathobiology are not yet clear; therefore the incidence, diagnostic criteria, or treatment methods have not been clearly defined. Recently, the working group on this area proposed a new consensus definition and diagnostic criteria of AEx-IPF[3] based on the available evidences published after the first "Consensus Definition for AE-IPF" proposed by Collard et al. in 2007.[4] This new report is the most up-to-date and extensive review, which was performed by 21 pulmonologists, 3 radiologists, and 2 pathologists; more detailed information is available there.[3]

Although a diffuse alveolar damage (DAD) pattern superimposed on usual interstitial pneumonia (UIP) was recognized among the pathologists many years ago and Kondoh et al. first reported three cases of AEx-IPF in 1993,[5] not much interest was paid to AEx-IPF until Martinez and colleagues found an apparently acute and rapid progression of lung disease in almost half of the patients who died of an IPF-related cause among the placebo group of the randomized clinical trial of interferon-$\gamma$ in 2005.[6] In 2006, Kim et al. reported the clinical, radiologic, and pathologic features of 11 cases of AEx-IPF among 147 patients with IPF,[7] and several other studies reported the significance of AEx-IPF. These studies provoked interest and resulted in the first consensus definition and diagnostic criteria, proposed by an expert committee sponsored by the IPF Clinical Research Network and the National Heart Lung and Blood Institute (NHLBI), in an attempt to standardize future research.[4] Because AEx-IPF has been thought of as an idiopathic acute worsening of respiratory condition in patients with IPF, having a different pathobiology and different outcomes from the worsening caused by known causes, exclusion of other known causes such as infection, which requires an invasive procedure such as bronchoalveolar lavage (BAL), was thought to be the most important step for the diagnosis of AEx-IPF. Therefore the committee defined AEx-IPF as an acute, clinically significant deterioration of unidentifiable cause and proposed five diagnostic criteria including (1) the presence of IPF, (2) a clinical worsening of less than 30 days' duration, (3) the presence of new radiologic abnormality on high-resolution computed tomography (HRCT) (i.e., bilateral ground-glass opacification/consolidation), (4) no evidence of pulmonary infection by endotracheal aspirate or BAL, and (5) the exclusion of alternative etiologies (e.g., heart failure, pulmonary embolism, or identifiable cause of acute lung injury). Only when all five requirements are satisfied is the diagnosis definite AEx-IPF, and if not, the diagnosis is suspected AEx-IPF.[4] However, in clinical practice, such an invasive procedure is not feasible in many critically ill patients. Therefore, it is very important to clarify the exact nature of AEx-IPF for the diagnosis and the treatment.

The key question is: "What is the real nature-pathobiology of AEx-IPF? Is it an acceleration of the original disease process or other clinically occult, unrecognized secondary conditions such as infection or aspiration?"[4]

## ACUTE EXACERBATION OF IDIOPATHIC PULMONARY FIBROSIS: UNRECOGNIZED OTHER CONDITIONS?

### An Occult Infection?

Because of the similarity in clinical features between infection and AEx-IPF and also the potentially increased susceptibility to infection in these patients secondary to therapy or underlying disease, it is difficult to exclude the possibility of infection at the time of diagnosis of AEx-IPF; it may be unrecognized viral infection. Furthermore, epidemiologic studies showed that AEx-IPF is more frequent in patients taking immunosuppressive drugs[8,9] and in winter and spring[8,10] seasons, when respiratory viral infection is common. To confirm this hypothesis, Wooten et al. studied the presence of virus in prospectively collected BAL fluid of 43 AEx-IPF patients using multiplex polymerase chain reaction, panviral microarray, and high-throughput cDNA sequencing and found respiratory viruses in only six patients (two rhinoviruses and one each of parainfluenza, coronavirus, herpes simplex, and Epstein-Barr virus) and torque teno virus in 12 patients, but the significance of torque teno virus was not certain because it was detected in a similar percentage of the samples of an acute lung injury control group.[11] Later, Bando et al. reported that it seemed to be unlikely that torque teno virus would be directly involved in the onset of AEx-IPF but it could reflect the immunosuppressive state of the host because of treatment.[12] Several other studies also confirmed the low prevalence of infective organism in AEx-IPF.[12–15] These results suggest that the majority of AEx-IPF is not infection, although there is still a possibility of viral triggering of acute lung injury and disappearance at the time of clinical presentation.

### Silent Aspiration of Gastric Contents?

Because aspiration of gastric contents can cause acute lung injury, manifested by DAD on lung biopsy,[16] occult aspiration of gastric contents has been proposed as one possible cause of AEx-IPF.[4,17] Joyce Lee et al. measured the BAL pepsin level of 24 patients with AEx-IPF and 30 stable IPF controls and showed measurable BAL pepsin in most patients with stable IPF, suggesting that occult aspiration is common in IPF. Eight (33%) of the AEx-IPF patients had high BAL pepsin levels, suggesting that occult aspiration may play a role in some

cases.[18] Another study showed a significantly higher rate of gastroesophageal reflux and acute exacerbations in patients with asymmetric IPF, and most of the exacerbation occurred in the more affected side (right lung), the dependent side during sleep.[19] A post hoc analysis of the placebo arms from three clinical trials showed that AEx-IPF occurred only in those subjects not on antacid therapy (proton pump inhibitor or H2 blocker), presumably because antacid therapy reduces the potential for microaspiration-related lung injury.[17] Furthermore, among the 242 patients assigned to the placebo groups of the three trials, 124 patients taking antacid treatment at baseline had a smaller decrease in forced vital capacity (FVC) at 30 weeks, suggesting that antacid treatment could be beneficial in patients with IPF, and abnormal acid gastroesophageal reflux seems to contribute to disease progression.[20] However, recent post hoc analyses of the INPULSIS clinical trials showed that the incidence of AEx-IPF among the placebo group who were taking antacids at baseline was very high compared with other groups[21] and FVC had declined in greater degree compared with the patients who received no antacid medication at baseline, suggesting that patients treated with antacid at baseline may actually do worse.[21] The reason for this contradictory result is not certain; it may be due to the persistent acid gastroesophageal reflux after antacid therapy and/or the nonacid components present in the refluxate. These results suggest that although in some patients aspiration may trigger AEx-IPF, the majority of AEx-IPF cases are not caused by aspiration. The role of gastroesophageal reflux in AEx-IPF and IPF itself is not certain, and further prospective study to verify the efficacy of antacid is warranted.

Therefore, it is reasonable to think that most acute exacerbations of IPF are not clinically unrecognized secondary conditions, although those conditions may act as triggering factors.

## ACUTE EXACERBATION OF IDIOPATHIC PULMONARY FIBROSIS: AN ACCELERATION OF IDIOPATHIC PULMONARY FIBROSIS PROCESS?

The next possibility is that AEx-IPF may be an acceleration of an underlying disease process, enhanced fibroproliferation. Although research is ongoing, the molecular mechanisms underlying AEx-IPF remain poorly understood. Activation of the immune system, disordered coagulation/fibrinolysis, and oxidative stress may all contribute to the pathophysiology of AEx-IPF.[22] Because AEx-IPF is similar to acute respiratory distress syndrome (ARDS) clinically, radiologically, and pathologically, the pathobiology may also be similar. To investigate this possibility, Collard et al. compared the biomarker profile of stable IPF, AEx-IPF, and ARDS. In ARDS, the levels of the receptor for advanced glycation end-products (RAGE), a marker of type I alveolar epithelial cell (AEC) injury/proliferation, proinflammatory cytokines, markers of endothelial dysfunction, activated coagulation, and inhibited fibrinolysis were all elevated, whereas the AEx-IPF group had lower levels of RAGE and higher levels of Krebs von Lungen-6 (KL-6) and surfactant protein-D (markers of type II AEC proliferation and/or injury), which was similar to stable IPF but in greater degree.[23] The absence of a type I cell injury signature combined with an exuberant elevation of type II cell markers provides support for the hypothesis that AEx-IPF is predominantly a manifestation of the acceleration of an underlying disease process, rather than the result of a second, different kind of injury.

This hypothesis was also supported by a gene expression study by Konishi et al. They found that the global gene expression patterns of AEx-IPF were almost identical to those of stable IPF. AEx-IPF exhibited a fibrosis signature that was identical to stable IPF, no dramatic shift indicating a new process, and no dramatic shift in cellular phenotype. Only 579 genes related to stress response were significantly differentially expressed.[24] There was no indication of any infectious etiology or overwhelming inflammatory response.

These results suggest that the basic pathologic process of AEx-IPF is the same as or similar to that of stable IPF, but more enhanced in degree.

Then what triggers the acute acceleration of IPF disease process?

## TRIGGERING FACTORS

As discussed previously, infection or aspiration can be triggering factors, although they cannot be the main pathobiologic process of AEx-IPF itself.

1. Infection
2. Aspiration of gastric content
3. Surgery and other procedures

There are many reports about the development of AEx-IPF after the surgery, not only lung resection, but also extrathoracic, and even surgical lung biopsy, or BAL.[25–30] The mechanism is not certain, but a surgical procedure or mechanical stress by high tidal volume, high oxygen flow, or intraoperative fluid imbalance may trigger AEx-IPF.[31]

4. Air pollution

The relationship between ambient air pollution and exacerbation of respiratory diseases such as asthma and chronic obstructive pulmonary disease is well established,[32,33] and AEx-IPF may be caused by air pollution. Johansen et al. studied the relationship between the development of AEx-IPF and exposure to air pollution using the data collected by a fixed telemonitoring system situated throughout Korea since 2000 in 505 patients with IPF. They found a significant relationship between AEx-IPF and exposure to ozone and $NO_2$ during 42 days prior to AE-IPF but not to other pollutants, suggesting that increased exposure to ozone and $NO_2$ contributes to the development of AEx in some patients.[34]

5. Drugs

Many biologic (etanercept and infliximab) and non-biologic (ambrisentan) agents, immunomodulatory agents (interferon α/β, everolimus, and leflunomide), and antineoplastic therapies[35–39] can provoke interstitial pneumonia and may mimic AEx in the patients with preexisting IPF. Minegishi and colleagues reported that the incidence of acute respiratory deterioration related to anticancer treatment was 22.7% among 120 patients with lung cancer accompanied by idiopathic interstitial pneumonia.[37]

Therefore, it seems that AEx-IPF may be the acute acceleration of an underlying fibroproliferative process triggered by these extrinsic or unknown insults in patients with IPF, who already have a predisposition of exaggerated fibrosis secondary to abnormal wound healing. Several studies reported increased incidence of AEx-IPF and/or higher mortality in patients with IPF after lung cancer surgery or major thoracic surgery compared with the patients without IPF,[25,40–45] which suggests the increased susceptibility of IPF patients to extrinsic insults. Voltolini et al. reported that patients with interstitial lung disease (ILD), mostly IPF, had a higher incidence of postoperative ARDS (presumable AEx-IPF) compared with patients without ILD (13% vs. 1.8%, $P < .01$).[41]

## RISK FACTORS

Most of the studies showed that AEx-IPF is more common in patients with advanced disease,[2,8,46–48] low FVC, low diffusing capacity for carbon monoxide, low 6-min walk distance, pulmonary hypertension,[49] poor baseline oxygenation,[8,50] increased dyspnea score,[8,46] and recent decline in FVC.[46,51] Younger age,[52] comorbid coronary artery disease,[8] higher body mass index,[46] a history of AEx,[34,51] and elevated serum level of KL-6 at baseline[53] have been reported to be associated with increased risk for AEx-IPF.

## BIOMARKERS

In addition to serum KL-6, neutrophil elastase, and lactate dehydrogenase levels, which have been suggested as markers of AEx-IPF,[4,31,53–55] there are several new possible biomarkers. The levels of α-defensins,[24] circulating fibrocytes,[56] high-mobility group box-1,[57] monocyte chemotactic protein-1, soluble ST2 protein,[58] annexin-1,[59] markers of oxidative stress,[60,61] heat shock protein 47,[62] heat shock protein 70,[63] galectin-3, a mediator of fibrosis induced by TGF-β, and intercellular adhesion molecule-1[64] were reported to be elevated in the peripheral blood of patients with AEx-IPF. Tachibana et al. demonstrated in 19 patients with AEx-IPF that increased serum IL-7, an inhibitor of transforming growth factor-β production and fibroblast signaling, was associated with better prognosis in AEx-IPF.[65]

## NEW DEFINITION FOR ACUTE RESPIRATORY DETERIORATION IN IDIOPATHIC PULMONARY FIBROSIS

The consensus opinion of the international working group was that the definition should include any acute respiratory event characterized by new bilateral ground-glass opacification/consolidation not fully explained by cardiac failure or fluid overload, because there is little clinical or biologic support for distinguishing idiopathic from nonidiopathic respiratory events.[3] However, cardiogenic pulmonary edema is believed to have a distinct pathobiology and favorable prognosis compared with other causes of acute respiratory deterioration with bilateral radiologic involvement, which parallels the Berlin criteria for ARDS[66] and excludes isolated congestive heart failure. Therefore the revised definition of AEx of IPF is: an acute, clinically significant, respiratory deterioration characterized by evidence of new, widespread alveolar abnormality in patients with IPF. It is more inclusive and results in diagnostic criteria that are more feasible for clinicians and clinical trialists, who have had difficulty in the requirement for invasive microbiologic evaluation of the 2007 criteria.

## NEW DIAGNOSTIC CRITERIA

There are two changes from the previous 2007 consensus diagnostic criteria.

1. Removing "idiopathic" from the diagnostic criteria of acute exacerbation

   Because of the changing definition of AEx-IPF, the exclusion of infection or other potential triggers is no longer required.[3] However, the committee stated that this change should not discount the clinical relevance of identifying infection when present, because its

treatment may be important to the overall management of the patient.[3] In addition, they suggested that future studies are needed to test whether aggressive investigation (e.g., BAL, bronchoscopic cryobiopsy, surgical lung biopsy) of patients with AEx-IPF improves outcomes.

2. Changing the time interval from 30 days to "typically less than 1 month"

   There was a majority opinion that the 30-day time period was arbitrary and should be made more flexible to allow for cases that fall outside the time window by a few days to weeks. The phrase "typically less than 1 month" seems to retain precision but allow for the inclusion of exceptions that physicians feel clinically represent acute exacerbations.[3] A more flexible time interval than this may lead to heterogeneity among clinical trial endpoint definitions for AEx and that this could complicate comparisons between trials.

   The new consensus report emphasized the importance of HRCT in the diagnosis of AEx-IPF and stated that HRCT of the chest should be obtained in all patients in whom it can be safely performed.[3] Transbronchial biopsy is of limited utility, and surgical lung biopsy should generally be avoided because of its high morbidity in the nonelective setting.[67]

   Although the new consensus criteria excluded the workup for infection for the diagnosis,[3] it is still important to exclude the possibility of the presence of active infection, not as a triggering factor, because the treatment is different. Considering that corticosteroid is still widely used for AEx-IPF and also one therapeutic candidate for future clinical trial, misdiagnosis of infection as AEx-IPF can be a big mistake. Furthermore, clinical and radiologic features of infection, especially viral infection, are similar to AEx-IPF, and actually Song et al. reported that almost half of the patients with acute respiratory deterioration among those with IPF had infection.[2] Recently Moua et al. also reported the high frequency of infection (20%) among the patients admitted because of acute respiratory worsening.[68]

## MANAGEMENT

Supportive care remains the mainstay of treatment for AEx-IPF, focused on palliation of symptoms and correction of hypoxemia with supplemental oxygen.[1] Because of high in-hospital mortality (90%) of the patients with respiratory failure, the international guidelines on the management of IPF made a weak recommendation against the use of mechanical ventilation in these patients, although it is "a value-laden decision that is best made by the patient, clinician, and family ahead of time" based on a firm understanding of the patient's goals of care.[1]

The guidelines also give a weak recommendation of corticosteroids for the majority of patients with AEx-IPF, based on a high value on anecdotal reports of benefit and the high mortality associated with AEx-IPF.[1] There are some data suggesting that response to high-dose corticosteroid treatment may depend on the type of HRCT lesion, with better responses achieved in those with a peripheral pattern[69] and the organizing pneumonia pattern of pathology compared with the DAD pattern.[70,71] Because of the difficulty in exclusion of infection, especially in the early phase, broad-spectrum antibiotics are commonly used.

Kubo et al. reported better survival in the anticoagulation group, mostly due to reduced mortality associated with AEx-IPF, suggesting the efficacy of anticoagulation in the treatment of AEx-IPF[72]; however, because of the small sample size and methodologic limitations of this study, the benefit of anticoagulation therapy is controversial and a recent clinical trial of anticoagulation in patients with IPF showed, actually, increased mortality in the warfarin-treated group.[73]

There are several innovative treatments for AEx-IPF mostly tried in Japan, including polymyxin B–immobilized fiber column (PMX) hemoperfusion[74,75] and tacrolimus,[76] intravenous thrombomodulin,[77–79] rituximab combined with plasma exchange,[80] and intravenous immunoglobulin,[81] usually administered in addition to corticosteroids. However, these studies are mostly small and uncontrolled, using historical data or a parallel, untreated control arm.

## PROGNOSIS

AEx-IPF is certainly a leading cause of hospitalization and death[46,82] among patients with IPF, and up to 46% of deaths in IPF are preceded by an AEx.[46,83,84] In a retrospective review of 461 patients with IPF, 96 (21%) patients were hospitalized for AEx-IPF over a median follow-up period of 22.9 months.[2] Patients with an AEx-IPF had a lower median survival time than those who had not suffered an AEx-IPF (15.5 vs. 60.6 months from the diagnosis of IPF) and lower 5-year survival rates (18.4% vs. 50.0%). Collard et al. reported that patients with both definite AEx-IPF and suspected AEx-IPF have a similar prognosis.[8,14]

## PREVENTION

Clinical trials of several investigational treatments for IPF suggested that chronic treatment of IPF might reduce the incidence of AEx-IPF. A trial of sildenafil, a phosphodiesterase-5 inhibitor, showed a numerical reduction in AEx-IPF in patients given sildenafil versus placebo (3.4% vs. 7.6%),[85] but the number of events was small and the difference was not statistically significant. A Phase II study of pirfenidone in Japanese patients with IPF was terminated early based on a higher frequency of AEx-IPF in the placebo group than in the pirfenidone group.[86] However, in a Phase III trial in Japan, no significant differences were observed.[87] The definitive Phase III clinical trials of pirfenidone did not report acute exacerbations as an endpoint.[88,89] Pirfenidone has been suggested to reduce the risk of AEx postoperatively, but these data are only observational and therefore are at high risk for confounding.[90] All three placebo-controlled clinical trials of nintedanib included AEx as a key secondary endpoint. In a Phase II trial of nintedanib, time to first investigator-reported AEx was delayed in the nintedanib group.[91] However, in Phase III trials, one trial demonstrated a significant reduction in the risk of acute exacerbations with nintedanib, but the other trial showed no significant difference.[92] Pooled data demonstrated a 68% reduction in the risk of an adjudicated confirmed or suspected AEx with nintedanib therapy (5.7% on placebo vs. 1.9% on nintedanib, $P = .01$).[92] Pooled data and metaanalyses of data from the Phase II TOMORROW trial and two Phase III INPULSIS trials including 1231 patients (nintedanib n = 723, placebo n = 508) showed the hazard ratio for time to first AEx was 0.53 (95% CI: 0.34, 0.83; $P = .0047$) in favor of nintedanib.[93] No other trial drugs (acetylcysteine monotherapy, bosentan, interferon-γ, sildenafil) showed impact on prevention of AEx-IPF, and ambrisentan, imatinib, "triple therapy" (combination of prednisone, azathioprine, and acetylcysteine), and warfarin actually increased the risk of IPF.[72,73,85,94–100]

## CONCLUSION

AEx-IPF is an important event exerting a critical impact on the prognosis of patients with IPF, but the real nature, etiology, pathobiology, and therapy are not yet clear. Many studies performed after the 2007 consensus report suggested that AEx-IPF may be an acute acceleration of an underlying fibroproliferative process triggered by various extrinsic or unknown insults in patients with IPF, who already have a predisposition to exaggerated fibrosis due to abnormal wound healing. Previously, it was defined as an idiopathic acute worsening of respiratory condition in patients with IPF, but recently an international working group proposed a new definition, which removes "idiopathic" and thus excludes the necessity of invasive procedures for the diagnosis, because there is little clinical or biologic support for distinguishing idiopathic from nonidiopathic respiratory events. It is hoped that this new definition and diagnostic criteria will improve the feasibility of future research to find effective treatment.

## REFERENCES

1. Raghu G, Collard HR, Egan JJ, et al. An official ATS/ERS/JRS/ALAT statement: idiopathic pulmonary fibrosis: evidence-based guidelines for diagnosis and management. *Am J Respir Crit Care Med.* 2011;183:788–824.
2. Song JW, Hong SB, Lim CM, Koh Y, Kim DS. Acute exacerbation of idiopathic pulmonary fibrosis: incidence, risk factors and outcome. *Eur Respir J.* 2011;37:356–363.
3. Collard HR, Ryerson CJ, Corte TJ, et al. Acute exacerbation of idiopathic pulmonary fibrosis: an international working group report. *Am J Respir Crit Care Med.* 2016;194(3):265–275.
4. Collard HR, Moore BB, Flaherty KR, et al. Acute exacerbations of idiopathic pulmonary fibrosis. *Am J Respir Crit Care Med.* 2007;176:636–643.
5. Kondoh Y, Taniguchi H, Kawabata Y, Yokoi T, Suzuki K, Takagi K. Acute exacerbation in idiopathic pulmonary fibrosis. Analysis of clinical and pathologic findings in three cases. *Chest.* 1993;103:1808–1812.
6. Martinez FJ, Safrin S, Weycker D, et al. The clinical course of patients with idiopathic pulmonary fibrosis. *Ann Intern Med.* 2005;142:963–967.
7. Kim DS, Park JH, Park BK, Lee JS, Nicholson AG, Colby T. Acute exacerbation of idiopathic pulmonary fibrosis: frequency and clinical features. *Eur Respir J.* 2006;27:143–150.
8. Collard HR, Yow E, Richeldi L, Anstrom KJ, Glazer C, IPFnet Investigators. Suspected acute exacerbation of idiopathic pulmonary fibrosis as an outcome measure in clinical trials. *Respir Res.* 2013;14:73.
9. Petrosyan F, Culver DA, Reddy AJ. Role of bronchoalveolar lavage in the diagnosis of acute exacerbations of idiopathic pulmonary fibrosis: a retrospective study. *BMC Pulm Med.* 2015;15:70.
10. Simon-Blancal V, Freynet O, Nunes H, et al. Acute exacerbation of idiopathic pulmonary fibrosis: outcome and prognostic factors. *Respiration.* 2012;83:28–35.
11. Wootton SC, Kim DS, Kondoh Y, et al. Viral infection in acute exacerbation of idiopathic pulmonary fibrosis. *Am J Respir Crit Care Med.* 2011;183:1698–1702.
12. Bando M, Nakayama M, Takahashi M, et al. Serum torque teno virus DNA titer in idiopathic pulmonary fibrosis patients with acute respiratory worsening. *Intern Med.* 2015;54:1015–1019.
13. Ushiki A, Yamazaki Y, Hama M, Yasuo M, Hanaoka M, Kubo K. Viral infections in patients with an acute exacerbation of idiopathic interstitial pneumonia. *Respir Invest.* 2014;52:65–70.
14. Huie TJ, Olson AL, Cosgrove GP, et al. A detailed evaluation of acute respiratory decline in patients with fibrotic lung disease: aetiology and outcomes. *Respirology.* 2010; 15:909–917.
15. Tomioka H, Sakurai T, Hashimoto K, Iwasaki H. Acute exacerbation of idiopathic pulmonary fibrosis: role of *Chlamydophila pneumoniae* infection. *Respirology.* 2007;12:700–706.
16. Ware LB, Matthay MA. The acute respiratory distress syndrome. *N Engl J Med.* 2000;342:1334–1349.
17. Lee JS, Collard HR, Raghu G, et al. Does chronic microaspiration cause idiopathic pulmonary fibrosis? *Am J Med.* 2010;123:304–311.
18. Lee JS, Song JW, Wolters PJ, et al. Bronchoalveolar lavage pepsin in acute exacerbation of idiopathic pulmonary fibrosis. *Eur Respir J.* 2012;39:352–358.
19. Tcherakian C, Cottin V, Brillet PY, et al. Progression of idiopathic pulmonary fibrosis: lessons from asymmetrical disease. *Thorax.* 2011;66:226–231.
20. Lee JS, Collard HR, Anstrom KJ, et al. Anti-acid treatment and disease progression in idiopathic pulmonary fibrosis: an analysis of data from three randomised controlled trials. *Lancet Respir Med.* 2013;1:369–376.
21. Raghu G, Wells AU, Nicholson AG, et al. Effect of nintedanib in subgroups of idiopathic pulmonary fibrosis by diagnostic criteria. *Am J Respir Crit Care Med.* 2016.
22. Antoniou KM, Wells AU. Acute exacerbations of idiopathic pulmonary fibrosis. *Respiration.* 2013;86:265–274.
23. Collard HR, Calfee CS, Wolters PJ, et al. Plasma biomarker profiles in acute exacerbation of idiopathic pulmonary fibrosis. *Am J Physiol Lung Cell Mol Physiol.* 2010;299:L3–L7.
24. Konishi K, Gibson KF, Lindell KO, et al. Gene expression profiles of acute exacerbations of idiopathic pulmonary fibrosis. *Am J Respir Crit Care Med.* 2009;180:167–175.
25. Bando M, Ohno S, Hosono T, et al. Risk of acute exacerbation after video-assisted thoracoscopic lung biopsy for interstitial lung disease. *J Bronchol Interventional Pulmonol.* 2009;16:229–235.
26. Ghatol A, Ruhl AP, Danoff SK. Exacerbations in idiopathic pulmonary fibrosis triggered by pulmonary and nonpulmonary surgery: a case series and comprehensive review of the literature. *Lung.* 2012;190:373–380.
27. Sakamoto S, Homma S, Mun M, Fujii T, Kurosaki A, Yoshimura K. Acute exacerbation of idiopathic interstitial pneumonia following lung surgery in 3 of 68 consecutive patients: a retrospective study. *Intern Med.* 2011;50:77–85.
28. Samejima J, Tajiri M, Ogura T, et al. Thoracoscopic lung biopsy in 285 patients with diffuse pulmonary disease. *Asian Cardiovasc Thorac Ann.* 2015;23:191–197.
29. Sakamoto K, Taniguchi H, Kondoh Y, et al. Acute exacerbation of IPF following diagnostic bronchoalveolar lavage procedures. *Respir Med.* 2012;106:436–442.
30. Hiwatari N, Shimura S, Takishima T, Shirato K. Bronchoalveolar lavage as a possible cause of acute exacerbation in idiopathic pulmonary fibrosis patients. *Tohoku J Exp Med.* 1994;174:379–386.
31. Mizuno Y, Iwata H, Shirahashi K, et al. The importance of intraoperative fluid balance for the prevention of postoperative acute exacerbation of idiopathic pulmonary fibrosis after pulmonary resection for primary lung cancer. *Eur J Cardiothorac Surg.* 2012;41:e161–e165.
32. MacNee W, Donaldson K. Exacerbations of COPD: environmental mechanisms. *Chest.* 2000;117:390S–397S.
33. Andersen ZJ, Bonnelykke K, Hvidberg M, et al. Long-term exposure to air pollution and asthma hospitalisations in older adults: a cohort study. *Thorax.* 2012;67:6–11.

34. Johannson KA, Balmes JR, Collard HR. Air pollution exposure: a novel environmental risk factor for interstitial lung disease? *Chest*. 2015;147:1161–1167.

35. Malouf MA, Hopkins P, Snell G, Glanville AR. Everolimus in IPFSI. An investigator-driven study of everolimus in surgical lung biopsy confirmed idiopathic pulmonary fibrosis. *Respirology*. 2011;16:776–783.

36. Perez-Alvarez R, Perez-de-Lis M, Diaz-Lagares C, et al. Interstitial lung disease induced or exacerbated by TNF-targeted therapies: analysis of 122 cases. *Semin Arthritis Rheum*. 2011;41:256–264.

37. Minegishi Y, Takenaka K, Mizutani H, et al. Exacerbation of idiopathic interstitial pneumonias associated with lung cancer therapy. *Intern Med*. 2009;48:665–672.

38. Honore I, Nunes H, Groussard O, et al. Acute respiratory failure after interferon-gamma therapy of end-stage pulmonary fibrosis. *Am J Respir Crit Care Med*. 2003;167:953–957.

39. Yamasawa H, Sugiyama Y, Bando M, Ohno S. Drug-induced pneumonitis associated with imatinib mesylate in a patient with idiopathic pulmonary fibrosis. *Respiration*. 2008;75:350–354.

40. Watanabe A, Higami T, Ohori S, Koyanagi T, Nakashima S, Mawatari T. Is lung cancer resection indicated in patients with idiopathic pulmonary fibrosis. *J Thorac Cardiovasc Surg*. 2008;136(5):1357–1363. 1363.e1351.

41. Voltolini L, Bongiolatti S, Luzzi L, et al. Impact of interstitial lung disease on short-term and long-term survival of patients undergoing surgery for non-small-cell lung cancer: analysis of risk factors. *Eur J Cardiothorac Surg*. 2013;43:e17–e23.

42. Choi SM, Lee J, Park YS, et al. Postoperative pulmonary complications after surgery in patients with interstitial lung disease. *Respiration*. 2014;87:287–293.

43. Sato T, Teramukai S, Kondo H, et al. Impact and predictors of acute exacerbation of interstitial lung diseases after pulmonary resection for lung cancer. *J Thorac Cardiovasc Surg*. 2014;147:1604–1611.e1603.

44. Kawasaki H, Nagai K, Yoshida J, Nishimura M, Nishiwaki Y. Postoperative morbidity, mortality, and survival in lung cancer associated with idiopathic pulmonary fibrosis. *J Surg Oncol*. 2002;81:33–37.

45. Suzuki H, Sekine Y, Yoshida S, et al. Risk of acute exacerbation of interstitial pneumonia after pulmonary resection for lung cancer in patients with idiopathic pulmonary fibrosis based on preoperative high-resolution computed tomography. *Surg Today*. 2011;41:914–921.

46. Kondoh Y, Taniguchi H, Katsuta T, et al. Risk factors of acute exacerbation of idiopathic pulmonary fibrosis. *Sarcoidosis Vasculitis Diffuse Lung Dis*. 2010;27:103–110.

47. Kishaba T, Tamaki H, Shimaoka Y, Fukuyama H, Yamashiro S. Staging of acute exacerbation in patients with idiopathic pulmonary fibrosis. *Lung*. 2014;192:141–149.

48. Costabel U, Inoue Y, Richeldi L, et al. Efficacy of nintedanib in idiopathic pulmonary fibrosis across prespecified subgroups in inpulsis. *Am J Respir Crit Care Med*. 2016;193:178–185.

49. Judge EP, Fabre A, Adamali HI, Egan JJ. Acute exacerbations and pulmonary hypertension in advanced idiopathic pulmonary fibrosis. *Eur Respir J*. 2012;40:93–100.

50. Kondoh Y, Taniguchi H, Ebina M, et al. Risk factors for acute exacerbation of idiopathic pulmonary fibrosis–extended analysis of pirfenidone trial in japan. *Respir Invest*. 2015;53:271–278.

51. Reichmann WM, Yu YF, Macaulay D, Wu EQ, Nathan SD. Change in forced vital capacity and associated subsequent outcomes in patients with newly diagnosed idiopathic pulmonary fibrosis. *BMC Pulm Med*. 2015;15:167.

52. Schupp JC, Binder H, Jager B, et al. Macrophage activation in acute exacerbation of idiopathic pulmonary fibrosis. *PLoS One*. 2015;10:e0116775.

53. Ohshimo S, Ishikawa N, Horimasu Y, et al. Baseline kl-6 predicts increased risk for acute exacerbation of idiopathic pulmonary fibrosis. *Respir Med*. 2014;108:1031–1039.

54. Yokoyama A, Kohno N, Hamada H, et al. Circulating kl-6 predicts the outcome of rapidly progressive idiopathic pulmonary fibrosis. *Am J Respir Crit Care Med*. 1998;158:1680–1684.

55. Kakugawa T, Yokota S, Ishimatsu Y, et al. Serum heat shock protein 47 levels in patients with drug-induced lung disease. *Respir Res*. 2013;14:133.

56. Moeller A, Gilpin SE, Ask K, et al. Circulating fibrocytes are an indicator of poor prognosis in idiopathic pulmonary fibrosis. *Am J Respir Crit Care Med*. 2009;179:588–594.

57. Ebina M, Taniguchi H, Miyasho T, et al. Gradual increase of high mobility group protein b1 in the lungs after the onset of acute exacerbation of idiopathic pulmonary fibrosis. *Pulm Med*. 2011;2011:916486.

58. Tajima S, Oshikawa K, Tominaga S, Sugiyama Y. The increase in serum soluble ST2 protein upon acute exacerbation of idiopathic pulmonary fibrosis. *Chest*. 2003;124:1206–1214.

59. Kurosu K, Takiguchi Y, Okada O, et al. Identification of annexin 1 as a novel autoantigen in acute exacerbation of idiopathic pulmonary fibrosis. *J Immunol*. 2008;181:756–767.

60. Iwata Y, Okamoto M, Hoshino T, et al. Elevated levels of thioredoxin 1 in the lungs and sera of idiopathic pulmonary fibrosis, non-specific interstitial pneumonia and cryptogenic organizing pneumonia. *Intern Med*. 2010;49:2393–2400.

61. Matsuzawa Y, Kawashima T, Kuwabara R, et al. Change in serum marker of oxidative stress in the progression of idiopathic pulmonary fibrosis. *Pulm Pharmacol Ther*. 2015;32:1–6.

62. Kakugawa T, Yokota S, Ishimatsu Y, et al. Serum heat shock protein 47 levels are elevated in acute exacerbation of idiopathic pulmonary fibrosis. *Cell Stress Chaperones*. 2013;18:581–590.

63. Kahloon RA, Xue J, Bhargava A, et al. Patients with idiopathic pulmonary fibrosis with antibodies to heat shock protein 70 have poor prognoses. *Am J Respir Crit Care Med*. 2013;187:768–775.

64. Okuda R, Matsushima H, Aoshiba K, et al. Soluble intercellular adhesion molecule-1 for stable and acute phases of idiopathic pulmonary fibrosis. *SpringerPlus.* 2015;4:657.

65. Tachibana K, Inoue Y, Nishiyama A, et al. Polymyxin-b hemoperfusion for acute exacerbation of idiopathic pulmonary fibrosis: serum il-7 as a prognostic marker. *Sarcoidosis, Vasculitis Diffuse Lung Dis.* 2011;28:113–122.

66. Force ADT, Ranieri VM, Rubenfeld GD, et al. Acute respiratory distress syndrome: the berlin definition. *JAMA.* 2012;307:2526–2533.

67. Hutchinson JP, Fogarty AW, McKeever TM, Hubbard RB. In-hospital mortality following surgical lung biopsy for interstitial lung disease in the USA: 2000-2011. *Am J Respir Crit Care Med.* 2015.

68. Moua T, Westerly BD, Dulohery MM, Daniels CE, Ryu JH, Lim KG. Patients with fibrotic interstitial lung disease hospitalized for acute respiratory worsening: a large cohort analysis. *Chest.* 2016;149:1205–1214.

69. Akira M, Kozuka T, Yamamoto S, Sakatani M. Computed tomography findings in acute exacerbation of idiopathic pulmonary fibrosis. *Am J Respir Crit Care Med.* 2008;178:372–378.

70. Churg A, Muller NL, Silva CI, Wright JL. Acute exacerbation (acute lung injury of unknown cause) in UIP and other forms of fibrotic interstitial pneumonias. *Am J Surg Pathol.* 2007;31:277–284.

71. Silva CI, Muller NL, Fujimoto K, et al. Acute exacerbation of chronic interstitial pneumonia: high-resolution computed tomography and pathologic findings. *J Thorac Imaging.* 2007;22:221–229.

72. Kubo H, Nakayama K, Yanai M, et al. Anticoagulant therapy for idiopathic pulmonary fibrosis. *Chest.* 2005;128:1475–1482.

73. Noth I, Anstrom KJ, Calvert SB, et al. A placebo-controlled randomized trial of warfarin in idiopathic pulmonary fibrosis. *Am J Respir Crit Care Med.* 2012;186:88–95.

74. Abe S, Hayashi H, Seo Y, et al. Reduction in serum high mobility group box-1 level by polymyxin b-immobilized fiber column in patients with idiopathic pulmonary fibrosis with acute exacerbation. *Blood Purif.* 2011;32:310–316.

75. Oishi K, Mimura-Kimura Y, Miyasho T, et al. Association between cytokine removal by polymyxin b hemoperfusion and improved pulmonary oxygenation in patients with acute exacerbation of idiopathic pulmonary fibrosis. *Cytokine.* 2013;61:84–89.

76. Horita N, Akahane M, Okada Y, et al. Tacrolimus and steroid treatment for acute exacerbation of idiopathic pulmonary fibrosis. *Intern Med.* 2011;50:189–195.

77. Kataoka K, Taniguchi H, Kondoh Y, et al. Recombinant human thrombomodulin in acute exacerbation of idiopathic pulmonary fibrosis. *Chest.* 2015;148:436–443.

78. Tsushima K, Yamaguchi K, Kono Y, et al. Thrombomodulin for acute exacerbations of idiopathic pulmonary fibrosis: a proof of concept study. *Pulm Pharmacol Ther.* 2014;29:233–240.

79. Isshiki T, Sakamoto S, Kinoshita A, Sugino K, Kurosaki A, Homma S. Recombinant human soluble thrombomodulin treatment for acute exacerbation of idiopathic pulmonary fibrosis: a retrospective study. *Respiration.* 2015;89:201–207.

80. Donahoe M, Valentine VG, Chien N, et al. Correction: autoantibody-targeted treatments for acute exacerbations of idiopathic pulmonary fibrosis. *PLoS One.* 2015;10:e0133684.

81. Donahoe M, Valentine VG, Chien N, et al. Autoantibody-targeted treatments for acute exacerbations of idiopathic pulmonary fibrosis. *PLoS One.* 2015;10:e0127771.

82. Daniels CE, Yi ES, Ryu JH. Autopsy findings in 42 consecutive patients with idiopathic pulmonary fibrosis. *Eur Respir J.* 2008;32:170–174.

83. Jeon K, Chung MP, Lee KS, et al. Prognostic factors and causes of death in Korean patients with idiopathic pulmonary fibrosis. *Respir Med.* 2006;100:451–457.

84. Natsuizaka M, Chiba H, Kuronuma K, et al. Epidemiologic survey of Japanese patients with idiopathic pulmonary fibrosis and investigation of ethnic differences. *Am J Respir Crit Care Med.* 2014;190:773–779.

85. Idiopathic Pulmonary Fibrosis Clinical Research N, Zisman DA, Schwarz M, et al. A controlled trial of sildenafil in advanced idiopathic pulmonary fibrosis. *N Engl J Med.* 2010;363:620–628.

86. Azuma A, Nukiwa T, Tsuboi E, et al. Double-blind, placebo-controlled trial of pirfenidone in patients with idiopathic pulmonary fibrosis. *Am J Respir Crit Care Med.* 2005;171:1040–1047.

87. Taniguchi H, Ebina M, Kondoh Y, et al. Pirfenidone in idiopathic pulmonary fibrosis. *Eur Respir J.* 2010;35:821–829.

88. King Jr TE, Bradford WZ, Castro-Bernardini S, et al. A phase 3 trial of pirfenidone in patients with idiopathic pulmonary fibrosis. *N Engl J Med.* 2014;370:2083–2092.

89. Noble PW, Albera C, Bradford WZ, et al. Pirfenidone in patients with idiopathic pulmonary fibrosis (capacity): two randomised trials. *Lancet.* 2011;377:1760–1769.

90. Iwata T, Yoshida S, Nagato K, et al. Experience with perioperative pirfenidone for lung cancer surgery in patients with idiopathic pulmonary fibrosis. *Surg Today.* 2015;45:1263–1270.

91. Richeldi L, Costabel U, Selman M, et al. Efficacy of a tyrosine kinase inhibitor in idiopathic pulmonary fibrosis. *N Engl J Med.* 2011;365:1079–1087.

92. Richeldi L, du Bois RM, Raghu G, et al. Efficacy and safety of nintedanib in idiopathic pulmonary fibrosis. *N Engl J Med.* 2014;370:2071–2082.

93. Richeldi L, Cottin V, du Bois RM, et al. Nintedanib in patients with idiopathic pulmonary fibrosis: combined evidence from the tomorrow and inpulsis((r)) trials. *Respir Med.* 2016;113:74–79.

94. Idiopathic Pulmonary Fibrosis Clinical Research N, Martinez FJ, de Andrade JA, Anstrom KJ, King Jr TE, Raghu G. Randomized trial of acetylcysteine in idiopathic pulmonary fibrosis. *N Engl J Med.* 2014;370:2093–2101.

95. Idiopathic Pulmonary Fibrosis Clinical Research N, Raghu G, Anstrom KJ, King Jr TE, Lasky JA, Martinez FJ. Prednisone, azathioprine, and n-acetylcysteine for pulmonary fibrosis. *N Engl J Med.* 2012;366:1968–1977.

96. King Jr TE, Albera C, Bradford WZ, et al. Effect of interferon gamma-1b on survival in patients with idiopathic pulmonary fibrosis (inspire): a multicentre, randomised, placebo-controlled trial. *Lancet.* 2009;374:222–228.

97. King Jr TE, Brown KK, Raghu G, et al. Build-3: a randomized, controlled trial of bosentan in idiopathic pulmonary fibrosis. *Am J Respir Crit Care Med.* 2011;184:92–99.

98. Raghu G, Behr J, Brown KK, et al. Treatment of idiopathic pulmonary fibrosis with ambrisentan: a parallel, randomized trial. *Ann Intern Med.* 2013;158:641–649.

99. Bando M, Hosono T, Mato N, et al. Long-term efficacy of inhaled n-acetylcysteine in patients with idiopathic pulmonary fibrosis. *Intern Med.* 2010;49:2289–2296.

100. Daniels CE, Lasky JA, Limper AH, et al. Imatinib treatment for idiopathic pulmonary fibrosis: randomized placebo-controlled trial results. *Am J Respir Crit Care Med.* 2010;181:604–610.

# CHAPTER 12

# Histopathologic Approach to the Surgical Lung Biopsy in Interstitial Lung Disease

KIRK D. JONES • ANATOLY URISMAN

---

**KEY POINTS**

- Knowledge of normal anatomy can aid in the diagnosis of pulmonary interstitial disease.
- Recognition of patterns of fibrosis is important in generating a differential diagnosis.
- Evaluation of all compartments of the lung is essential in establishing a correct pathologic diagnosis.
- Clinical and radiologic correlation can aid the pathologist and refine the diagnosis.

---

Interpretation of lung biopsy specimens is an integral part in the diagnosis of interstitial lung disease. The process of evaluating a surgical lung biopsy for disease involves answering several questions. Unlike much of surgical pathology of neoplastic lung disease, arriving at the correct diagnosis in nonneoplastic lung disease often requires correlation with clinical and radiologic findings. The topic of interstitial lung disease or diffuse infiltrative lung disease covers several hundred entities, and the pathology of interstitial lung disease has been the topic of several comprehensive textbooks. This chapter is not meant to be an encyclopedic overview of the topic but is rather meant to be a launching point in the clinician's approach to the histologic evaluation of lung disease.

## WHAT DOES NORMAL LOOK LIKE?

The first step in evaluating abnormal lung tissue is to understand the normal appearance of the lung. Just as the pulmonologist knows the difference between a healthy and sick patient, so the pathologist must know the difference between normal and diseased tissue when evaluating factors such as inflammation and fibrosis.

The lung can be divided into separate anatomic compartments of alveolar spaces, alveolar interstitium, large airways, small airways, pulmonary vessels, and pleura. When examining the lung, it is important to recognize the possibility of disease in any and all of these components. In addition, the alveolar parenchyma can be divided into various zones that can aid in generation of differential diagnoses. Several definitions are required here. A primary lobule is defined as that portion of the lung supplied by one respiratory bronchiole. A secondary lobule is defined as a region of lung, centered on a respiratory bronchiole, bound on its peripheral margins by fibrous interlobular septa, and extending distally to the pleural surface (Fig. 12.1). This histologic construct is more easily recognized microscopically than the primary lobule; therefore, pathologists (and radiologists) often use the term lobule interchangeably with secondary lobule.

Much of the histologic assessment of the lung is performed by evaluation of the structures of the secondary lobule. The central portion of a secondary lobule contains the bronchovascular bundle, consisting of a small airway with associated pulmonary artery. The surrounding tissue consists of alveolar spaces and alveolar septa. The interlobular septa, at the periphery of the lobule, contain the pulmonary veins. The distal boundary of the lobule consists of the visceral pleura. The pulmonary lymphatics are present in the bronchovascular bundles, the interlobular septa, and the subpleural connective tissue. Using the structural unit of the lobule, several patterns of distribution can be described. A diffuse

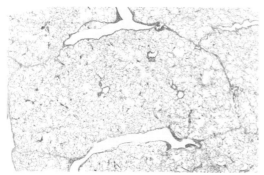

FIG. 12.1 The secondary lobule. Low-magnification image of normal lung parenchyma highlights the pulmonary lobular architecture. Bronchioles and paired branches of pulmonary artery compose the center of the lobule. The peripheral boundaries are delineated by the interlobular septa containing pulmonary veins and lymphatics and the visceral pleura.

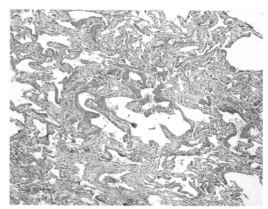

FIG. 12.2 Diffuse alveolar damage. Alveolar septa are thickened by edema and a sparse lymphocytic infiltrate. Alveolar spaces contain hyaline membranes, brightly eosinophilic filmlike material accumulating along alveolar septa.

interstitial process involves the majority of the alveolar septa within the lobule. A bronchiolocentric process shows accentuation of the disease in the tissue surrounding the small airways. A peripheral lobular pattern shows accentuation of inflammation or fibrosis in the subpleural and paraseptal regions. A lymphatic pattern shows a distribution of disease involving the subpleural regions, the interlobular septa, and the bronchovascular bundles. Other patterns of disease include angiocentric and random distribution. Several of these distribution patterns can also describe consolidative processes in which there is alveolar filling.

Once one is familiar with normal tissue, there are a series of questions that can be asked to help define the disease process within the lung biopsy.

## IS THIS ACUTE LUNG INJURY?

Two common patterns of acute lung injury include diffuse alveolar damage and organizing pneumonia. Because these diseases can mimic other chronic fibrosing diseases, the first question to ask when evaluating a biopsy is if this can all be an acute process.

Diffuse alveolar damage is a histologic pattern of lung injury that results from damage to the endothelial and epithelial component of the alveolus: the alveolar capillary and type 1 pneumocyte. Histologically, the appearance of diffuse alveolar damage varies based on the time from the initial injury.[1,2] In the first hours after injury, the leaky alveolar vascular-epithelial barrier results in an accumulation of proteinaceous fluid within the alveolar spaces. Over

the course of 12–24 h, the alveolar septa become thickened by edema and minimal acute and chronic inflammation. As the injury progresses, the alveolar walls have the appearance of granulation tissue–like fibrosis with proliferating fibroblasts within a myxoid matrix. The alveolar spaces show additional filling by hyaline membranes (Fig. 12.2). These hyaline membranes appear homogenously eosinophilic with a slight waxy appearance (the term is based on *hyalos*, Greek for glass). They are present in close apposition to the alveolar surface. Although appearing quite uniform on light microscopy, when viewed ultrastructurally, these hyaline membranes appear to be composed of a porridge of nucleoplasm, cytoplasm, fibrin, and other proteins secondary to the cell death that resulted from the acute injury. Often small vessels (usually pulmonary arteries ≤2 mm) show small luminal fibrin thrombi. This is thought to be secondary to activation of the coagulation cascade due to tissue damage.[3]

Over the course of days to weeks, the lung begins the process of attempted healing. This is termed organization and is characterized histologically by thickened alveolar septa, often with a sparse chronic inflammatory infiltrate, with a loose granulation tissuelike fibrosis. The alveolar walls are lined by type 2 pneumocytes, and there may be an increase in alveolar macrophages (Fig. 12.3). Often squamous metaplastic changes are observed in the distal bronchioles. The histologic changes of acute lung injury are summarized in Box 12.1.

The differential diagnosis in cases of acute lung injury includes infection, drug reaction, connective tissue disease, and fume inhalation injury. Many cases

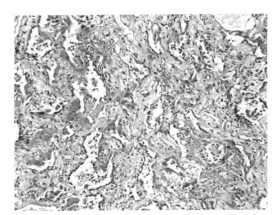

FIG. 12.3 Organizing diffuse alveolar damage. Alveolar septa are markedly thickened by granulation tissue–like fibrosis and mild chronic inflammation. There is prominent type 2 pneumocyte hyperplasia. The alveolar spaces contain increased alveolar macrophages as well as focal fibrinous material.

---

**BOX 12.1**
**Features of Acute Lung Injury**

Uniform alveolar septal thickening (may occasionally spare adjacent lobules)

Alveolar septal edema

Granulation tissue–like fibrosis

Hyaline membranes (pathognomonic of diffuse alveolar damage)

Fibrin and edema in airspaces

Type 2 pneumocyte hyperplasia

Small vessel thrombi

Squamous metaplasia of distal airways and alveolar ducts

Clinical picture of acute respiratory compromise

---

are idiopathic. Despite the prominence of neutrophils in alveolar lavage in patients with diffuse alveolar damage, most cases lack marked histologic neutrophilia. In patients with increased neutrophil levels, the differential diagnosis includes pulmonary infection, sepsis, trauma, and transfusion-related acute lung injury.

Organizing pneumonia is characterized histologically by alveolar filling with polypoid plugs of granulation tissue (Fig. 12.4A).[4,5] These plugs are rounded, are often branching, and have a myxoid edematous quality. One can usually identify a separation from the alveolar septa at the periphery of these regions of airspace organization, a feature that differentiates them from interstitial fibroplasia. The term bronchiolitis "obliterans organizing pneumonia" has been used synonymously with organizing pneumonia, but this has been discouraged because of its confusion with bronchiolitis obliterans (also known as constrictive bronchiolitis or cicatricial bronchiolitis), a disease characterized by circumferential scarring of small airways and physiologic obstruction.[6,7] In organizing pneumonia, the airspace polyps are often present within the bronchiolar lumens, mimicking bronchiolar obliteration. Often the central portion of the polypoid plug contains the organized contents of the alveolar space. These may be chronic inflammatory cells, macrophages, or aspirated foreign material. Although etiologic clues may sometimes be found within these cores (Fig. 12.4B), most often the polyps have only the appearance of bland granulation tissue. In these cases, histologic separation of cryptogenic organizing from an organizing infectious pneumonia or some other secondary organizing pneumonia (e.g., from connective tissue disease) can be a futile task.

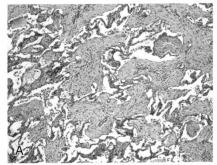
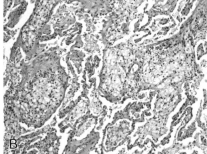

FIG. 12.4 Organizing pneumonia. (A) Cryptogenic organizing pneumonia. Alveolar spaces are consolidated by prominent rounded and branching polypoid plugs of granulation tissue. (B) Secondary organizing pneumonia due to amiodarone toxicity. Alveolar spaces are expanded by rounded aggregates of foamy macrophages containing lipidlike material. Focally, the foam cells are being incorporated into the interstitium. Type 2 pneumocyte hyperplasia is prominent.

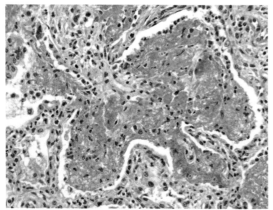

FIG. 12.5 Acute fibrinous organizing pneumonia. The alveolar duct shows a rounded branching polypoid plug of organizing fibrin with sparse mixed inflammatory cells.

A third pattern of acute lung injury is acute fibrinous organizing pneumonia.[8] This pattern has a hybrid appearance between diffuse alveolar damage and organizing pneumonia and is characterized histologically by polypoid plugs of fibrin within airspaces (Fig. 12.5).

## IS THERE FIBROSIS?

Lung fibrosis can be simply defined as excess collagen deposition in the lung. This can be in the form of loose edematous granulation tissue–like fibrosis, as in organizing diffuse alveolar damage or organizing pneumonia, or dense collagenous fibrosis, as in fibrosing interstitial pneumonias.

Fibrotic lung disease can be evaluated using a pattern-based system categorized by the distribution within the secondary lobule. Certain diseases tend to follow a characteristic pattern of fibrosis. Whether the disease shows a peripheral lobular pattern, a diffuse pattern, a bronchiolocentric pattern, or a combination of these patterns can help establish a diagnosis or differential diagnosis (Fig. 12.6).

## IS THIS USUAL INTERSTITIAL PNEUMONIA?

Usual interstitial pneumonia (UIP) is characterized by peripheral lobular fibrosis such that the fibrosis is accentuated subpleurally and along interlobular septa. The histologic diagnosis is more accurately made when evidence of chronic active disease is seen; the chronicity is represented by fibrosis and microscopic honeycombing and the activity is represented by fibroblast foci.[9,10] Microscopic honeycombing really does not look much

like honeycomb. Honeycomb, the wax structure made by bees, consists of a series of uniform hexagonal cells with thin partitions. Microscopic honeycombing of the sort observed in UIP is rarely uniform appearing and is characterized by irregular enlarged airspaces, lined by bronchiolar or cuboidal epithelium, frequently filled with mucin-containing occasional macrophages and neutrophils, surrounded by dense collagenous fibrosis often with interspersed smooth muscle. Fibroblast foci are usually present at the interface between the dense peripheral fibrosis and the central less involved lung tissue. These foci are composed of fibroblasts within an edematous myxoid matrix. The fibroblasts are often arranged with their spindled nuclei parallel to the alveolar surface. An overlying layer of plump reactive epithelial cells is frequently present at the alveolar border. Fibroblast foci can occasionally be difficult to separate from organizing pneumonia but can be recognized by histologic clues and a clinical history of chronicity (Table 12.1). This variation in the stage of fibrosis from chronic to active within the same biopsy specimen has been termed temporal heterogeneity. This term has to be used with caution, however, for not everything that shows temporal heterogeneity is UIP (e.g., a patient with fibrosis from smoking who has an acute pneumonia shows temporal heterogeneity). The temporal heterogeneity of UIP is often stereotypical with the worst fibrosis in subpleural regions, normal lung adjacent to bronchovascular bundles, and fibroblast foci at the interface between the two (Fig. 12.7). When one sees this classic temporal heterogeneity, the diagnosis is UIP and often correlates with the clinical entity idiopathic pulmonary fibrosis (IPF).

There are other diseases that may show similar histology, and it is important to look for clues that might separate them from IPF (Box 12.2).[11] Chronic hypersensitivity pneumonia may show peripheral fibrosis but is often also associated with bronchiolocentric fibrosis and poorly formed granulomas. Connective tissue disease may show a partial UIP pattern, but often the more central tissue is not normal and will have a uniform alveolar septal thickening (combining this UIP pattern with a nonspecific interstitial pneumonia [NSIP] pattern).[12,13] Connective tissue disease may also show pleural inflammation or prominent parenchymal lymphoid aggregates. Other diseases may show similar peripheral lobular fibrosis, but the distribution within the lung may be wrong. Examples of this include apical fibrous cap, subpleural fibrosis in a patient with prior spontaneous pneumothorax, or idiopathic pleuroparenchymal fibroelastosis (PPFE). Similar to UIP, PPFE can show extensive subpleural

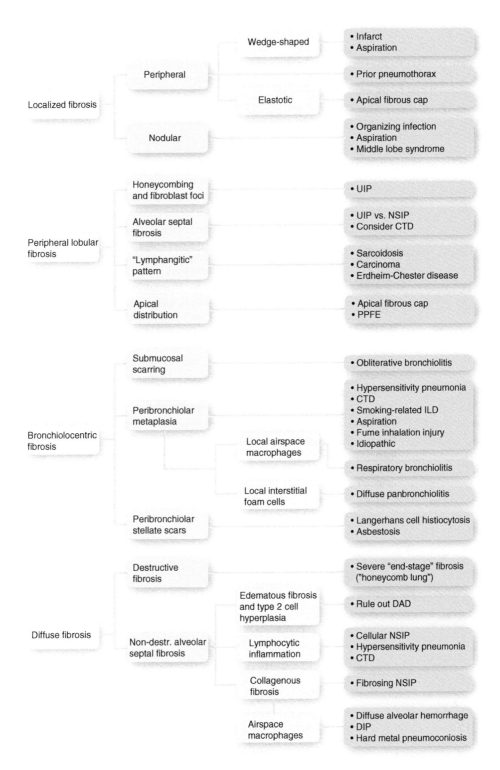

FIG. 12.6 Flow chart for lung fibrosis evaluation.

fibrosis; however, both the distribution and the character of the fibrosis differ from UIP[41]. In PPFE, the fibrosis appears slightly paler on H&E stain, and an elastic tissue stain reveals that the tissue does not show marked alveolar septal destruction but rather appears slightly collapsed and filled with fibrous tissue (atelectatic fibroelastosis) (Fig. 12.8). This last point emphasizes why it is important to correlate all histologic findings with the imaging data.

When the biopsy consists of microscopic honeycombing and there is diffuse destructive fibrosis, it is tempting to use the term end-stage fibrotic lung or honeycomb lung. This may be acceptable in cases in which the pathologist knows the extent of disease by computed tomographic scan (and there is widespread uniform fibrosis), but occasionally this is not the case, and a biopsy report of end-stage lung is overzealously given to a localized region of scarring. It is preferable to be descriptive in these cases and to make the diagnosis

### TABLE 12.1
### Differentiation of Organizing Pneumonia From Fibroblast Foci

| Organizing Pneumonia | Fibroblast Foci |
| --- | --- |
| Rounded or polypoid appearance | Bulgelike or crescentic |
| Airspace visible on most surfaces | Dense collagen present along half of surface |
| Located within airway or airspace | Located within interstitium |
| Branching common | Branching rare |
| Thin or absent surface epithelial layer | Reactive surface epithelial layer |
| Haphazardly arranged fibroblasts | Fibroblasts often parallel to alveolar surface |

### BOX 12.2
### Diagnosis of Usual Interstitial Pneumonia

**Pathologic findings**

Basilar and peripheral fibrosis grossly/radiographically

Subpleural and paraseptal fibrosis microscopically

Microscopic honeycombing subpleurally

Fibroblast foci at interface between fibrotic and less involved lung

Normal appearance of the lung in centrilobular regions

**Clues for alternative diagnoses**

Bronchiolocentric fibrosis: chronic HP, CTD, smoking-related lung disease

Granulomas: chronic HP

Centrilobular lung shows diffuse NSIP-like thickening: CTD

Pleural inflammation/fibrosis: CTD

Apical distribution: apical fibrous cap, prior pneumothorax, pneumoconiosis

Alveolar macrophage accumulation: smoking-related lung disease, drug reaction

Age <50 years: CTD, familial interstitial fibrosis (surfactant C mutations, telomerase mutations)

*CTD*, connective tissue disease; *HP*, hypersensitivity pneumonia; *NSIP*, nonspecific interstitial pneumonia.

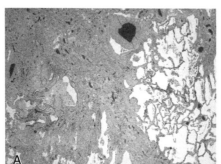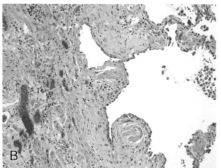

FIG. 12.7 Usual interstitial pneumonia (UIP). (A) Low-magnification image shows the classical temporal heterogeneity of UIP. Marked interstitial fibrosis with subpleural microscopic honeycombing is present at lower left, while relatively normal-appearing parenchyma is seen more centrally at lower right. (B) High-magnification view of an area at the interface between fibrotic and less involved parenchyma shows several fibroblast foci. Note the presence of type 2 cell hyperplasia in the overlying epithelium.

of extensive interstitial fibrosis with a comment explaining that a scarring process is present throughout the biopsy. If clinical and radiologic data are available, it can be stated whether the histologic features are consistent with the clinical diagnosis. In many of these cases, the clinical data support a diagnosis of UIP.

## IS THIS NONSPECIFIC INTERSTITIAL PNEUMONIA?

Diffuse widening of the alveolar septa without significant architectural destruction is referred to as NSIP. NSIP pattern can be further classified as cellular, in which inflammatory cells are the source of alveolar septal thickening,

or fibrotic, in which collagen deposition is the cause of alveolar septal thickening.[14] The pattern of fibrosis in NSIP has been described as dusty cobweb fibrosis (Fig. 12.9). This is an easy description to remember, and it effectively describes the uniform alveolar septal thickening that is observed. The alveolar architecture remains relatively intact in this nondestructive type of fibrosis until fairly late in the disease when there is often alveolar simplification. The prognosis in NSIP is related to the extent of fibrosis, with cellular cases having a favorable prognosis and fibrotic cases showing decreased survival (although still somewhat better than UIP).[10,14]

Several pulmonary diseases show an NSIP pattern (Box 12.3). The most common entities with this

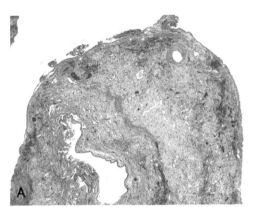
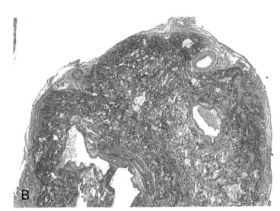

FIG. 12.8 Pleuroparenchymal fibroelastosis. (A) There is marked subpleural fibrosis. Entrapped small compressed bronchioles are observed, and there is extension of the fibrosis around bronchovascular bundles. (B) An elastic tissue stain reveals underlying intact alveolar architecture with filling of collapsed alveolar spaces by fibrosis (atelectatic fibroelastosis).

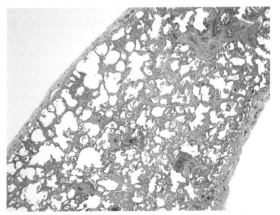

FIG. 12.9 Fibrotic nonspecific interstitial pneumonia. Low-magnification view of lung parenchyma shows variable but diffuse alveolar septal thickening by collagenous fibrosis. Patchy chronic interstitial inflammation and peribronchiolar metaplasia are present.

---

> **BOX 12.3**
> **Diagnosis of Nonspecific Interstitial Pneumonia**
>
> **Pathologic findings**
> Uniform alveolar septal thickening (i.e., there are similar degrees of inflammation or fibrosis in peripheral, central, and transitional zones within the lobule)
>
> **Clues for alternative diagnoses**
> Bronchiolocentric fibrosis: chronic HP, CTD, smoking-related ILD
> Granulomas: chronic HP
> Pleural inflammation/fibrosis: CTD
> Lymphoid aggregates/germinal centers: CTD, smoking-related ILD

*CTD,* connective tissue disease; *HP,* hypersensitivity pneumonia; *ILD,* interstitial lung disease.

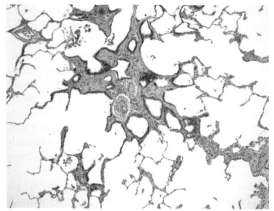

FIG. 12.10 Bronchiolocentric fibrosis. The alveolar septa surrounding a central bronchiole show mild thickening by collagenous fibrosis. The fibrosis is associated with prominent peribronchiolar metaplasia. Note the normal delicate alveolar septa more distally.

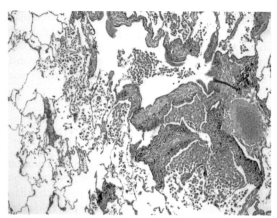

FIG. 12.11 Respiratory bronchiolitis. Alveolar spaces surrounding an airway are filled with lightly pigmented (smoker's) macrophages. Subtle bronchiolocentric fibrosis with mild chronic inflammation and peribronchiolar metaplasia are also present.

pattern are connective tissue disease, drug reactions, and hypersensitivity pneumonia. Other diseases that show diffuse alveolar septal widening that can mimic NSIP include acute diseases such as organizing diffuse alveolar damage,[2] fibrotic diseases such as smoking-related interstitial fibrosis,[15] and more unusual diseases such as the alveolar septal pattern of amyloidosis.[16]

## IS THE FIBROSIS BRONCHIOLOCENTRIC?

There are two forms of bronchiolocentric fibrosis. In the first, the fibrosis extends along the alveolar ducts and peribronchiolar alveolar septa without significant architectural destruction. This peribronchiolar fibrosis is often accompanied by a change in the alveolar lining from type 1 pneumocytes to a cuboidal or respiratory epithelium. This process is known as peribronchiolar metaplasia, bronchiolization of alveolar ducts, or lambertosis (Fig. 12.10). This peribronchiolar metaplasia often results in a lacy appearance in the central portion of the secondary lobule, which can be appreciated at low power. The second type of bronchiolocentric fibrosis, obliterative bronchiolitis, is often more difficult to identify histologically and is described later.

Peribronchiolar fibrosis is present in several conditions, most of which share a common etiology of chronic bronchiolar irritation or inflammation.[17-19] The differential diagnosis includes smoking-related interstitial lung disease (respiratory bronchiolitis [Fig. 12.11], pulmonary Langerhans cell histiocytosis), connective tissue disease, chronic hypersensitivity pneumonia, pneumoconiosis, fume inhalation injury, chronic aspiration, infection, and diffuse panbronchiolitis.

## IS THE BIOPSY TOO CELLULAR OR INFLAMED?

The normal alveolar septum is a delicate-appearing structure with only a few visible nuclei. Across the length of an alveolar wall, there are distinct spaces between nuclei, and only rare back-to-back nuclei are noted across its width. If nuclear crowding is observed with several nuclei touching each other along the length, or several septa thicker than two cells, then the interstitium is too cellular. In the normal septum, the nuclei are derived from capillary endothelial cells and pneumocytes. When the septa are too cellular, the cause is often lymphocytic inflammation. As the inflammatory infiltrate increases within the alveolar septa, the diagnosis moves from cellular nonspecific pneumonia (or cellular interstitial pneumonia) to lymphocytic interstitial pneumonia.[20] If the cellularity is accentuated around bronchioles in lymphoid follicles, the term "follicular bronchiolitis" is used.

## IS THIS CELLULAR NONSPECIFIC INTERSTITIAL PNEUMONIA?

Cellular NSIP is characterized by uniform alveolar septal thickening by mild to moderate chronic inflammation composed of lymphocytes and plasma cells.[14] The differential diagnosis in cellular NSIP is similar

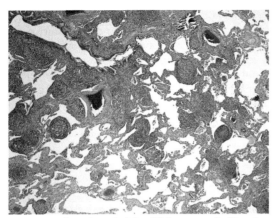

FIG. 12.12 Lymphocytic interstitial pneumonia. The alveolar septa show prominent diffuse thickening by lymphocytes, occasionally forming rounded lymphoid aggregates with germinal center formation.

to that for fibrotic NSIP. When a diagnosis of cellular NSIP is made, connective tissue disease, drug reaction, hypersensitivity pneumonia, and infection should be considered.

As the number of lymphoid aggregates and density of the lymphocytic infiltrate increase, the term lymphocytic interstitial pneumonia may be more appropriate (Fig. 12.12).[20] The question how dense should the infiltrate be tends to be subjective. Most cases tend to show alveolar septa that are at least half as wide as the adjacent alveolar space. The differential diagnosis includes connective tissue disease (e.g., Sjögren syndrome, rheumatoid arthritis), immune deficiency states (e.g., congenital human immunodeficiency viral infection, common variable immunodeficiency), and lymphoma. Lymphomas are often identified by the presence of a dominant nodule with lymphangitic extension of the inflammatory infiltrate along interlobular septa and subpleural regions. They are also more commonly of B-lymphocytic origin, whereas most cases of lymphocytic interstitial pneumonia are rich in T lymphocytes. Flow cytometric analysis of lymphocyte surface markers or immunohistochemical staining for B and T lymphocyte markers may be used to separate neoplastic lymphoproliferative disorders from nonneoplastic processes.

## ARE THERE GRANULOMAS?

Granulomas are aggregates of inflammatory cells (particularly histiocytes) that form as a result of chronic irritation, infection, inflammation, or immune stimulation. Within the lung, solitary localized granulomatous nodules or diffuse granulomatous diseases can be observed.

## HOW CAN THE GRANULOMAS BE FURTHER CLASSIFIED?

The pathologist assesses several histologic features of the granuloma simultaneously to make a correct diagnosis.[21–24] These features include aspects of distribution (e.g., random, lymphangitic), quantity (frequent or rare), and quality of the granulomas (e.g., necrosis, coalescence). In practice, most pathologists are familiar with several histologic patterns that characterize granuloma types, including sarcoidal granulomas, necrotizing granulomas, and scattered small granulomas within a background of interstitial inflammation or fibrosis (Box 12.4).

### Sarcoidal Granulomas

Sarcoidal granulomas show several classic histologic features. The granulomas are composed of tightly packed histiocytes, many of which show a characteristic boomerang-shaped nucleus. There is little to no lymphocytic inflammatory cuff (thus the designation of naked granuloma) (Fig. 12.13A). Rather the granulomas, as they age, often obtain a cuff of hyaline collagenous fibrosis. The distribution is characteristically in a lymphangitic pattern, present in bronchovascular bundles, along the pleura, and in interlobular septa (Fig. 12.13B). In addition, the granulomas frequently merge into each other, making a coalescent multinodular beading along the routes mentioned earlier. Although the classic description of sarcoidosis is nonnecrotizing, small central areas of fibrinoid necrosis can occasionally be observed, which can mimic caseation.

Sarcoidal granulomas are present in the multisystemic inflammatory disease sarcoidosis. They can also be observed in metal-related sarcoid reactions as in chronic beryllium disease and rare earth metal exposure, in drug reactions as in interferon-α or antiretroviral therapy, or in infection. Infectious granulomas often show a prominent dominant necrotic granuloma with satellite sarcoidal granulomas in the adjacent tissue.

Although the granulomas of sarcoidosis have several distinct qualities that make them some of the more easily recognizable granulomatous illnesses, most pathologists and pulmonologists have heard the mantra that sarcoidosis is a diagnosis of exclusion. The pathologist should recognize the features that make a biopsy likely to represent sarcoidosis and then give a descriptive diagnosis, such as nonnecrotizing granulomas. Then the diagnosis can be qualified with the statement "consistent with sarcoidosis" in either the diagnosis line or in a diagnostic comment.

## Necrotizing Granulomas

Granulomatous inflammation with (usually central) necrosis is referred to as necrotizing. This term is not precisely synonymous with caseating, although it is often used as such. If used accurately, the term "caseous" applies only to the gross pathologic cheeselike appearance of several necrotic lesions, including granulomas or neoplasms. There is no defined microscopic appearance that corresponds to the gross appearance of caseation; however, it usually has an eosinophilic granular quality and tends to destroy the underlying parenchymal architecture. Most necrotizing granulomas are caused by infection. Cultures should be sent at the time of surgery (either by the surgeon or by the pathologist after identification of a gross lesion). When

---

**BOX 12.4**
**Differential Diagnosis for Granulomatous Diseases**

**Sarcoidal granulomas**: Characterized by rounded, coalescent, well-defined granulomas with sparse inflammation and no necrosis

　Sarcoidosis

　Metal-related sarcoid reaction (e.g., chronic beryllium disease)

　Drug reaction (e.g., interferon-α therapy)

　Infection (sarcoidal granulomas are often present at the periphery of necrotic granulomas)

**Necrotizing granulomas**: Characterized by central necrosis with surrounding histiocytic inflammation

　With granular necrosis (caseation): mycobacterial infection, fungal infection

　With infarctlike necrosis: parasite (e.g., *Dirofilaria*), mycobacteria, fungus

　With prominent eosinophils: coccidioidomycosis, parasite

　With prominent neutrophils: blastomycosis, aspiration, actinomycosis, nocardiosis

**Interstitial pneumonias with granulomas**: Characterized by interstitial inflammation or fibrosis with small nonnecrotizing granulomas

　Hypersensitivity pneumonia

　Atypical mycobacteria (e.g., hot tub lung, Lady Windermere syndrome)

　Drug reaction (e.g., methotrexate)

　Connective tissue disease (especially Sjögren syndrome)

　Inflammatory bowel disease

　Common variable immunodeficiency (granulomatous lymphocytic interstitial lung disease)

**Mimics and granuloma-like diseases**: Characterized by histiocyte-rich inflammation or nodular necrosis

　Wegener granulomatosis

　Rheumatoid nodule

　Lymphomatoid granulomatosis

　Pulmonary venous infarction

　Malakoplakia

---

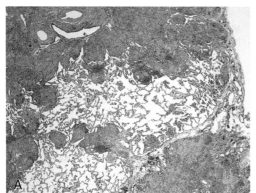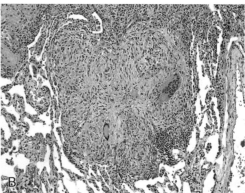

FIG. 12.13 (A) Sarcoidosis. In this low-power view, the lymphangitic distribution of coalescent rounded granulomas is observed with aggregation around bronchovascular bundle (*upper left*) and interlobular septum (*lower right*). The pleura shows mild involvement in this section. (B) Sarcoidosis. This high-power view shows a rounded single granuloma composed of epithelioid histiocytes with occasional curved nuclei and occasional multinucleate giant cells.

confronted by necrotizing granulomas, staining for fungus and staining for acid-fast bacilli should be performed. Grocott methenamine silver stain is preferred for fungi because the periodic acid–Schiff stain tends not to stain two common lung pathogens: *Pneumocystis jiroveci* and *Histoplasma capsulatum*. In a study of solitary necrotizing granulomas, El-Zammar and Katzenstein[23] noted that in cases of tuberculosis (as well as histoplasmosis) the organisms were identified only in the central necrotic portions of the granuloma. In other fungal diseases, the organisms were more randomly distributed throughout the granuloma. This information is helpful, as the biggest deterrent to identification of microorganisms on special stains is time. If the lesions appear suspect for infection, two or more blocks should be stained for microorganisms; however, pathologists should not perform stains on more blocks than they have time to carefully examine. The absence of identifiable organisms is not equivalent to the absence of infectious disease, and all cases should be correlated with clinical data and microbiologic cultures.

A small number of necrotizing granulomas are secondary to aspiration. The easiest method of recognizing such a process is when there are food particles within the granuloma. One of the more characteristic particles is leguminous pulse (Fig. 12.14). The cellulose shells and cotyledons form a rounded structure with internal smaller rounded starch granules. A vigorous giant cell reaction may be present in cases of aspiration. Acutely, one sees numerous neutrophils adjacent to the foreign material.

## Interstitial Lung Disease With Associated Small Granulomas

Several diseases are characterized by the pattern of a diffuse or bronchiolocentric alveolar septal inflammatory infiltrate (NSIP or bronchiolocentric pattern) with scattered granulomas within the interstitium. The two most common diagnoses in this scenario are hypersensitivity pneumonia and atypical mycobacterial infection in an immunocompetent host (i.e., hot tub lung).

Hypersensitivity pneumonia is an immunologically mediated pulmonary disease that results from a reaction to inhaled organic dusts.[11,25,26] The most common causes are molds, animal dander (bird antigens such as bloom), bacteria, and chemicals. The histologic findings in hypersensitivity pneumonia consist of what is sometimes referred to as a triad of four findings: (1a) a diffuse lymphoplasmacytic interstitial infiltrate, (1b) with bronchiolocentric accentuation, (2) poorly formed granulomas, and (3) foci of organizing pneumonia. The poorly formed granulomas of hypersensitivity pneumonia consist of loose aggregates of epithelioid histiocytes with or without multinucleate giant cells (Fig. 12.15). Their edges are poorly defined, and they tend to blend into the adjacent interstitium. Cholesterol clefts within giant cells are a common, but nonspecific, finding in hypersensitivity pneumonia, within granulomas or singly. Giant cells with cholesterol clefts are common in the airspaces in patients with physiologic obstruction. However, when present in the interstitium, they are more specific for hypersensitivity pneumonia.

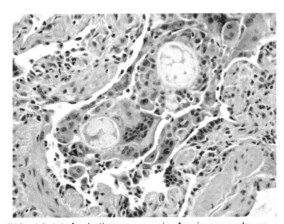

FIG. 12.14 Aspiration pneumonia. An airspace, shown at high magnification, contains several macrophages and multinucleated giant cells aggregating around aspirated foreign material with the characteristic appearance of leguminous pulse (bits of bean). Alveolar septa show mild chronic inflammation and type 2 pneumocyte hyperplasia.

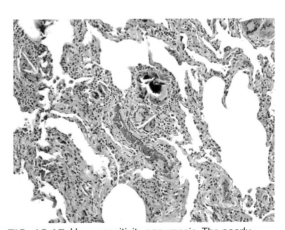

FIG. 12.15 Hypersensitivity pneumonia. The poorly formed granuloma of hypersensitivity pneumonia consists of a loose interstitial aggregate of multinucleate histiocytes with mild associated lymphocytic inflammation. One giant cell contains a chunky Schaumann body (cytoplasmic calcium carbonate), whereas another shows an acicular cleft consistent with cholesterol crystal.

Hot tub lung is a combination immunologic reaction and infection resulting from inhalation of aerosolized *Mycobacterium avium–intracellulare* complex (MAC), usually from indoor spas with Jacuzzi-like jets but also from contaminated showerheads in poorly ventilated rooms.[27,28] The biopsy in hot tub lung overlaps histologically with sarcoidosis and hypersensitivity pneumonia. The granulomas tend to be randomly distributed throughout the lung parenchyma, are usually well formed, and often occur as solitary granulomas rather than coalescent nodules. The granulomas of hot tub lung also commonly show a mild to moderate cuff of lymphocytes, unlike the usually naked granulomas of sarcoidosis. The results of special staining techniques for mycobacteria are almost always negative, but the techniques should be performed. Cultures of lung tissue or bronchial washings frequently reveal the organism; however, they may take weeks to grow out.

There are several other scenarios in which one sees MAC in immunocompetent patients: in patients with chronic obstructive pulmonary disease or bronchiectasis and in those with middle lobe syndrome (Lady Windermere syndrome).[29] In both settings, there is probable colonization and infection secondary to abnormal clearance of secretions.

## OTHER CAUSES OF CELLULAR INTERSTITIAL PNEUMONIA WITH GRANULOMAS

Several drugs may result in a histologic picture indistinguishable from hypersensitivity pneumonitis. Some of the more common culprits are methotrexate,[30] nitrofurantoin,[31] and mesalazine.[32] A useful resource when investigating whether a particular drug may result in lung injury is the website of the Groupe d'Etudes de la Pathologie Pulmonaire Iatrogène (www.pneumotox.com).[33] Necrosis within the granulomas essentially eliminates drug reaction from the differential and makes infection the likely cause. Granulomas in cases of collagen vascular disease are relatively unusual; however, in cases in which there is an extensive lymphocytic infiltrate, one can find small scattered granulomas.[34] This is most common in cases of Sjögren syndrome. Necrotic nodules with peripheral palisading histiocytes may be observed in rheumatoid nodules as part of rheumatoid arthritis. Patients with inflammatory bowel disease may have small airway involvement with or without granulomatous inflammation.[35] Lung involvement is described in both patients with

ulcerative colitis and those with Crohn disease, but granulomatous inflammation is more common in the latter. It is important to rule out a drug reaction in these patients because mesalazine (also known as mesalamine or 5-aminosalicylic acid) may also cause this histologic picture. Patients with common variable immunodeficiency often show lymphocytic interstitial pneumonia. Occasional cases will show small poorly formed granulomas. This pattern of lung disease has been recently termed granulomatous lymphocytic interstitial lung disease.[36,37] Finding a rare nonnecrotizing granuloma in specimens resected for malignancy is relatively common. They may be a result of antigen stimulation by the tumor or may be related to prior infection or immune reaction. In these cases, obtaining stains on a single block is sufficient.

## THIS LOOKS NORMAL, WHAT AM I MISSING?

It is well known that when a person is concentrating on a specific problem, other obvious changes can occur without notice. This inattentional blindness[38] can occur in the interpretation of lung biopsies when the pathologist is focused on alveolar spaces and interstitium and the other compartments of the lung, particularly small airways and blood vessels, are ignored.

### Obliterative Bronchiolitis

Obliterative bronchiolitis, also called constrictive bronchiolitis or cicatricial bronchiolitis, is a small airway disease characterized by concentric subepithelial scarring with narrowing of the bronchiolar lumens (Fig. 12.16).[17–19] In these cases, there are two primary difficulties in recognition. First, the bronchioles do not show extended long segments of fibrosis but rather show focal stenotic scarring. This leads to underrecognition due to the paucity of identifiable lesions. Second, the fibrotic lesions may completely obscure the normal appearance of the bronchiole, replacing it with a small nodular scar. To overcome these difficulties, two strategies may be used. First, multiple step sections may be obtained to increase the likelihood of observing pathologic changes, and, second, elastic tissue stains may be obtained to help identify the epithelial elastica within the scar. It is also helpful to remember that pulmonary arteries run alongside bronchioles in the centrilobular bronchovascular bundle. The identification of a scar adjacent to an artery is a clue to the diagnosis of obliterative bronchiolitis. Other histologic changes of obstruction may also be observed, including

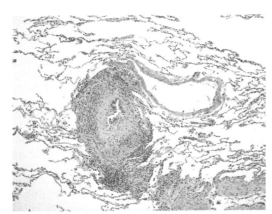

FIG. 12.16 Obliterative bronchiolitis. This bronchiole, present adjacent to its partnering pulmonary artery, shows luminal narrowing due to subepithelial scarring. The original diameter of the airway is approximated by the ring of surrounding submucosal smooth muscle.

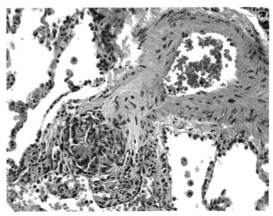

FIG. 12.17 Plexiform arteriopathy. A pulmonary artery shows mural disruption and emergence of a plexiform lesion characterized by a tangle collection of thin-walled vessels.

peribronchiolar foam cell accumulation and airspace cholesterol granuloma formation. Obliterative bronchiolitis is observed in chronic pulmonary transplant rejection, graft-versus-host disease, connective tissue disease, drug reactions, and postinfectious scarring.

### Pulmonary Hypertension

Pulmonary hypertension may result from arterial or venous abnormalities. Pulmonary arterial disease is more common and is more readily identified histologically than its venous counterpart. The pulmonary arteries show luminal narrowing characterized by several histologic patterns. Plexiform arteriopathy is recognized by bulgelike tangled small vascular channels within or adjacent to small pulmonary arteries (Fig. 12.17). Thrombotic arteriopathy shows intimal thickening and luminal occlusion with histologic changes of recanalization. Other cases show only medial and intimal thickening. Elastic tissue stains may be helpful in identifying these lesions.

Pulmonary venous hypertension tends to be a more histologically subtle finding. Although pulmonary venoocclusive disease or occlusive venopathy may rarely be seen within the large veins in the interlobular septa, it is most often present in the smaller postcapillary venules within the lung parenchyma.[39] These small veins show intimal thickening by fibrosis. Elastic tissue stains are useful in these cases both to demonstrate the degree of fibrosis and to differentiate pulmonary veins (which have a single elastic layer) from pulmonary arteries (which have a dual elastic layer). As in other

---

**BOX 12.5**
**Clues for Vascular Disease**

**Pulmonary arterial hypertension**
  Pulmonary atherosclerosis
  Plexiform lesions
**Pulmonary venous disease**
  Increased airspace siderophages
  Encrustation of vascular elastica
  Mild increase in alveolar septal cellularity
  Pulmonary capillary hemangiomatosis-like changes
  Pulmonary venous intimal sclerosis

---

causes of increased pulmonary venous pressures (e.g., sclerosing mediastinitis, congestive heart failure, mitral valve disease), there are additional histologic clues to prompt the pathologist to consider occlusive venopathy (Box 12.5).[40]

### IS THERE A DIAGNOSIS THAT I AM FORGETTING?

Absolutely. We cannot emphasize enough the value of putting together a strong team of clinicians, radiologists, and pathologists to minimize the chance of missing a diagnosis. A good clinician and radiologist can perform as the pathologist's alchemists; their data can turn a leaden descriptive diagnosis into a golden specific diagnosis.

# REFERENCES

1. Tomashefski Jr JF. Pulmonary pathology of acute respiratory distress syndrome. *Clin Chest Med.* 2000;21:435–466.
2. Beasley MB. The pathologist's approach to acute lung injury. *Arch Pathol Lab Med.* 2010;134:719–727.
3. Ware LB, Matthay MA. The acute respiratory distress syndrome. *N Engl J Med.* 2000;342:1334–1349.
4. Epler GR. Bronchiolitis obliterans organizing pneumonia: definition and clinical features. *Chest.* 1992;102(suppl 1):2S–6S.
5. Epler GR, Colby TV, McLoud TC, et al. Bronchiolitis obliterans organizing pneumonia. *N Engl J Med.* 1985;312:152–158.
6. American Thoracic Society/European Respiratory Society International Multidisciplinary Consensus Classification of the Idiopathic Interstitial Pneumonias. This joint statement of the American Thoracic Society (ATS), and the European Respiratory Society (ERS) was adopted by the ATS board of directors, June 2001 and by the ERS Executive Committee, June 2001. *Am J Respir Crit Care Med.* 2002;165:277–304.
7. Nicholson AG. Classification of idiopathic interstitial pneumonias: making sense of the alphabet soup. *Histopathology.* 2002;41:381–391.
8. Beasley MB, Franks TJ, Galvin JR, et al. Acute fibrinous and organizing pneumonia: a histological pattern of lung injury and possible variant of diffuse alveolar damage. *Arch Pathol Lab Med.* 2002;126:1064–1070.
9. Katzenstein AL, Myers JL. Idiopathic pulmonary fibrosis: clinical relevance of pathologic classification. *Am J Respir Crit Care Med.* 1998;157:1301–1315.
10. Travis WD, Matsui K, Moss J, et al. Idiopathic nonspecific interstitial pneumonia: prognostic significance of cellular and fibrosing patterns: survival comparison with usual interstitial pneumonia and desquamative interstitial pneumonia. *Am J Surg Pathol.* 2000;24:19–33.
11. Trahan S, Hanak V, Ryu JH, et al. Role of surgical lung biopsy in separating chronic hypersensitivity pneumonia from usual interstitial pneumonia/idiopathic pulmonary fibrosis: analysis of 31 biopsies from 15 patients. *Chest.* 2008;134:126–132.
12. Nicholson AG, Colby TV, Wells AU. Histopathological approach to patterns of interstitial pneumonia in patient with connective tissue disorders. *Sarcoidosis Vasc Diffuse Lung Dis.* 2002;19:10–17.
13. Nakamura Y, Chida K, Suda T, et al. Nonspecific interstitial pneumonia in collagen vascular diseases: comparison of the clinical characteristics and prognostic significance with usual interstitial pneumonia. *Sarcoidosis Vasc Diffuse Lung Dis.* 2003;20(3):235–241.
14. Katzenstein AL, Fiorelli RF. Nonspecific interstitial pneumonia/fibrosis. Histologic features and clinical significance. *Am J Surg Pathol.* 1994;18:136–147.
15. Katzenstein AL, Mukhopadhyay S, Zanardi C, et al. Clinically occult interstitial fibrosis in smokers: classification and significance of a surprisingly common finding in lobectomy specimens. *Hum Pathol.* 2010;41:316–325.
16. Utz JP, Swensen SJ, Gertz MA. Pulmonary amyloidosis. The Mayo Clinic experience from 1980 to 1993. *Ann Intern Med.* 1996;124:407–413.
17. Couture C, Colby TV. Histopathology of bronchiolar disorders. *Semin Respir Crit Care Med.* 2003;24:489–498.
18. Cordier JF. Challenges in pulmonary fibrosis. 2: bronchiolocentric fibrosis. *Thorax.* 2007;62:638–649.
19. Visscher DW, Myers JL. Bronchiolitis: the pathologist's perspective. *Proc Am Thorac Soc.* 2006;3:41–47.
20. Swigris JJ, Berry GJ, Raffin TA, et al. Lymphoid interstitial pneumonia: a narrative review. *Chest.* 2002;122:2150–2164.
21. Hutton Klein JR, Tazelaar HD, Leslie KO, et al. One hundred consecutive granulomas in a pulmonary pathology consultation practice. *Am J Surg Pathol.* 2010;34:1456–1464.
22. Cheung OY, Muhm JR, Helmers RA, et al. Surgical pathology of granulomatous interstitial pneumonia. *Ann Diagn Pathol.* 2003;7:127–138.
23. El-Zammar OA, Katzenstein AL. Pathological diagnosis of granulomatous lung disease: a review. *Histopathology.* 2007;50:289–310.
24. Mukhopadhyay S, Gal AA. Granulomatous lung disease: an approach to the differential diagnosis. *Arch Pathol Lab Med.* 2010;134:667–690.
25. Patel AM, Ryu JH, Reed CE. Hypersensitivity pneumonitis: current concepts and future questions. *J Allergy Clin Immunol.* 2001;108:661–670.
26. Coleman A, Colby TV. Histologic diagnosis of extrinsic allergic alveolitis. *Am J Surg Pathol.* 1988;12:514–518.
27. Agarwal R, Nath A. Hot-tub lung: hypersensitivity to *Mycobacterium avium* but not hypersensitivity pneumonitis. *Respir Med.* 2006;100:1478.
28. Hanak V, Kalra S, Aksamit TR, et al. Hot tub lung: presenting features and clinical course of 21 patients. *Respir Med.* 2006;100:610–615.
29. Kwon KY, Myers JL, Swensen SJ, et al. Middle lobe syndrome: a clinicopathological study of 21 patients. *Hum Pathol.* 1995;26:302–307.
30. Imokawa S, Colby TV, Leslie KO, et al. Methotrexate pneumonitis: review of the literature and histopathological findings in nine patients. *Eur Respir J.* 2000;15:373–381.
31. Taskinen E, Tukiainen P, Sovijarvi AR. Nitrofurantoin-induced alterations in pulmonary tissue. A report on five patients with acute or subacute reactions. *Acta Pathol Microbiol Scand A.* 1977;85(5):713–720.
32. Foster RA, Zander DS, Mergo PJ, et al. Mesalamine-related lung disease: clinical, radiographic, and pathologic manifestations. *Inflamm Bowel Dis.* 2003;9(5):308–315.
33. Camus P, Fanton A, Bonniaud P, et al. Interstitial lung disease induced by drugs and radiation. *Respiration.* 2004;71:301–326.
34. Colby TV. Pulmonary pathology in patients with systemic autoimmune diseases. *Clin Chest Med.* 1998;19:587–612.vii.
35. Camus P, Colby TV. The lung in inflammatory bowel disease. *Eur Respir J.* 2000;15:5–10.

36. Bates CA, Ellison MC, Lynch DA, et al. Granulomatous-lymphocytic lung disease shortens survival in common variable immunodeficiency. *J Allergy Clin Immunol.* 2004;114(2):415–421.

37. Park JH, Levinson AI. Granulomatous-lymphocytic interstitial lung disease (GLILD) in common variable immunodeficiency (CVID). *Clin Immunol.* 2010;134:97–103.

38. Simons DJ, Chabris CF. Gorillas in our midst: sustained inattentional blindness for dynamic events. *Perception.* 1999;28:1059–1074.

39. Montani D, O'Callaghan DS, Savale L, et al. Pulmonary veno-occlusive disease: recent progress and current challenges. *Respir Med.* 2010;104(suppl 1):S23–S32.

40. Lantuejoul S, Sheppard MN, Corrin B, et al. Pulmonary veno-occlusive disease and pulmonary capillary hemangiomatosis: a clinicopathologic study of 35 cases. *Am J Surg Pathol.* 2006;30:850–857.

41. Frankel SK, Cool CD, Lynch DA, Brown KK. Idiopathic pleuroparenchymal fibroelastosis: description of a novel clinicopathologic entity. *Chest.* 2004:2007–2013.

# CHAPTER 13

# Interstitial Lung Disease in the Connective Tissue Diseases

DANIELLE ANTIN-OZERKIS • AMI RUBINOWITZ • JANINE EVANS • ROBERT J. HOMER • RICHARD A. MATTHAY

---

### KEY POINTS

- Lung disease is a common manifestation of the connective tissue diseases and may be a presenting feature.
- Clinically apparent disease is often slowly progressive but may present acutely, contributing to high morbidity and mortality.
- Infection and drug reaction often share clinical features with CTD-ILD and should be considered when evaluating the patient with dyspnea and abnormal radiographic findings.
- Treatment of CTD-ILD is not well studied but typically includes corticosteroid therapy and immunosuppressive agents, as well as careful supportive care.
- Further study is needed for the many unanswered questions in this field.

---

Connective tissue diseases (CTDs) are a group of inflammatory, immune-mediated disorders in which a failure of self-tolerance leads to autoimmunity and subsequent tissue injury. Involvement of the respiratory system, particularly interstitial lung disease (ILD), is common and is an important contributor to morbidity and mortality. The presentation of ILD within the context of clinically established underlying CTD is a well-recognized complication and will be reviewed in detail later in this chapter. The CTDs in which ILD is most commonly observed include rheumatoid arthritis (RA), systemic sclerosis/scleroderma (SSc), polymyositis/dermatomyositis (PM/DM), Sjögren syndrome, and systemic lupus erythematosus (SLE). Among patients with known CTD, subclinical disease is common and raises difficult questions regarding screening, diagnosis, treatment, and the safety of disease-modifying therapies aimed at systemic extrathoracic features of disease. Other causes of parenchymal abnormalities such as drug toxicity and opportunistic infection may also masquerade as ILD and must be carefully considered before an attribution of ILD to the underlying CTD.

ILD may also be the first manifestation of systemic rheumatic disease in a previously healthy patient. Before making a diagnosis of idiopathic interstitial pneumonia, careful evaluation for possible CTD is required, as the prognosis and therapy are markedly altered. Serologic testing may offer clues. Although the radiographic findings and histopathologic appearance of connective tissue disease–associated interstitial lung disease (CTD-ILD) closely resemble those of the idiopathic interstitial pneumonias, certain features may offer clues to a previously unrecognized diagnosis of underlying CTD. Some patients do not fit into a well-defined CTD, but rheumatologic disease is suggested by symptoms and laboratory abnormalities. This group of patients has been described in various ways, including "undifferentiated CTD–associated interstitial lung disease," "lung-dominant CTD," and "autoimmune-featured ILD."[1-3] More recently a European Respiratory Society (ERS)/American Thoracic Society (ATS) research statement described this group of patients as having "interstitial pneumonia with autoimmune features."[4] Information regarding this group of patients is evolving.[5] Long-term follow-up of patients with idiopathic disease should include repeated rheumatologic evaluation as new symptoms evolve.

Few controlled trials address primary therapy aimed at the lung disease, although corticosteroids and immunosuppressive agents are often utilized. Response to therapy and prognosis vary with the underlying CTD as well as with the histopathologic pattern, although further study on these issues is needed, as data are limited.

## GENERAL APPROACH
### Respiratory Symptoms

Patients with CTD-ILD are often asymptomatic early in the disease course, and symptoms are usually nonspecific. Many patients present with dyspnea on exertion, fatigue, or cough. However, CTD-ILD in an asymptomatic patient may be discovered incidentally through radiographic abnormalities. Once lung function is significantly impaired, progressive dyspnea often develops. Over time, diffusion defects lead to exertional hypoxemia. Increased dead space ventilation also may contribute to breathlessness. Ultimately, progressive fibrosis leads to increased work of breathing due to high static recoil of the lung.[6]

The diagnosis of CTD-ILD may be delayed if patients attribute mild dyspnea to deconditioning and age. Limited functional status in patients with severe joint disease or significant muscle weakness may also contribute to delays in diagnosis. Conversely, the early onset of cough may lead to an earlier pulmonary evaluation. Other symptoms referable to the respiratory system include pleuritic chest pain secondary to serositis and other pleural involvement, or rarely the development of pneumothorax.[7,8] With advanced pulmonary fibrosis, pulmonary hypertension may develop, leading to symptoms of cor pulmonale, such as lower extremity edema and exertional chest discomfort or syncope.

### Other Review of Systems

In patients with recent-onset ILD without a known CTD diagnosis, a detailed clinical history can uncover symptoms suggestive of underlying CTD. For example, careful questioning regarding rashes may lead to the discovery of a heliotrope rash, Gottron papules, or "mechanic's hands" in DM.[9] A history of skin thickening, telangiectasias, or digital nail pitting may suggest SSc.[10] Symptoms of acid reflux or regurgitation of food or a history of dysphagia may reflect underlying esophageal dysmotility and dysfunction, as seen in SSc and PM.[9,10] Musculoskeletal system complaints such as joint pain, swelling, and inflammation, as well as morning stiffness, may lead to a diagnosis of RA, while muscle pain and proximal muscle weakness could indicate PM.[11-13] Swollen, tight skin on the fingers may be observed in SSc and PM, and a history of Raynaud

phenomenon is suggestive of underlying SSc, mixed connective tissue disease (MCTD), SLE, or PM.[10,14,15] Any new symptoms can be suggestive, and open-ended questions may lead to a definitive diagnosis.

### Physical Examination

Physical examination findings are often nonspecific but may include bibasilar fine, dry, "Velcro" crackles in patients with underlying lung fibrosis.[16] Late signs of CTD-ILD may include digital clubbing and evidence of right-sided heart failure. Notably, dermatologic and musculoskeletal signs of CTD, including rashes, sclerodactyly, skin thickening, "mechanic's hands," synovitis, joint deformities, Raynaud phenomenon, and telangiectasias, may assist in uncovering primary or mixed diagnoses. Involvement of rheumatologists accustomed to nailfold capillaroscopy and detailed joint assessments may lead to the discovery of early signs of CTD.[17]

### Serologic Testing

Serologic testing in patients with idiopathic ILD has historically been limited to antinuclear antibodies (ANA) and rheumatoid factor (RF). The most recent ATS guidelines on idiopathic pulmonary fibrosis (IPF) cite only weak evidence in support of recommendations to test ANA, RF, and anticyclic citrullinated peptide (anti-CCP) antibodies, but nonetheless recommend serologic testing in the majority of patients.[18] Distinguishing idiopathic from CTD-associated fibrotic lung disease is clinically important, particularly as new information has emerged on the treatment of IPF. In particular, immunosuppressive therapy such as with corticosteroids and azathioprine is often used in CTD-ILD but is now thought to be contraindicated in IPF patients because of increased mortality.[19] New antifibrotic medications are indicated in the treatment of IPF but are not approved for CTD-ILD.[20,21]

When careful evaluation for subtle historical and physical examination features is undertaken, it is estimated that at least 15% of patients will have evidence of underlying CTD.[22] Nearly a quarter of patients in one series who presented with presumed idiopathic interstitial pneumonia and negative ANA, but who had clinical findings of antisynthetase syndrome, were found to have antisynthetase antibodies.[23] Adjunct testing is often utilized in a search for systemic manifestations of CTD. Examples include the use of muscle enzymes (creatine kinase and aldolase), electromyography, magnetic resonance imaging (MRI) of the proximal skeletal muscles, and muscle biopsy in the evaluation of

**TABLE 13.1**
Autoantibody Testing in the Evaluation of Interstitial Lung Disease (ILD)

| Autoantibody | Type | Association With CTD |
|---|---|---|
| ANA | Antinuclear antibody | May be seen in various CTDs (SLE, SSc, SS, PM/DM) Nucleolar staining suggests SSc |
| dsDNA | Anti–double-stranded DNA antibody | Highly specific for SLE |
| SS-A | Anti-Ro antibody | SLE, SS, myositis-associated |
| SS-B | Anti-La antibody | Common in SS, 15% in SLE |
| Scl-70 | Anti-DNA topoisomerase 1 | Common in SSc (70% prevalence); high association with ILD |
| RF | Rheumatoid factor | Sensitivity 60–80% and specificity 60–85% for RA |
| CCP | Anticyclic citrullinated peptide antibody | Sensitivity 68% and specificity 96% for RA |
| RNP | Anti-U1 small nuclear ribonucleoprotein | High titers seen in MCTD |
| Jo-1, EJ, PL7, PL12, OJ | Anti-tRNA synthetases | Seen in DM/PM/antisynthetase syndrome |

*ANA*, antinuclear antibody; *CCP*, cyclic citrullinated peptide; *CTD*, connective tissue disease; *DM*, dermatomyositis; *dsDNA*, double-stranded DNA; *MCTD*, mixed connective tissue disease; *PM*, polymyositis; *RA*, rheumatoid arthritis; *RF*, rheumatoid factor; *RNP*, ribonucleoprotein; *SSc*, systemic sclerosis; *SLE*, systemic lupus erythematosus; *SS*, Sjögren syndrome.
Data from Fischer A, et al. Connective tissue disease-associated interstitial lung disease: a call for clarification. *Chest*. 2010;138(2):251–256; Duskin A, Eisenberg RA. The role of antibodies in inflammatory arthritis. *Immunol Rev*. 2010;233(1):112–125; Self SE. Autoantibody testing for autoimmune disease. *Clin Chest Med*. 2010;31(3):415–422; Peng S, Craft J. *Anti-nuclear Antibodies, in Kelley's Textbook of Rheumatology*. 8th ed. Firestein GS, ed. Saunders Elsevier: Philadelphia; 2008:741–754.

possible PM as well as barium esophagram and other motility testing in the search for evidence of dysmotility in SSc and MCTD.[24,25] Although based on small case series, many centers that specialize in the evaluation of ILD patients routinely test for autoantibodies to Ro (anti-SSA) and La (anti-SSB), topoisomerase antibodies (anti-Scl-70), antisynthetase antibodies, antiribonucleoprotein antibodies, and anti-CCP antibodies, in addition to ANA and RF (Table 13.1).[2] Extended myositis antibody panels at some centers may include anti-MDA5 (also known as CADM-140 and associated with amyopathic dermatomyositis [ADM]), PMScl (associated with PM/SSc overlap), and Ro-52 (associated with more aggressive lung disease).[26-28]

### Pulmonary Function Tests

Typical pulmonary function test (PFT) abnormalities include restrictive physiology and diffusion impairment, the latter often predating other defects.[29,30] Exercise testing is an important if underutilized modality of testing patients with ILD, frequently unmasking exertional desaturation in the patient with a normal resting arterial saturation. Desaturation with exercise may be predicted by abnormalities in lung function.[31,32] It can be explained by a combination of inadequate

pulmonary capillary recruitment with reduced time available for gas exchange, as well as reduced mixed venous oxygen content due to areas of V/Q mismatch and intrapulmonary shunt.[33,34] In more advanced fibrosis, pulmonary vascular obliteration leads to resting arterial hypoxemia and profound exertional desaturation. Oxygen desaturation with activity is common among patients with ILD.[35]

### Chest Imaging

The first suggestion of underlying ILD may arise from an abnormal chest radiograph, typically demonstrating basilar, peripheral reticular, or reticulonodular opacities.[36] However, particularly in early disease, the chest radiograph may be normal.[37] High-resolution computed tomography (HRCT) of the chest is more sensitive than the chest radiograph, particularly in the evaluation of CTD-ILD. Other thoracic features of CTD may also suggest the underlying diagnosis, if not previously known, including pleural and pericardial effusions or thickening and esophageal dilation.[38,39]

In some cases of CTD-ILD, the pattern and distribution of radiographic abnormalities observed on HRCT accurately predict the pathologic findings.[40] Common features that may be present on HRCT include ground-glass opacities (hazy areas of increased parenchymal density that do not obscure the underlying lung markings), reticulation (a series of crisscrossing lines resulting in a weblike pattern), bronchiectasis, and centrilobular nodules.[36,41,42] The abnormalities in chronic, fibrotic CTD-ILD occur predominantly at the periphery and the bases of the lung and are often associated with architectural distortion, traction bronchiectasis, and honeycombing. HRCT findings in CTD-ILD are indistinguishable from those of the idiopathic interstitial pneumonias.[43] The radiographic differential diagnosis most often includes usual interstitial pneumonia (UIP), nonspecific interstitial pneumonia (NSIP), desquamative interstitial pneumonia, and organizing pneumonia (OP), as well as mosaic, heterogeneous lung attenuation due to air trapping from obstructive small airways disease, as seen with bronchiolitis

obliterans. Mixed or unclassifiable patterns are common and should suggest a diagnosis of CTD-ILD if not previously suspected (Table 13.2).[44,45]

Among patients with idiopathic ILD, certain HRCT features predict the histopathologic findings of UIP, which is the pathologic equivalent of IPF.[41,46] In particular, the characteristic "radiographic UIP pattern" consists of peripheral, subpleural, basilar-predominant, reticular opacities in combination with basilar honeycombing, but without features, such as ground-glass opacities, that might suggest another form of ILD (Fig. 13.1). When present, these features have been demonstrated to confidently predict the presence of pathologic UIP when surgical biopsy is obtained in idiopathic ILD.[47–49] The same correlation between radiographic and pathologic UIP is assumed to occur in patients with CTD-ILD.[50]

**TABLE 13.2**

**Features of the Common Radiographic and Pathologic Patterns Observed in Connective Tissue Disease–Associated Interstitial Lung Disease**

| | Distribution on HRCT | Typical Radiographic Features | Typical Pathologic Features |
|---|---|---|---|
| **UIP** | Peripheral, subpleural<br>Basilar<br>Bilateral | Reticular markings<br>Traction bronchiectasis<br>Honeycombing<br>Minimal ground-glass opacities | Fibrosis with microscopic honeycombing<br>Fibroblastic foci<br>Heterogeneous lung involvement<br>Subpleural distribution<br>Absence of features suggesting alternative diagnosis |
| **NSIP** | Peripheral, subpleural<br>Basilar<br>Bilateral | Ground-glass opacities<br>Reticular markings<br>"NSIP line"<br>Minimal or no honeycombing | Homogeneous interstitial fibrosis and/or inflammation<br>Rare honeycombing |
| **OP** | Diffuse<br>Often peripheral and patchy<br>Occasionally peribronchovascular | Patchy ground-glass opacity and consolidation<br>Sometimes nodular | Plugs of connective tissue in small airways<br>Patchy distribution<br>Little or no fibrosis<br>Preservation of lung architecture<br>Mild interstitial chronic inflammation |
| **DAD** | Diffuse | Ground-glass opacities<br>Airspace consolidation | Hyaline membranes<br>Edema<br>Diffuse distribution<br>Uniform temporal appearance |
| **LIP** | Diffuse | Ground-glass opacities<br>Centrilobular nodules<br>Septal and bronchovascular thickening<br>Thin-walled cysts | Diffuse interstitial infiltration by T lymphocytes, plasma cells, macrophages<br>Alveolar septal distribution<br>Lymphoid hyperplasia |

*DAD*, diffuse alveolar damage; *HRCT*, high-resolution computed tomography; *LIP*, lymphoid interstitial pneumonia; *NSIP*, nonspecific interstitial pneumonia; *OP*, organizing pneumonia; *UIP*, usual interstitial pneumonia.
Data from American Thoracic Society/European Respiratory Society International Multidisciplinary Consensus Classification of the Idiopathic Interstitial Pneumonias. *Am J Respir Crit Care Med.* 2002;165(2):277–304.

A "radiographic NSIP pattern" has also been described, in which the ILD is lower lobe predominant, often sparing the immediate subpleural lung and consisting of bilateral, patchy areas of ground-glass opacity with reticulation, architectural distortion, and traction bronchiectasis but without significant honeycombing (Fig. 13.2).[44,51–53] Correlation between this radiographic pattern and the histopathologic pattern of NSIP is not reliable, as biopsies will commonly show histologic patterns other than NSIP, including UIP.[52] Some characteristics in the inflammatory forms of CTD-ILD may be suggestive of underlying pathology, such as the peripheral, patchy alveolar opacities in OP, which are sometimes peribronchovascular and migratory, but the radiographic appearance in such cases is not specific and tissue may be required for diagnosis.[54] In CTD, it is common to see multiple radiographic patterns simultaneously. When observed over time, HRCT manifestations in CTD-ILD typically demonstrate progressive reticular and honeycomb change, with occasional acute exacerbations of disease, in which diffuse ground-glass opacities are superimposed on underlying fibrotic lung disease.[55] Progressive fibrosis on HRCT is associated with worse prognosis.[56] Despite the inability to clearly predict histology through the use of HRCT in all cases, many patients with CTD do not undergo surgical lung biopsy, as histopathologic diagnosis is believed unlikely to change management. Biopsy may be considered in the setting of atypical CT findings or

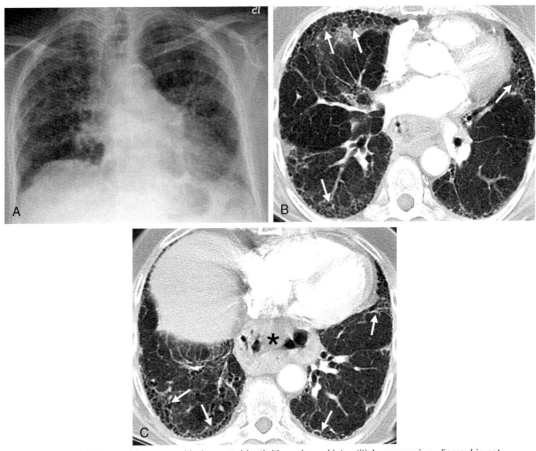

FIG. 13.1 A 73-year-old woman with rheumatoid arthritis and usual interstitial pneumonia radiographic pattern. Frontal chest radiograph (A) demonstrates reduced lung volumes with lower lobe–predominant coarse interstitial markings compatible with pulmonary fibrosis. High-resolution (1.25-mm-thick sections) CT images at the level of the midthorax (B) and lower thorax (C) show peripheral reticular markings with architectural distortion and small subpleural cysts/honeycombing (*arrows*). The patient also has a large hiatal hernia (*asterisk*).

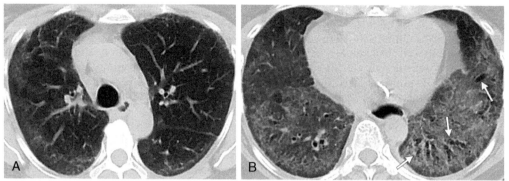

FIG. 13.2 High-resolution (1.25-mm-thick sections) CT images obtained through the midthorax (A) and lower thorax (B) in a 57-year-old woman with scleroderma who presented with cough and shortness of breath. There are bilateral areas of ground-glass opacity with a peripheral distribution (A) and lower lobe predominance (B), as well as reticular markings and traction bronchiectasis (*arrows*), all compatible with a nonspecific interstitial pneumonia pattern.

to help with prognostication, but the decision should be individualized with an assessment of risk and benefit in each individual case.[57]

### Bronchoalveolar Lavage

Bronchoalveolar lavage (BAL) has long been advocated in the evaluation of CTD-ILD because it offers a relatively noninvasive way to sample the cellular and protein composition of the lower respiratory tract in the absence of lung biopsy. Saline is instilled into the distal airways with the bronchoscope wedged in a subsegmental bronchus. Aliquots of fluid are then aspirated, forming the BAL fluid sample. The cellular differential in healthy adults consists predominantly of alveolar macrophages. Other leukocytes are present in smaller numbers, usually <15% lymphocytes, <3% neutrophils, and <2% eosinophils.[58] Research has focused on correlations between fluid characteristics and clinical features, including the presence or absence of ILD, the severity of ILD, progression of disease, and overall prognosis, as well as response to therapy.

Although BAL fluid analysis has been performed in all of the CTDs, it has received particular attention in SSc. In particular, the presence or absence of "alveolitis" has been described to reflect local inflammation, in which neutrophils and eosinophils are predominant. Despite the correlation between BAL alveolitis and severity of lung disease in SSc, BAL cytology has not been consistently demonstrated to correlate well with prognosis or response to therapy.[59] Similarly, in many of the other CTD-ILDs, BAL neutrophilia seems to correlate with poorer lung function but has not consistently proven useful for diagnosis or assessing

prognosis and response to therapy.[60–63] Multiple biomarkers in BAL fluid have been proposed to give prognostic information, but no individual finding has been adequately replicated in larger studies.[64]

The promise of BAL sampling to give clinical information is likely limited by several issues. The largest constraint is a lack of standardization in the performance of the procedure. Some of the many variables between operators include the amount of fluid instilled, the pressure with which the fluid is aspirated, the location sampled and whether this is guided by HRCT abnormalities, which aliquots are examined and whether the first is discarded, and the skill of the technician examining the fluid.[65,66] Despite published guidelines, wide variability continues to exist and likely explains much of the inconsistent data that have resulted.[67,68] Another major factor in the inconsistent interpretation of BAL fluid results is that there are other explanations relevant to the CTD-ILD population for alterations in BAL cellularity, including infection, smoking, and recurrent aspiration.[66]

Despite these issues, BAL is an important adjunct in the evaluation of radiographic abnormalities, primarily in ruling out alternative diagnoses to CTD-ILD, including eosinophilia observed in some drug reactions, diffuse alveolar hemorrhage (DAH), and opportunistic infection.[69–71] Bronchoscopy with BAL should be considered in the evaluation of new airspace opacities in any patient receiving immunosuppressive therapy to exclude infection.

### Pathology

The major pathologic patterns recognized in CTD-ILD are the same as those recognized by the 2002

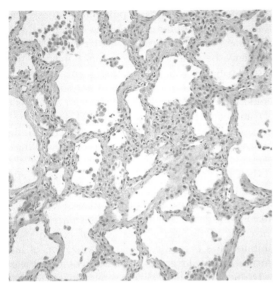

FIG. 13.3 Nonspecific interstitial pneumonia. There is diffuse septal fibrosis with a mild mononuclear infiltrate, as well as mild diffuse type II cell hypertrophy. No organizing pneumonitis or fibroblast foci are seen. No granulomas or eosinophilic infiltrate is present. Honeycombing is absent. There is a very mild accumulation of alveolar macrophages in the alveoli. 20× objective.

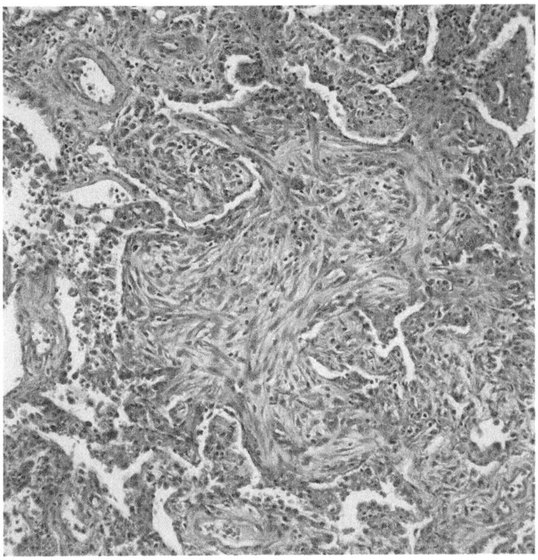

FIG. 13.4 Organizing pneumonia. There is florid fibromyxoid granulation tissue within alveolar ducts and a moderate lymphoplasmacytic infiltrate. No hyaline membranes; necrosis, neutrophilic, or eosinophilic infiltrate; or granulomas are seen. Established "collagen" fibrosis is not present, including lack of honeycombing. 10× objective.

ERS/ATS reclassification of the idiopathic interstitial pneumonias (Table 13.2).[72] UIP may be more common than NSIP in RA.[73] In other CTDs, particularly SSc and PM/DM, the NSIP pattern is the most common form (Fig. 13.3).[74,75] OP is more commonly observed in RA and PM/DM but may be present in SLE, Sjögren syndrome, and SSc (Fig. 13.4).[40] Diffuse alveolar damage (DAD), lymphoid interstitial pneumonia (LIP), and follicular bronchiolitis are less commonly observed patterns, but can complicate CTD.[7] Other findings, such as lymphoid hyperplasia and plasma cell infiltration, are more common in CTD-ILD, and when present pathologically should suggest the diagnosis if CTD has not previously been suspected.[76] Another notable feature of CTD-ILD is that several pathologic patterns may be present in the same biopsy specimen.[7,77]

Prognosis in the idiopathic interstitial pneumonias is linked with histopathologic pattern. UIP (IPF) carries a poor prognosis, while NSIP in general carries a significantly better prognosis.[31,49,78] Despite radiographic and pathologic characteristics similar to the idiopathic interstitial pneumonias, most forms of CTD-ILD have been demonstrated to carry a better prognosis than idiopathic ILD.[43,79,80] Among the CTD-ILDs, however,

RA may be the exception to this finding. Recent data suggest that the course of UIP in RA-ILD may be similar to that of IPF.[81]

## Treatment of Connective Tissue Disease–Associated Interstitial Lung Disease

### Immunosuppressive therapy

Many forms of CTD-ILD show responsiveness to immunosuppression. The decision to initiate immunosuppressive therapy should include an assessment of the likelihood of response as well as the risks and side effects of the medications. Corticosteroids have many potential toxicities, including glucose intolerance, bone loss, cataract development, delirium, and mood instability.[82] Underlying clinical characteristics, such as the patient's age and comorbidities (diabetes mellitus, osteoporosis, psychiatric disease), should be strongly considered. Frequently in CTD-ILD, a more prolonged course of therapy is warranted, and the early addition of steroid-sparing medications can allow for lower doses of corticosteroids. Severity of disease, or particular CTD (such as SSc), may dictate the use of cytotoxic agents such as cyclophosphamide or mycophenolate mofetil (MMF). These medications should be prescribed only by physicians familiar with their use and potential toxicities. Measures of objective improvement, including PFTs, exercise oximetry, and radiographic studies should be utilized. This is particularly true with the use of corticosteroids, which lead to an increase in energy level and mood, making subjective measures of patient assessment problematic. When patients either demonstrate progression despite ongoing therapy or show no improvement in the rate of decline in lung function after 6 months of therapy, discontinuation should be considered to avoid toxicity without the likelihood of benefit.

### Supportive therapy

Measures aimed at improving quality of life and decreasing respiratory symptoms should be considered in all patients with CTD-ILD. Pulse oximetry testing can uncover resting and exertional hypoxemia. Even simple ambulation in the hallway can unmask exertional desaturation and the need for supplemental oxygen. Oxygen use has not been well studied in CTD-ILD, but the use of supplemental oxygen and correction of exertional hypoxemia have been demonstrated to improve exercise capacity.[83,84] It is recommended to maintain saturations >90% at rest or with exercise while further study regarding mortality benefit is ongoing.[85] Similarly, nocturnal oxygen is utilized, based on data demonstrating the negative impact nocturnal hypoxemia has on quality of life.[86] A wide variety of options are available to provide convenient, portable systems.

A large body of evidence demonstrates that a structured form of exercise such as pulmonary rehabilitation clearly improves muscle strength and endurance in chronic obstructive pulmonary disease.[87,88] Compelling data supporting the use of pulmonary rehabilitation in ILD are now increasing.[89–94] In addition to the benefits of improved exercise tolerance, patients with ILD may also benefit from education regarding oxygen use, breathing and pacing techniques, and social support.[87] Pulmonary rehabilitation can assist in the identification of anxiety and depression, a common problem for patients with chronic lung disease.[95]

### Treatment of comorbidities

Patients with CTD-ILD frequently have comorbid conditions, which need to be addressed. Particularly in dyspneic patients, investigations for the presence of ischemic heart disease should be undertaken in patients with other cardiovascular risk factors. The risk for ischemic heart disease is increased among patients with ILD, and patients with SLE and RA are at risk for premature atherosclerosis.[96,97] Patients should also be counseled regarding smoking cessation. In particular,

patients with some forms of pulmonary fibrosis have an increased risk of developing lung cancer, and CTD itself may carry some risk for malignancy.[85,98,99] The prevalence of obstructive sleep apnea may be high among patients with ILD, even in the absence of excessive sleepiness or obesity, and polysomnography should be considered.[100–102] Patients with all forms of ILD, and particularly patients with CTD, seem to be at increased risk for development of thromboembolic disease and should have new complaints of leg swelling or shortness of breath evaluated with this in mind.[103–107]

There is a high prevalence of gastroesophageal reflux disease (GERD), often asymptomatic, among patients with IPF.[108,109] Some data suggest that GERD may be linked to the development of IPF and is correlated with worsening of disease, whereas use of proton pump inhibitors has been linked with stabilization of lung function, reduced risk for exacerbation of lung disease, and reduced mortality.[110,111] Close ties between SSc lung disease and GERD are also suspected and many forms of CTD may be strongly associated with GERD.[112–114] The question of when to seek evidence of and to treat asymptomatic GERD is less clear.[85] Lifestyle modifications such as specific trigger food avoidance, taking smaller, more frequent meals, avoiding late eating, and elevation of the head of bed can all be attempted.[115] Medications such as H2-receptor antagonists and proton pump inhibitors may be required, and promotility agents such as domperidone are utilized in some cases.[116] Surgical interventions are rarely considered, often in the setting of lung transplantation.[117]

Pulmonary hypertension develops in a significant proportion of patients with ILD, often because of the effects of chronic hypoxia and the destruction of capillaries by the fibrotic process.[118] Additionally, pulmonary arterial hypertension (PAH) may complicate several of the CTDs, particularly scleroderma, MCTD, SLE, PM/DM, and more rarely RA.[119] PH contributes to diffusion impairment and symptoms. Right-sided heart catheterization may be needed to further characterize the nature of the pulmonary hypertension, as well as to assess any role of left-sided heart dysfunction.[118,120] Therapy for the combination of ILD and PH is controversial but may be considered.[121–123]

### Lung transplantation

Lung transplantation should be considered for patients with advanced, progressive CTD-ILD. Data suggest that carefully selected patients with CTD may have equivalent survival to other patients undergoing lung transplantation, particularly if esophageal dysfunction is addressed.[124–127] The lung allocation score tends to prioritize patients with advanced ILD.[128] Decisions regarding whether and when to list are challenging in CTD-ILD because the rate of progression is difficult to predict, and a sudden, unanticipated exacerbation of disease may occur.[129] In the idiopathic ILDs, fibrotic lung disease with a severely impaired diffusing capacity of the lungs for carbon monoxide (DLCO) (less than 39% predicted) predicts poor survival due to the underlying disease, and this measure is one often used to prompt evaluation for listing.[130] Lung transplantation requires the emotional and physical ability to tolerate a complex medical regimen of immunosuppressive therapy.[131]

## RHEUMATOID ARTHRITIS

RA is a chronic inflammatory disease affecting the synovial lined joints and symmetrically involves the small joints of the hands and feet.[11] The diagnosis of RA has typically been made with the use of criteria proposed by the American Rheumatism Association in 1987.[11] However, the use of newer molecular markers such as anti-CCP antibodies has led to earlier diagnosis, reflected in the criteria proposed in 2010 by the American College of Rheumatology (ACR) and European League Against Rheumatism (EULAR) (Table 13.3).[132,133] RA occurs most commonly in women between the ages of 35 and 50 years, although men are also affected.[134,135]

Pulmonary disease is a major source of morbidity and mortality in RA, manifesting most commonly as ILD, obstructive airways disease, and pleural involvement.[134] Rheumatoid nodules are more rare, seen in men with advanced RA. RA-associated ILD (RA-ILD) is often diagnosed in the setting of long-standing RA, but may present before or at the same time as arthritis and other rheumatologic complaints.[136] In general, RA-ILD tends to be slowly progressive; however, some patients may experience periods of sudden deterioration and ~10% of patients die of progressive respiratory failure.[55,137,138] Hospitalization for a respiratory cause predicts high mortality over the subsequent 5 years.[139] Risk factors for the development of RA-ILD include anti-CCP antibody titers, older age, male sex, and a history of cigarette smoking.[140,141]

Early reports prompted increased awareness of ILD in RA.[142–145] Estimates of its prevalence vary, largely because of variations in the sensitivity of the modalities used. For example, ILD identified by chest radiograph alone in patients with RA was present in fewer than 5% of patients.[37] Studies utilizing PFTs identified ILD in 33–41% of RA patients and HRCT identified

---

**TABLE 13.3**

**2010 ACR/EULAR Criteria for the Diagnosis of Rheumatoid Arthritis**

1. Presence of synovitis in at least one joint
2. Absence of an alternative diagnosis to explain the synovitis
3. Score of at least 6 out of 10 from the following list
4. Evidence of long-standing or inactive disease with previous fulfillment of criteria

**1. JOINTS**

| | |
|---|---|
| 2–10 large joints (shoulder, elbow, hip, knee, ankle) | 1 point |
| 1–3 small joints | 2 points |
| 4–10 small joints | 3 points |
| More than 10 joints (at least one small joint) | 5 points |

**2. SEROLOGY**

| | |
|---|---|
| Low-positive RF or anti-CCP | 2 points |
| High-positive RF or anti-CCP | 3 points |

**3. ACUTE PHASE REACTANTS**

| | |
|---|---|
| Elevated CRP or ESR | 1 point |

**4. DURATION OF SYMPTOMS**

| | |
|---|---|
| At least 6 weeks | 1 point |

*anti-CCP*, anticyclic citrullinated peptide; *CRP*, C-reactive protein; *ESR*, erythrocyte sedimentation rate; *RF*, rheumatoid factor.
Adapted from Aletaha, D et al. Rheumatoid arthritis classification criteria: an American College of Rheumatology/European League Against Rheumatism collaborative initiative. *Arthritis Rheum.* 2010;62(9):2569–2581, with permission.

---

abnormalities in 20–63%, which have been confirmed by autopsy studies.[29,30,137,138,146–148] Retrospective population-based studies have estimated a much lower rate of clinically significant ILD among RA patients (6.3–9.4%).[149,150] Although it is possible that HRCT and PFT identify abnormalities without clinical significance, it is also likely that significant ILD is underrecognized in this population.

### Clinical Features

Generally, ILD occurs in patients with well-established RA.[151] However, up to 20% of patients have onset of ILD before the diagnosis of RA.[140] Among patients with idiopathic ILD who are found to have RA-related autoantibodies such as RF and anti-CCP but no articular findings of RA, some eventually develop clinical RA.[152] The delay between presentation of lung disease

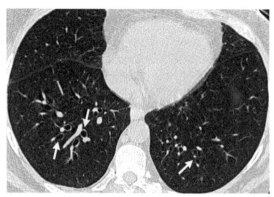

FIG. 13.5 56-year-old woman with rheumatoid arthritis and bronchiectasis. High-resolution (1.25-mm-thick sections) CT image through the lower thorax demonstrates mild, cylindrical bronchiectasis (*arrows*) in both lower lobes.

and subsequent joint symptoms can be as long as 6 years.[140,153] Similar to other forms of CTD, it is important to distinguish interstitial abnormalities related to drug toxicity or opportunistic infection before attributing the findings to RA-ILD. Often making this distinction is challenging and relies on the relationship between the time of medication exposure, response to withdrawal of the agent, and other adjunct testing, such as bronchoscopy with BAL.

RA-ILD typically presents with progressive dyspnea, although cough and pleuritic chest pain may occur.[8] Physical examination findings are often nonspecific and may include bibasilar fine, dry, "Velcro" crackles. Digital clubbing and evidence of right-sided heart failure are late signs of RA-ILD.

PFTs in RA-ILD typically demonstrate restrictive physiology and diffusion impairment. A defect in $D_{LCO}$ is often the earliest PFT finding in RA-ILD.[29,30] Exertional arterial oxygen desaturation may be present despite normal resting saturations and is predicted by abnormalities in lung function.[31,32]

### Radiographic Features

The most common features on HRCT in RA-ILD are ground-glass opacities, reticulation, bronchiectasis (Fig. 13.5), and micronodules.[36,41,42] In particular, the findings in RA-ILD have been grouped into four main patterns: a UIP pattern consisting of lower lobe–predominant subpleural reticulations and honeycombing; an NSIP pattern consisting of predominantly lower lobe reticulation and ground-glass opacities; a bronchiolitis pattern demonstrating centrilobular micronodules and bronchiectasis or bronchiolectasis; and an OP pattern consisting of largely peripheral airspace

consolidation and ground-glass opacities.[41] Based on several small studies, it is likely that the radiographic UIP pattern in RA-ILD predicts a pathologic finding of UIP.[50,73] The presence of a radiographic UIP pattern seems to predict increased mortality.[141] It is not clear that the radiographic NSIP pattern is similarly predictive of its pathologic correlate.[52,154] Patients with a ground-glass–predominant pattern may have a better prognosis than those with well-established fibrosis.[55] On serial HRCT, RA-ILD may manifest radiographically with acute exacerbations of disease characterized by the onset of diffuse ground-glass opacities, or with progressive reticulation, traction bronchiectasis, and honeycombing.[55] Care should be taken with the interpretation of ground-glass opacities when a mosaic pattern is present. Inspiratory and expiratory high-resolution images are useful to help distinguish ground-glass opacities from mosaic lung attenuation due to small airways obstruction, in which the denser areas reflect normal lung adjacent to radiolucent areas of air trapping. This finding is observed in RA-associated bronchiolitis obliterans (Fig. 13.6).

### Pathologic Features

In contrast to the other CTD-ILDs, the pathology of RA-ILD demonstrates a preponderance of UIP.[73] Certain features, such as lymphoid hyperplasia and plasma cell infiltration, as well as the presence of more than one pathologic process in the same biopsy specimen, are quite common in RA-ILD and should suggest the diagnosis (Fig. 13.7).[7,76,77] Some less common histopathologic patterns observed in RA include OP, follicular bronchiolitis, LIP, and DAD.[7] RA-ILD may not share the favorable prognosis some other forms of CTD-ILD seem to carry.[155] In fact, data suggest that the course of UIP in RA-ILD may be inexorable and fatal as seen in IPF (idiopathic UIP).[81]

Diagnostically, the differentiation between infection, drug reaction, and underlying RA-ILD can be difficult, as many of the drugs used to treat RA can cause pulmonary toxicity (e.g., methotrexate, leflunomide, and the tumor necrosis factor alpha [TNF-α] inhibitors [etanercept, infliximab, and adalimumab]) and can also predispose to opportunistic infection.[156–162] The diagnosis of RA-ILD should take into consideration the clinical features, the radiographic appearance, the pathology, and the temporal correlation with drug initiation or withdrawal.[163,164] Several different pathologic patterns may be consistent with drug toxicity, including cellular interstitial infiltrates, granulomas, tissue eosinophilia, and a DAD pattern with perivascular inflammation.[156,165]

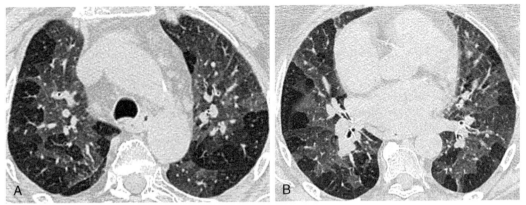

FIG. 13.6 65-year-old woman with rheumatoid arthritis and progressive shortness of breath secondary to bronchiolitis obliterans. High-resolution (1.25-mm sections) CT images performed during expiration at the level of the upper thorax (A) and midthorax (B) demonstrate multifocal lucent areas of moderate to severe air trapping. The *grayer areas* are normal lung at expiration.

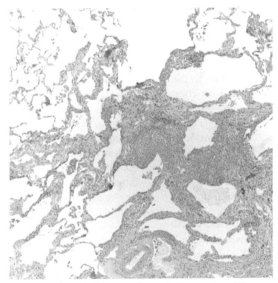

FIG. 13.7 Lymphoid hyperplasia. In the center of the image, there is a lymphoid follicle with a germinal center. Fibroblast foci and organizing pneumonitis are not present. There is established fibrosis. While lymphoid hyperplasia in end-stage lung is nonspecific, in areas away from end-stage lung, this finding suggests collagen vascular disease. 4× objective.

## Treatment

There are many unanswered questions pertaining to RA-ILD, in particular, whether to treat subclinical disease and which therapies should be utilized. However, progressive lung disease is typically treated aggressively because response has been reported with corticosteroids, azathioprine, cyclosporine, and cyclophosphamide.[16,166,167] If there is no response, therapy can be discontinued to avoid toxicity without hope of benefit. MMF has been reported to have a beneficial effect on CTD-ILD and may be considered in RA-ILD, although it does not generally treat the articular manifestations, necessitating that an additional agent be added.[167-169] Data for the use of rituximab in RA-ILD are mixed. Some reports have indicated safety and stabilization of disease, while others have been inconclusive.[170-172] Some reports suggest that TNF-α inhibitors may be effective in RA-ILD, but others report cases of pulmonary toxicity in patients with underlying ILD.[160,161,173] Limited data exist regarding the use of other biologics such as abatacept, tocilizumab, and anakinra.[174] Lung transplant referral should be considered in patients with severe fibrotic lung disease. Patients receiving lung transplants for RA-ILD seem to have survival rates similar to IPF patients and experience a significant improvement in quality of life with regard to respiratory symptoms.[175]

## SYSTEMIC SCLEROSIS (SCLERODERMA)

SSc is a multisystem disorder characterized by endothelial and epithelial cell injury, fibroblast dysregulation, and immune system abnormalities, which ultimately lead to systemic inflammation, fibrosis, and vascular injury.[176,177] Clinically, the disease is heterogeneous and may involve multiple organ systems, most commonly the respiratory system, the skin, and the digestive system. Pulmonary involvement is the leading cause of morbidity and mortality among SSc patients.[178] ILD is exceptionally common among patients with SSc, historically found in 28% of patients, and with the use of HRCT in more than 65% of all patients with SSc and up to 93% of patients with abnormal PFT results.[179,180] Clinically significant ILD is found in at least 40% of patients and is a major contributor to morbidity and mortality.[181] At autopsy, the vast majority of patients have microscopic evidence of lung fibrosis.[182] Clinically significant ILD is more commonly observed in diffuse SSc than in the limited form, but all types of SSc, including SSc sine scleroderma (SSc without skin involvement), may be complicated by ILD.[183,184] It is possible that this distinction is more closely related to antibody profile; the majority of patients with SCL-70 antibodies will develop ILD.[185,186] Progression of ILD itself is associated with a recent onset of disease and progression of disease, more severe pulmonary function impairment, and extent of radiographic fibrosis on HRCT.[187]

## Pulmonary Function Tests

Early ILD in SSc is often asymptomatic and is detected only by PFT and HRCT abnormalities. In particular, the earliest sign of SSc-associated ILD (SSc-ILD) on PFT is a decrement in $D_{LCO}$, which correlates better than other lung function parameters with the extent of radiographically evident ILD by HRCT.[188] In particular with SSc, decrements in $D_{LCO}$ can be reflective of concomitant pulmonary vascular disease, and evaluation should be undertaken to distinguish between ILD and PAH.[189] Declines in both forced vital capacity (FVC) and diffusion capacity ($D_{LCO}$) at diagnosis correlate well with severity of disease and with overall prognosis.[190] In particular, an FVC less than 80% predicted at diagnosis is highly predictive of both the severity of decline in FVC percent predicted over the subsequent 5 years, as well as time to decline in $D_{LCO} < 70$% predicted.[191] Additionally, among patients with early SSc, FVC <50% is highly predictive of mortality.[192] Most of the deterioration in FVC seems to occur in the first 2 years after diagnosis, making initial screening and follow-up PFTs particularly important during that period.[193] Patients with antitopoisomerase antibodies (anti-Scl-70) may be at higher risk for this more rapid decline.[194] Low 6-min walk distance correlates with functional impairment in SSc-ILD, but may not be an adequately reliable outcome measure for use in clinical trials, as it can be affected by musculoskeletal issues, including pain, weakness, and vascular insufficiency, as well as by concomitant PAH.[195]

## Radiographic Features

As with all CTD-ILD, HRCT is more sensitive than the chest radiograph at identifying ILD in SSc as well as in characterizing the extent of fibrosis.[196] Radiographic features in SSc-ILD typically resemble those described in NSIP, characterized by subpleural ground-glass opacities and fine reticular markings with traction bronchiectasis, but little or no honeycombing (Fig. 13.8).[197] The presence of ground-glass opacities on initial CT is a predictor for progression to more advanced fibrosis, whereas an initial CT without ground-glass opacities predicts a lack of progression for most patients.[198] Despite long-held presumptions that ground-glass opacities represent active alveolitis and inflammation, their presence may often reflect fine fibrosis and be irreversible despite therapy in SSc-ILD.[199] Intra- and interobserver variability has hampered the use of HRCT data for research and clinical assessment; however, computer-aided models may offer some improvement in reliability.[200,201] Combined staging systems, incorporating simple measurements of radiographic lung involvement with PFT data, may improve predictions of disease progression and mortality, but also require further study.[202]

Other clues to the presence of scleroderma that can be detected on chest CT include a dilated esophagus and the presence of tumoral calcinosis (soft tissue calcification) (Fig. 13.8).[203] Because esophageal dysmotility is common in these patients, they are also at increased risk of aspiration pneumonia, which can be seen at imaging as dependent areas of consolidation and ground-glass opacity, as well as small, clustered centrilobular nodules.[112]

## Pathologic Features

The most common histopathologic pattern in SSc-ILD is NSIP, with a minority of biopsies demonstrating UIP or end-stage fibrosis.[190] Unlike the marked contrast in survival seen between idiopathic UIP (IPF) and idiopathic NSIP, there seems to be little difference in mortality based on histopathologic subsets in SSc.[74,190] For this reason, surgical biopsy is generally not obtained in SSc-ILD unless atypical features are present. A central distribution of radiographic abnormalities on CT has been associated with the pathologic finding of centrilobular fibrosis and clinical evidence of esophageal reflux in SSc.[113] This finding suggests that there may be a causal link between subclinical aspiration and some forms of SSc-ILD. Abnormal esophageal motility, decreased lower esophageal sphincter pressure, and gastroparesis can all contribute to reflux in SSc, and chronic aspiration may occur.[204] Among patients with

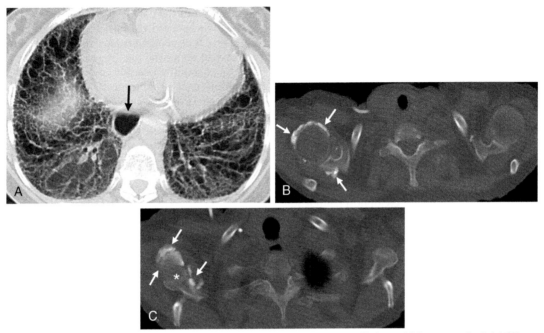

FIG. 13.8 A 58-year-old woman with scleroderma and fibrotic nonspecific interstitial pneumonia. Axial CT image through the lower thorax (A) shows reticular markings, architectural distortion, and extensive traction bronchiectasis compatible with pulmonary fibrosis. A dilated distal esophagus (*arrow*) is also present. Axial CT images through the upper thorax with bone windows show amorphous areas of calcification in the soft tissues surrounding the right shoulder (*arrows* in B) and anterior to the right scapula (*arrows* in C) due to calcinosis. The right scapula is denoted by the *asterisk* in (C).

more severe esophageal dysfunction, PFT parameters are more severely impaired, and there is an increased frequency of radiographically apparent ILD.[205–208] Over time, these patients seem to have more rapid progression of lung impairment.[208] It is not clear whether this association is causal for most patients or whether simultaneous worsening of lung and GI disease reflects progression of fibrosis in multiple organ systems.

## Treatment

Treatment in SSc-ILD has typically been targeted at the inflammatory component of the disease, although with only modest improvement in outcomes. Prednisone and other corticosteroids were used in the past, but with the discovery of a link between high-dose steroid use and scleroderma renal crisis, this has fallen out of favor.[209] Most studies of other immunosuppressive agents have included low dose of prednisone, and for this reason, it is often included in treatment regimens.

Multiple small, uncontrolled trials suggested a beneficial effect of cyclophosphamide on symptoms, lung function, radiographic abnormalities, and survival.[210–212] The Scleroderma Lung Study I was the first randomized, placebo-controlled trial to evaluate the effect of oral cyclophosphamide on lung function in SSc-ILD.[213] Cyclophosphamide had a statistically significant, although modest (2.53%), positive effect on the primary outcome of difference in FVC percent predicted at 1 year.[213] Some important secondary outcomes such as dyspnea, skin thickening, and health-related quality of life were also improved. Cyclophosphamide was associated with increased short-term toxicity in the study and is known to have long-term risks, including elevated risk for bladder cancer and other malignancies.[214] Subset analysis has suggested that the group most likely to benefit from treatment includes those patients with more severe restriction and fibrosis at baseline.[213,215] Long-term follow-up demonstrated that the beneficial effects of cyclophosphamide on lung function were lost by 24 months.[215] Despite the small absolute change in FVC percent predicted, it has been suggested that the stability of lung function attained in treated patients may represent the true success in SSc-ILD and that immunosuppressive therapy to prevent progression of disease may be required long term.[216]

Methods to diminish the toxicity of treatment include alteration in the administration of cyclophosphamide from daily oral administration to monthly infusions, which minimize the cumulative dose; switching from cyclophosphamide after 6 to 12 months to another, less toxic agent such as azathioprine or MMF; or replacing cyclophosphamide entirely by initiating therapy with such agents.[216–218] MMF demonstrated some early promising results.[219–221] The Scleroderma Lung Study II, the results of which were released in abstract form only as of this writing, examines the role of MMF as primary therapy for SSc-ILD compared with cyclophosphamide. Patients were randomized to 2 years of MMF as compared with 1 year of oral cyclophosphamide followed by 1 year of placebo. Both treatment arms experienced the same 5% increase in FVC, but adverse events and withdrawal from study were more common in the cyclophosphamide arm.[222] Azathioprine has similarly been used when less severe disease is present, or when the side effects of cyclophosphamide are prohibitive. This agent may offer some efficacy but is not well studied and is limited by side effects in a substantial minority of patients.[223] It can be used for maintenance after cyclophosphamide and seems to offer some utility in this regard.[224]

Other agents have been evaluated as potential alternatives to cyclophosphamide; however, none has fulfilled its promise. The endothelin-1 inhibitor bosentan was proposed for its antifibrotic effects in SSc skin and lungs, but failed to show treatment efficacy in SSc-ILD.[225] Imatinib mesylate, a tyrosine kinase inhibitor, interferes in several profibrotic pathways and has been proposed for use in SSc. Uncontrolled trials suggest improvement in skin scores with modest improvement in FVC as well.[226] Further study is needed to assess the role of imatinib in SSc-ILD; however, no effect was seen in a recent study in IPF.[227] Rituximab, an inhibitor of B-cell proliferation, has been demonstrated in a small study of SSc-ILD patients to improve FVC and D$_{LCO}$, and reports of safety with increased use have made a case for further study.[228–230] However, concerns regarding its potential for lung toxicity do exist.[231] Other biologic agents and newer therapies require further study, including pirfenidone and anticonnective tissue growth factor antibodies.[232,233] Early data have supported the role of stem cell transplantation in SSc, with improvement in ground-glass opacities on HRCT as well as FVC.[234] Trials in the United States and Europe have enrolled patients to examine this high-risk strategy more fully, and further data are awaited.[235]

Lung transplantation may be considered for advanced fibrotic lung disease but has been controversial in the past. SSc is considered a systemic disease, which may increase overall morbidity and mortality after transplantation. In particular, concern has been raised about the role of gastroesophageal reflux because of motility issues in SSc that may predispose to chronic graft dysfunction. However, among carefully selected patients, early (1-year) and late (5-year) mortality seems to be similar to that of other groups, even with severe esophageal dysfunction; patients with severe fibrotic lung disease should be referred for evaluation.[124,126,127,236,237]

## IDIOPATHIC INFLAMMATORY MYOPATHIES

The idiopathic inflammatory myopathies (IIMs) are autoimmune disorders typically affecting the skeletal muscle, leading to inflammation and proximal muscle weakness.[12,13] Systemic involvement, including inflammation of the skin, lung, joints, and gastrointestinal tract, may be present.[238] In particular, the presence of ILD has long been recognized and contributes significantly to morbidity and mortality.[239–241] There are several subtypes of the IIMs, all of which may be complicated by ILD, including PM, DM, ADM, and the antisynthetase syndrome.

Criteria for classification of the IIMs are still in evolution. Initial diagnostic criteria proposed by Bohan and Peter included the presence of symmetric proximal muscle weakness in combination with elevated serum muscle enzymes, typical EMG and muscle biopsy findings, and typical rash; these criteria continue to be clinically useful.[12,13] However, evolving immunohistochemical and pathologic features, as well as the discovery of myositis-related autoantibodies such as the anti-tRNA synthetase Jo-1, have led to the proposal of other classification schemes, although none is universally accepted.[242,243]

### Clinical Features

The clinical presentation of PM/DM typically involves the subacute onset of proximal muscle symptoms, which may include myalgias, muscle fatigue, or frank weakness, in which patients complain of difficulty rising from a chair or lifting objects. In cases of DM, skin manifestations are present and may include the heliotrope rash, a violaceous discoloration of the eyelids; periorbital edema; Gottron papules, maculopapular erythematous lesions present on the extensor surface of the metacarpophalangeal and proximal interphalangeal joints of the hands; the shawl sign, poikilodermatous macules on the shoulders, arms, or upper back; and "mechanic's hands," a scaly, cracked, hyperkeratotic erythema found on the lateral and palmar surfaces of hands and fingers, which has specific histopathologic features.[244,245]

Several pulmonary manifestations may be seen in the IIMs and are a major contributor to morbidity and mortality.[246,247] Primary muscle weakness may lead to hypoventilation and respiratory failure and may be complicated by pneumonia because of weak cough and poor airway clearance.[248–250] Aspiration pneumonia may occur due to respiratory muscle weakness but most commonly reflects the presence of skeletal muscle dysfunction in the pharynx and upper esophagus.[249]

ILD is the most common pulmonary complication of the IIMs, although like other CTD-ILDs, the incidence of myositis-associated ILD (MA-ILD) is greatly affected by the mode of ascertainment, with high rates observed with the combined use of PFTs and HRCT. The presence of ILD in this population contributes significant to mortality from the disease.[251] In a prospective study of patients with a new diagnosis of PM or DM, many of whom had no respiratory symptoms, 78% of patients were demonstrated to have some lung involvement as defined by radiographic evidence (chest radiograph or HRCT abnormalities) or restrictive physiology and diffusion impairment on PFTs (total lung capacity and $D_{LCO} < 80\%$ predicted).[252] Among a population of patients with anti-Jo-1 antibodies, 86% were demonstrated to have ILD.[253] These numbers may be overestimates based on the lack of HRCT evidence of ILD for all patients, but they do suggest that parenchymal involvement is common and should be aggressively sought.

MA-ILD may occur concomitantly with the onset of myositis or rash but may precede the diagnosis of IIM.[241,254] Cases of DM with typical skin rash in association with ILD may occur without biochemical evidence for muscle involvement, known as ADM.[255] The clinical course of MA-ILD is variable, ranging from a total lack of symptoms to fulminant hypoxemic respiratory failure, although many patients present subacutely and experience chronic, progressive disease.[246] Dyspnea and cough are the most common symptoms reported in MA-ILD. Notably, almost one-third of patients with MA-ILD are asymptomatic, demonstrating the need for evaluation of these patients with PFTs and chest imaging.[256] DM and particularly ADM may be more associated with an acute and fatal presentation, which is characterized by histopathologic findings of DAD, and resistance to treatment.[26,255,257] The strongest predictor for the onset of ILD in IIM is the presence of antisynthetase antibodies, particularly anti-Jo-1.[256,258]

The "antisynthetase syndrome" has been described to include ILD, myositis, arthritis, fever, Raynaud phenomenon, and "mechanic's hands."[259] In many cases, only a few features are present, and in many the lung manifestations may predominate. In addition to anti-Jo-1, other antisynthetase antibodies (such as anti-PL7, anti-PL12, anti-EJ) have been associated with the development of ILD with IIM.[260] Particular antibodies may be more or less strongly associated with the development of ILD or myositis, and subtypes based on antibody specificity may predict the clinical course.[261,262] Among the myositis-associated antibodies, the presence of anti-SSA in conjunction with anti-Jo-1 has been associated with more severe and progressive ILD.[28,263]

### Pulmonary Function Testing

PFTs are important in the assessment of MA-ILD and help assess disease severity and response to therapy. They also help to distinguish between the role of MA-ILD and diaphragmatic weakness, although this may not be straightforward.[264] Like other forms of ILD, PFTs in MA-ILD demonstrate restrictive physiology and reduced $D_{LCO}$. However, respiratory muscle insufficiency is also characterized by reductions in FVC and total lung capacity as well as reduction in other tests such as the maximum voluntary ventilation and maximal inspiratory and expiratory pressures.[250] Reductions in the $D_{LCO}$ may also be the result of pulmonary hypertension, which can coexist with ILD, or due to atelectasis from diaphragmatic weakness.[264]

### Radiographic Features

HRCT findings are similar to those in other forms of CTD-ILD. In MA-ILD, the most common abnormalities are ground-glass opacities, reticular markings, and airspace consolidation (Fig. 13.9).[265] Honeycombing is less common. The radiographic findings suggest the underlying pathology (i.e., dense consolidation reflecting DAD and OP; honeycombing reflecting UIP); however, these findings are not specific.[265] Centrilobular nodules, linear opacities, and traction bronchiectasis may also be observed.[265] Some studies have suggested that dense, peripheral consolidation in a pattern consistent with OP is associated with a better prognosis, while ground-glass opacities predict a worse outcome.[266,267]

### Pathologic Features

Surgical lung biopsy is not typically obtained in the diagnosis of MA-ILD, and the role of pathologic diagnosis remains controversial. In studies reporting pathologic findings in MA-ILD, the majority of patients have NSIP, with UIP and OP as the next most frequent

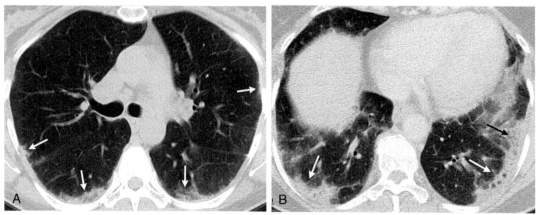

**FIG. 13.9** 58-year-old woman with organizing pneumonia secondary to polymyositis. Axial images at the level of the midthorax (A) and lower thorax (B) demonstrate peripheral, subpleural areas of consolidation.

possibilities, and DAD in a minority of patients.[264] Although some studies have suggested that DAD carries a poorer prognosis than either OP or cellular NSIP, it is not clear that pathologic pattern alters treatment choice, and other studies have not confirmed an impact of histopathologic pattern on overall survival.[75,241,246,268] In the setting of rapid onset ILD, surgical biopsy may not be clinically feasible and may lead to postoperative complications in a patient who will likely receive high-dose corticosteroids and other immunosuppressive agents.

### Treatment

All treatment is empiric in MA-ILD, as no controlled studies exist to guide treatment decisions. MA-ILD seems responsive to corticosteroids, but high doses may be required.[239,269] Corticosteroids continue to be the most common and widely accepted therapy for MA-ILD.[270] In acute, life-threatening disease, pulse dose regimens (1 g/day) of methylprednisolone may be required. Additional therapy is often needed in MA-ILD and may be added either for steroid-sparing effect or for additional efficacy. In particular, some forms of MA-ILD with low creatine kinase levels may respond poorly to corticosteroids alone and require treatment with other agents.[271] Choice of agent often depends on clinician familiarity as well as on the severity of illness.

Azathioprine, an inhibitor of purine synthesis, is efficacious in treating myositis in the IIMs.[270] It is a commonly used agent in many CTD-ILDs and is often used in MA-ILD, although with few reports in the literature.[75,272] Cyclophosphamide is typically chosen for rapidly progressive or severe MA-ILD, via either

monthly IV pulse infusions or oral therapy.[273] Pulse dosage between 300 and 800 mg/m$^2$ has been described to improve MA-ILD in treatment-resistant disease.[274] Methotrexate has long been used in the treatment of myositis in the IIMs and has been utilized in the treatment of MA-ILD.[270] However, the known pulmonary toxicity, which may occur with this drug, can be difficult to distinguish from progressive MA-ILD, making choice of this agent less ideal.[275] Other agents such as cyclosporine, tacrolimus, MMF, intravenous immune globulin, and rituximab have all been used in small numbers of patients with refractory disease and may be utilized in select situations.[271,276-281] There is increasing experience with rituximab, but controlled trials are still needed.[282-284]

### SJÖGREN SYNDROME

Sjögren syndrome is characterized by lymphocytic infiltration of the exocrine glands and marked B-cell hyperreactivity.[285] In particular, the salivary and lacrimal glands are affected, leading to the sicca syndrome characterized by dry eye (keratoconjunctivitis sicca) and dry mouth (xerostomia), often accompanied by arthritis.[286] When Sjögren syndrome is seen in isolation, it is called primary Sjögren syndrome. Secondary Sjögren syndrome may accompany other CTDs such as RA, SSc, SLE, and PM/DM.[287] In addition to the main sicca symptoms of Sjögren syndrome, involvement of the stomach, pancreas, kidney, and peripheral nervous system may occur.[287,288] Middle-aged women are most commonly affected.[289] The diagnosis depends on a combination of ocular and oral symptoms of dryness, objective testing for xerophthalmia and xerostomia,

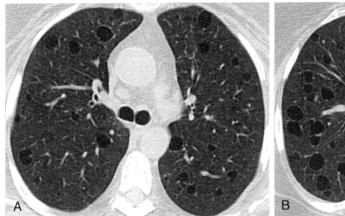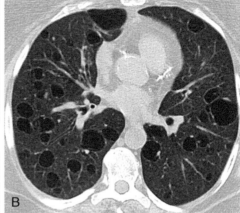

FIG. 13.10 63-year-old woman with Sjögren syndrome and lymphoid interstitial pneumonia. Axial CT images through the upper thorax (A) and midthorax (B) show multiple thin-walled cysts of varying sizes scattered throughout the lungs.

histopathologic features on minor salivary gland biopsy, and autoantibodies to Ro (anti-SSA) and/or La (anti-SSB).[290]

## Clinical Features

Like other forms of CTD-ILD, the prevalence of lung involvement in Sjögren syndrome depends on the methodology used to determine active disease and varies between 9% and 60%.[291] While radiographic abnormalities observed on HRCT may be common, the prevalence of clinically significant pulmonary disease was 11% in a large cohort of patients with Sjögren syndrome.[292] Many patients are asymptomatic, and lung involvement is mild and only slowly progressive.[291,293,294] Most commonly, lung involvement is manifested by both upper and lower airways disease, ILD, and lymphoproliferative disorders. Many patients complain of a dry cough ("sicca cough"), which is a result of xerosis of the airways due to involvement of the submucosal glands.[295]

Symptoms of ILD most often include dyspnea and cough, with a minority complaining of chest pain and wheezing.[296] Sicca symptoms are present in most patients.[296] Inspiratory crackles are commonly found, although wheezing may also be present. Clubbing is rare.[296] PFTs are most often normal in patients with Sjögren syndrome, but among those with ILD, restriction and diffusion abnormalities predominate.[285,296,297] Care with interpretation must be taken, as airways obstruction is common in Sjögren syndrome and may lead to mixed obstructive and restrictive physiology.[298]

## Radiographic Features

HRCT is abnormal in more than one-third of Sjögren syndrome patients.[299] Multiple abnormalities may be observed and include findings of large airways disease (bronchiectasis, bronchial wall thickening), small airways disease (air trapping, bronchiolectasis, centrilobular nodules, and tree-in-bud opacities), as well as interstitial disease (ground-glass opacities, airspace consolidation, interlobular septal thickening, honeycombing, and cysts).[286,299,300] The presence of thin-walled cysts suggests the diagnosis of LIP, which is a lymphoproliferative disorder common in Sjögren syndrome (Fig. 13.10).[301,302] LIP is considered to be a steroid-responsive lung disease but may rarely evolve into lymphoma.[301,302] Findings that may suggest lymphoma include nonresolving airspace consolidation, nodules greater than 1 cm in size, and enlarging lymph nodes.[303] If these features are present, biopsy should be considered. The presence of air trapping on expiratory films may be helpful in distinguishing small airways disease from ILD and may be present in the absence of PFT abnormalities.[304] In general, in Sjögren syndrome–associated ILD (SS-ILD), HRCT features and histopathology tend to correlate well, particularly for NSIP.[296,305]

## Pathologic Features

Older studies of histologic pattern in Sjögren syndrome reported LIP as the most common ILD.[306] More recent studies, using the newer ERS/ATS classification of ILD, describe a higher frequency of NSIP, although with UIP, OP, and LIP also observed.[296,305]

Rarely, primary pulmonary lymphoma and amyloidosis are found.[296] When CT features are typical for NSIP, biopsy need not be pursued, but when features suggestive of lymphoma are present tissue sampling is advisable.

### Treatment

Treatment in SS-ILD is most often initiated with corticosteroids, although little is known about the optimal treatment. In some milder cases of LIP, observation without therapy may be reasonable.[296] In the case of more advanced fibrotic lung disease, it is less clear that immunosuppressive therapy will reverse the underlying injury and may expose the patient to excessive risk without significant benefit. In general, SS-ILD seems to be treatment responsive. When SS-ILD is treated, symptoms can improve relatively rapidly, while objective treatment response may occur over months and may be incomplete.[296] The addition of steroid-sparing agents, such as azathioprine, may improve lung function but has not been rigorously studied, and use of these agents is largely anecdotal.[306] Early data suggest that B-cell depletion with rituximab may play some role in the treatment of SS-ILD and deserves further study.[307-309]

## SYSTEMIC LUPUS ERYTHEMATOSUS

SLE is an immune-mediated disease, which most commonly occurs in younger women.[310] It typically presents with malar, discoid, and photosensitivity rashes; oral ulcers; nonerosive arthritis; glomerulonephritis; and hematologic abnormalities.[311] Autoantibodies, including ANA, anti–double-stranded DNA, and anti-Smith, are commonly detected and are part of the diagnostic criteria.[311] The most common form of pulmonary involvement in SLE is pleuritis, but parenchymal lung disease, pulmonary vascular disease, airways disease, and respiratory muscle dysfunction may all occur.[310] Diffuse parenchymal lung disease in SLE may have either acute or chronic presentation.

### Acute Lupus Pneumonitis

One of the less common complications of SLE is acute lupus pneumonitis, which occurs in 1–12% of patients and which may be the presenting feature of SLE.[312] Patients present with acute onset of fever, cough, dyspnea, and hypoxemia.[312] Acute respiratory failure requiring mechanical ventilatory support may occur. Physical examination may demonstrate bibasilar rales, and radiographic findings are significant for diffuse ground-glass opacities and airspace consolidation on chest radiograph and HRCT.

In all forms of acute parenchymal lung disease in SLE, there is significant overlap in terms of presentation, with similar clinical history, radiographic findings, and progression. The most important piece of the clinical evaluation is to rule out infection. In particular, SLE patients are at high risk for both bacterial and opportunistic infection. In addition to the common use of immunosuppressive medications, SLE itself is associated with innate immune dysfunction resulting from complement deficiency, immunoglobulin deficiency, defects in chemotaxis and phagocytosis, as well as functional asplenia.[313] Empiric antibiotics are typically begun in an acutely ill patient, and BAL should be performed if clinically feasible, particularly in the patient already receiving immunosuppressive drugs.

Surgical lung biopsy is not always feasible or warranted in acute lupus pneumonitis but, when performed, is nonspecific and commonly demonstrates DAD characterized by hyaline membranes and type II pneumocyte proliferation and inflammation. Capillary inflammation and fibrin thrombi may be present, and immunofluorescence studies have demonstrated immune complement deposition.[314]

Prognosis for acute lupus pneumonitis is generally felt to be poor, with older studies reporting mortality rates of 50% and residual lung impairment among the survivors.[312] Newer data are not available to assess whether alterations in supportive care have changed these outcomes. Treatment is largely anecdotal, with emphasis on empiric antibiotics accompanied by a careful search for opportunistic infection, followed by corticosteroids. High doses are utilized for critically ill patients and include a 3-day pulse of methylprednisolone (1 g per day) followed by 1–2 mg/kg/day depending on clinical response. Additional cytotoxic therapies such as cyclophosphamide and azathioprine have been reported to improve lung function, but no well-controlled studies are available to guide practice.[315,316]

### Diffuse Alveolar Hemorrhage

DAH is also quite rare, but when it occurs, it contributes to high mortality and may be recurrent among survivors.[317,318] The clinical presentation is similar to that of acute lupus pneumonitis with the abrupt onset of dyspnea, cough, and hypoxemia. Fever may be present and hemoptysis may occur; however, at least half of patients may present without this feature.[317,319] Lupus nephritis or other active SLE involvement may be concomitant.

An acute drop in hematocrit may suggest the diagnosis. Radiographic findings may be initially unimpressive but can progress to diffuse ground-glass opacities and airspace consolidation and can be indistinguishable from acute lupus pneumonitis, infectious pneumonia, pulmonary edema, or the acute respiratory distress syndrome (ARDS).[319] BAL is a crucial diagnostic step in the evaluation of these patients, both for the exclusion of infection and the diagnosis of DAH, which can be made with the observation of progressively bloody lavage fluid and hemosiderin-laden macrophages in the fluid. Among more clinically stable patients, $D_{LCO}$ measurements obtained within the first 48 h after the hemorrhage have been reported to demonstrate a rise of 30% over baseline while the erythrocytes are still within the alveoli.[319] Surgical lung biopsies are not typically performed in acutely ill patients. Histopathologic findings in DAH most commonly demonstrate bland hemorrhage, but some cases of capillaritis with immune complex deposition as well as small vessel vasculitis and microangiitis have been reported.[313,318,320]

DAH may be triggered by infection, and initial treatment consists of empiric antibiotics, which may significantly improve survival.[319] High-dose corticosteroids are generally combined with intravenous cyclophosphamide.[317] Plasmapheresis may also improve survival.[321–323] MMF has been reported to be efficacious in maintaining remission from DAH episodes.[324] Rituximab may be emerging as a potential treatment option.[325,326]

### Chronic Interstitial Lung Disease in Systemic Lupus Erythematosus

Chronic ILD may be observed in SLE and has been reported as being less common than in other CTDs, with a reported prevalence of 3–13%.[327] However, subclinical disease is likely relatively common, based on HRCT studies, which estimate the prevalence of ILD at 38% among lupus patients without previously diagnosed lung disease.[328] In some cases, an association is seen between ILD and anti-SSA antibodies, but it is unclear whether this is pathogenic and whether such findings actually describe an overlap with Sjögren syndrome.[329,330]

Like other forms of ILD, SLE-associated ILD (SLE-ILD) commonly presents with the insidious onset of dyspnea and occasional nonproductive cough. ILD may present acutely as in acute lupus pneumonitis, and chronic lung disease may result from prior episodes of lupus pneumonitis.[312] ILD onset is associated with longer disease duration, male gender, and older age, as well as later onset of SLE.[331]

HRCT findings in SLE-ILD are similar to those of other chronic ILD and demonstrate bibasilar-predominant reticulations and ground-glass opacities with progression to traction bronchiectasis with some honeycombing. The most typical histopathologic patterns are NSIP, UIP, and LIP; however, surgical biopsy is rarely obtained.[80,332]

Treatment of SLE-ILD is not standardized and the choice to treat is an individualized decision based on clinical progression and radiographic findings. In particular, the presence of ground-glass opacities might suggest a more active alveolar inflammatory process with the possibility of treatment responsiveness. Corticosteroids are often utilized and, when chronic therapy is anticipated, steroid-sparing agents such as azathioprine and MMF are added. MMF has been demonstrated to have a reasonably good safety profile in patients with CTD-ILD.[168,333] Cyclophosphamide has been utilized for refractory disease.[316] Rituximab has been reported to have controlled progressive and refractory ILD in one case.[334]

### SUMMARY

Lung disease is a common manifestation of the CTDs and may be a presenting feature. Subclinical disease is common. Clinically apparent disease is often slowly progressive but may present acutely, contributing to high morbidity and mortality. Infection and drug reaction often share clinical features with CTD-ILD and should be considered when evaluating the patient with dyspnea and abnormal radiographic findings. Treatment of CTD-ILD is not well studied but typically includes corticosteroid therapy and immunosuppressive agents, as well as careful supportive care. Further study is needed for the many unanswered questions in this field.

### REFERENCES

1. Kinder BW, et al. Idiopathic nonspecific interstitial pneumonia: lung manifestation of undifferentiated connective tissue disease? *Am J Respir Crit Care Med.* 2007;176(7):691–697.
2. Fischer A, et al. Connective tissue disease-associated interstitial lung disease: a call for clarification. *Chest.* 2010;138(2):251–256.
3. Vij R, Noth I, Strek ME. Autoimmune-featured interstitial lung disease: a distinct entity. *Chest.* 2011;140(5): 1292–1299.
4. Fischer A, et al. An official European Respiratory Society/American Thoracic Society research statement: interstitial pneumonia with autoimmune features. *Eur Respir J.* 2015;46(4):976–987.

5. Oldham JM, et al. Characterisation of patients with interstitial pneumonia with autoimmune features. *Eur Respir J.* June 2016;47(6):1767–1775.

6. O'Donnell DE, et al. Mechanisms of activity-related dyspnea in pulmonary diseases. *Respir Physiol Neurobiol.* 2009;167(1):116–132.

7. Leslie KO, Trahan S, Gruden J. Pulmonary pathology of the rheumatic diseases. *Semin Respir Crit Care Med.* 2007;28(4):369–378.

8. Roschmann RA, Rothenberg RJ. Pulmonary fibrosis in rheumatoid arthritis: a review of clinical features and therapy. *Semin Arthritis Rheum.* 1987;16(3):174–185.

9. Khan S, Christopher-Stine L. Polymyositis, dermatomyositis, and autoimmune necrotizing myopathy: clinical features. *Rheum Dis Clin North Am.* 2011;37(2):143–158. v.

10. Hachulla E, Launay D. Diagnosis and classification of systemic sclerosis. *Clin Rev Allergy Immunol.* 2010;40(2):78–83.

11. Arnett FC, et al. The American Rheumatism Association 1987 revised criteria for the classification of rheumatoid arthritis. *Arthritis Rheum.* 1988;31(3):315–324.

12. Bohan A, Peter JB. Polymyositis and dermatomyositis (first of two parts). *N Engl J Med.* 1975;292(7):344–347.

13. Bohan A, Peter JB. Polymyositis and dermatomyositis (second of two parts). *N Engl J Med.* 1975;292(8):403–407.

14. Katzap E, Barilla-LaBarca ML, Marder G. Antisynthetase syndrome. *Curr Rheumatol Rep.* 2011;13(3):175–181.

15. Lambova SN, Muller-Ladner U. The role of capillaroscopy in differentiation of primary and secondary Raynaud's phenomenon in rheumatic diseases: a review of the literature and two case reports. *Rheumatol Int.* 2009;29(11):1263–1271.

16. Gauhar UA, Gaffo AL, Alarcon GS. Pulmonary manifestations of rheumatoid arthritis. *Semin Respir Crit Care Med.* 2007;28(4):430–440.

17. Minier T, et al. Preliminary analysis of the very early diagnosis of systemic sclerosis (VEDOSS) EUSTAR multicentre study: evidence for puffy fingers as a pivotal sign for suspicion of systemic sclerosis. *Ann Rheum Dis.* 2014;73(12):2087–2093.

18. Raghu G, et al. An official ATS/ERS/JRS/ALAT statement: idiopathic pulmonary fibrosis: evidence-based guidelines for diagnosis and management. *Am J Respir Crit Care Med.* 2011;183(6):788–824.

19. Idiopathic Pulmonary Fibrosis Clinical Research, N, et al. Prednisone, azathioprine, and N-acetylcysteine for pulmonary fibrosis. *N Engl J Med.* 2012;366(21):1968–1977.

20. Noble PW, et al. Pirfenidone for idiopathic pulmonary fibrosis: analysis of pooled data from three multinational phase 3 trials. *Eur Respir J.* 2016;47(1):243–253.

21. Richeldi L, et al. Nintedanib in patients with idiopathic pulmonary fibrosis: combined evidence from the TOMORROW and INPULSIS((R)) trials. *Respir Med.* 2016;113:74–79.

22. Strange C, Highland KB. Interstitial lung disease in the patient who has connective tissue disease. *Clin Chest Med.* 2004;25(3):549–559. vii.

23. Fischer A, et al. Anti-synthetase syndrome in ANA and anti-Jo-1 negative patients presenting with idiopathic interstitial pneumonia. *Respir Med.* 2009;103(11):1719–1724.

24. Malik A, et al. Idiopathic inflammatory myopathies: clinical approach and management. *Front Neurol.* 2016;7:64.

25. Carlson DA, Hinchcliff M, Pandolfino JE. Advances in the evaluation and management of esophageal disease of systemic sclerosis. *Curr Rheumatol Rep.* 2015;17(1):475.

26. Tanizawa K, et al. HRCT features of interstitial lung disease in dermatomyositis with anti-CADM-140 antibody. *Respir Med.* 2011;105(9):1380–1387.

27. Hanke K, et al. Antibodies against PM/Scl-75 and PM/Scl-100 are independent markers for different subsets of systemic sclerosis patients. *Arthritis Res Ther.* 2009;11(1):R22.

28. Vancsa A, et al. Characteristics of interstitial lung disease in SS-A positive/Jo-1 positive inflammatory myopathy patients. *Rheumatol Int.* 2009;29(9):989–994.

29. Popper MS, Bogdonoff ML, Hughes RL. Interstitial rheumatoid lung disease. A reassessment and review of the literature. *Chest.* 1972;62(3):243–250.

30. Frank ST, et al. Pulmonary dysfunction in rheumatoid disease. *Chest.* 1973;63(1):27–34.

31. Bjoraker JA, et al. Prognostic significance of histopathologic subsets in idiopathic pulmonary fibrosis. *Am J Respir Crit Care Med.* 1998;157(1):199–203.

32. Chetta A, et al. Relationship between outcome measures of six-minute walk test and baseline lung function in patients with interstitial lung disease. *Sarcoidosis Vasc Diffuse Lung Dis.* 2001;18(2):170–175.

33. O'Donnell D. Physiology of interstitial lung disease. In: Schwarz M, ed. *Interstitial Lung Disease.* Ontario: BC Decker; 2003.

34. Hughes JM, et al. DLCO/Q and diffusion limitation at rest and on exercise in patients with interstitial fibrosis. *Respir Physiol.* 1991;83(2):155–166.

35. Jenkins S, Cecins N. Six-minute walk test: observed adverse events and oxygen desaturation in a large cohort of patients with chronic lung disease. *Intern Med J.* 2011;41(5):416–422.

36. Miller W. *Diagnostic Thoracic Imaging.* McGraw-Hill; 2006.

37. Stack BH, Grant IW. Rheumatoid interstitial lung disease. *Br J Dis Chest.* 1965;59(4):202–211.

38. Silva CI, Muller NL. Interstitial lung disease in the setting of collagen vascular disease. *Semin Roentgenol.* 2010;45(1):22–28.

39. Hwang JH, et al. Computed tomographic features of idiopathic fibrosing interstitial pneumonia: comparison with pulmonary fibrosis related to collagen vascular disease. *J Comput Assist Tomogr.* 2009;33(3):410–415.

40. Kim EA, et al. Interstitial lung diseases associated with collagen vascular diseases: radiologic and histopathologic findings. *Radiographics.* 2002:S151–S165. 22 Spec No.

41. Tanaka N, et al. Rheumatokid arthritis-related lung diseases: CT findings. *Radiology.* 2004;232(1):81–91.

42. Mori S, et al. Comparison of pulmonary abnormalities on high-resolution computed tomography in patients with early versus longstanding rheumatoid arthritis. *J Rheumatol.* 2008;35(8):1513–1521.

43. Kocheril SV, et al. Comparison of disease progression and mortality of connective tissue disease-related interstitial lung disease and idiopathic interstitial pneumonia. *Arthritis Rheum.* 2005;53(4):549–557.

44. Travis WD, et al. Idiopathic nonspecific interstitial pneumonia: report of an American Thoracic Society project. *Am J Respir Crit Care Med.* 2008;177(12):1338–1347.

45. Walsh SL, Hansell DM. Diffuse interstitial lung disease: overlaps and uncertainties. *Eur Radiol.* 2010;20(8):1859–1867.

46. Hunninghake GW, et al. Utility of a lung biopsy for the diagnosis of idiopathic pulmonary fibrosis. *Am J Respir Crit Care Med.* 2001;164(2):193–196.

47. Schmidt SL, Sundaram B, Flaherty KR. Diagnosing fibrotic lung disease: when is high-resolution computed tomography sufficient to make a diagnosis of idiopathic pulmonary fibrosis? *Respirology.* 2009;14(7):934–939.

48. Hunninghake GW, et al. Radiologic findings are strongly associated with a pathologic diagnosis of usual interstitial pneumonia. *Chest.* 2003;124(4):1215–1223.

49. Flaherty KR, et al. Clinical significance of histological classification of idiopathic interstitial pneumonia. *Eur Respir J.* 2002;19(2):275–283.

50. Kim EJ, Collard HR, King Jr TE. Rheumatoid arthritis-associated interstitial lung disease: the relevance of histopathologic and radiographic pattern. *Chest.* 2009;136(5):1397–1405.

51. Kim TS, et al. Nonspecific interstitial pneumonia with fibrosis: high-resolution CT and pathologic findings. *AJR Am J Roentgenol.* 1998;171(6):1645–1650.

52. Kligerman SJ, et al. Nonspecific interstitial pneumonia: radiologic, clinical, and pathologic considerations. *Radiographics.* 2009;29(1):73–87.

53. Park JS, et al. Nonspecific interstitial pneumonia with fibrosis: radiographic and CT findings in seven patients. *Radiology.* 1995;195(3):645–648.

54. Lynch DA, et al. Idiopathic interstitial pneumonias: CT features. *Radiology.* 2005;236(1):10–21.

55. Dawson JK, et al. Predictors of progression of HRCT diagnosed fibrosing alveolitis in patients with rheumatoid arthritis. *Ann Rheum Dis.* 2002;61(6):517–521.

56. Shin KM, et al. Prognostic determinants among clinical, thin-section CT, and histopathologic findings for fibrotic idiopathic interstitial pneumonias: tertiary hospital study. *Radiology.* 2008;249(1):328–337.

57. Mathai SC, Danoff SK. Management of interstitial lung disease associated with connective tissue disease. *BMJ.* 2016;352:h6819.

58. Committee TBCGS. Bronchoalveolar lavage constituents in healthy individuals, idiopathic pulmonary fibrosis, and selected comparison groups. The BAL Cooperative Group Steering Committee. *Am Rev Respir Dis.* 1990;141(5 Pt 2):S169–S202.

59. Strange C, et al. Bronchoalveolar lavage and response to cyclophosphamide in scleroderma interstitial lung disease. *Am J Respir Crit Care Med.* 2008;177(1):91–98.

60. Nagasawa Y, et al. Inflammatory cells in lung disease associated with rheumatoid arthritis. *Intern Med.* 2009;48(14):1209–1217.

61. Biederer J, et al. Correlation between HRCT findings, pulmonary function tests and bronchoalveolar lavage cytology in interstitial lung disease associated with rheumatoid arthritis. *Eur Radiol.* 2004;14(2):272–280.

62. Garcia JG, et al. Lower respiratory tract abnormalities in rheumatoid interstitial lung disease. Potential role of neutrophils in lung injury. *Am Rev Respir Dis.* 1987;136(4):811–817.

63. Komocsi A, et al. Alveolitis may persist during treatment that sufficiently controls muscle inflammation in myositis. *Rheumatol Int.* 2001;20(3):113–118.

64. Silver RM, Wells AU. Histopathology and bronchoalveolar lavage. *Rheumatology (Oxford).* 2008;47(suppl 5):v62–v64.

65. Meyer KC, Raghu G. Bronchoalveolar lavage for the evaluation of interstitial lung disease: is it clinically useful? *Eur Respir J.* October 2011;38(4):761–769.

66. Kowal-Bielecka O, et al. Bronchoalveolar lavage fluid in scleroderma interstitial lung disease: technical aspects and clinical correlations: review of the literature. *Semin Arthritis Rheum.* 2010;40(1):73–88.

67. Haslam PL, Baughman RP. Report of ERS Task Force: guidelines for measurement of acellular components and standardization of BAL. *Eur Respir J.* 1999;14(2):245–248.

68. Baughman RP. Technical aspects of bronchoalveolar lavage: recommendations for a standard procedure. *Semin Respir Crit Care Med.* 2007;28(5):475–485.

69. Costabel U, et al. Bronchoalveolar lavage in other interstitial lung diseases. *Semin Respir Crit Care Med.* 2007;28(5):514–524.

70. Schnabel A, et al. Bronchoalveolar lavage cell profile in methotrexate induced pneumonitis. *Thorax.* 1997;52(4):377–379.

71. Ramirez P, Valencia M, Torres A. Bronchoalveolar lavage to diagnose respiratory infections. *Semin Respir Crit Care Med.* 2007;28(5):525–533.

72. American Thoracic Society/European Respiratory Society International Multidisciplinary Consensus Classification of the Idiopathic Interstitial Pneumonias. This joint statement of the American Thoracic Society (ATS), and the European Respiratory Society (ERS) was adopted by the ATS board of directors, June 2001 and by the ERS Executive Committee, June 2001. *Am J Respir Crit Care Med.* 2002;165(2):277–304.

73. Lee HK, et al. Histopathologic pattern and clinical features of rheumatoid arthritis-associated interstitial lung disease. *Chest.* 2005;127(6):2019–2027.

74. Kim DS, et al. The major histopathologic pattern of pulmonary fibrosis in scleroderma is nonspecific interstitial pneumonia. *Sarcoidosis Vasc Diffuse Lung Dis.* 2002;19(2):121–127.

75. Douglas WW, et al. Polymyositis-dermatomyositis-associated interstitial lung disease. *Am J Respir Crit Care Med.* 2001;164(7):1182–1185.

76. Kim DS. Interstitial lung disease in rheumatoid arthritis: recent advances. *Curr Opin Pulm Med.* 2006;12(5):346–353.

77. Yousem SA, Colby TV, Carrington CB. Lung biopsy in rheumatoid arthritis. *Am Rev Respir Dis.* 1985;131(5):770–777.

78. Riha RL, et al. Survival of patients with biopsy-proven usual interstitial pneumonia and nonspecific interstitial pneumonia. *Eur Respir J.* 2002;19(6):1114–1118.

79. Park JH, et al. Prognosis of fibrotic interstitial pneumonia: idiopathic versus collagen vascular disease-related subtypes. *Am J Respir Crit Care Med.* 2007;175(7):705–711.

80. Tansey D, et al. Variations in histological patterns of interstitial pneumonia between connective tissue disorders and their relationship to prognosis. *Histopathology.* 2004;44(6):585–596.

81. Kim EJ, et al. Usual interstitial pneumonia in rheumatoid arthritis-associated interstitial lung disease. *Eur Respir J.* 2010;35(6):1322–1328.

82. Moghadam-Kia S, Werth VP. Prevention and treatment of systemic glucocorticoid side effects. *Int J Dermatol.* 2010;49(3):239–248.

83. Harris-Eze AO, et al. Oxygen improves maximal exercise performance in interstitial lung disease. *Am J Respir Crit Care Med.* 1994;150(6 Pt 1):1616–1622.

84. Visca D, et al. Ambulatory oxygen in interstitial lung disease. *Eur Respir J.* 2011;38(4):987–990.

85. Bradley B, et al. Interstitial lung disease guideline: the British Thoracic Society in collaboration with the Thoracic Society of Australia and New Zealand and the Irish Thoracic Society. *Thorax.* 2008;63(suppl 5):v1–v58.

86. Clark M, et al. A survey of nocturnal hypoxaemia and health related quality of life in patients with cryptogenic fibrosing alveolitis. *Thorax.* 2001;56(6):482–486.

87. Nici L, et al. American Thoracic Society/European Respiratory Society statement on pulmonary rehabilitation. *Am J Respir Crit Care Med.* 2006;173(12):1390–1413.

88. Laviolette L, et al. Assessing the impact of pulmonary rehabilitation on functional status in COPD. *Thorax.* 2008;63(2):115–121.

89. Swigris JJ, et al. Pulmonary rehabilitation in idiopathic pulmonary fibrosis: a call for continued investigation. *Respir Med.* 2008;102(12):1675–1680.

90. Holland A, Hill C. Physical training for interstitial lung disease. *Cochrane Database Syst Rev.* 2008;(4):CD006322.

91. Garvey C. Interstitial lung disease and pulmonary rehabilitation. *J Cardiopulm Rehabil Prev.* 2010;30(3):141–146.

92. Salhi B, et al. Effects of pulmonary rehabilitation in patients with restrictive lung diseases. *Chest.* 2010;137(2):273–279.

93. Ryerson CJ, Garvey C, Collard HR. Pulmonary rehabilitation for interstitial lung disease. *Chest.* 2010;138(1):240–241. author reply 241–242.

94. Vainshelboim B, et al. Long-term effects of a 12-week exercise training program on clinical outcomes in idiopathic pulmonary fibrosis. *Lung.* 2015;193(3):345–354.

95. Singer HK, et al. The psychological impact of end-stage lung disease. *Chest.* 2001;120(4):1246–1252.

96. Ponnuswamy A, et al. Association between ischaemic heart disease and interstitial lung disease: a case-control study. *Respir Med.* 2009;103(4):503–507.

97. Nathan SD, et al. Prevalence and impact of coronary artery disease in idiopathic pulmonary fibrosis. *Respir Med.* 2010;104(7):1035–1041.

98. Adzic TN, et al. Clinical features of lung cancer in patients with connective tissue diseases: a 10-year hospital based study. *Respir Med.* 2008;102(4):620–624.

99. Khurana R, et al. Risk of development of lung cancer is increased in patients with rheumatoid arthritis: a large case control study in US veterans. *J Rheumatol.* 2008;35(9):1704–1708.

100. Lancaster LH, et al. Obstructive sleep apnea is common in idiopathic pulmonary fibrosis. *Chest.* 2009;136(3):772–778.

101. Mermigkis C, et al. How common is sleep-disordered breathing in patients with idiopathic pulmonary fibrosis? *Sleep Breath.* 2010;14(4):387–390.

102. Rasche K, Orth M. Sleep and breathing in idiopathic pulmonary fibrosis. *J Physiol Pharmacol.* 2009;60(suppl 5):13–14.

103. Sode BF, et al. Venous thromboembolism and risk of idiopathic interstitial pneumonia: a nationwide study. *Am J Respir Crit Care Med.* 2010;181(10):1085–1092.

104. Petri M. Update on anti-phospholipid antibodies in SLE: the Hopkins' Lupus Cohort. *Lupus.* 2010;19(4):419–423.

105. Ungprasert P, Sanguankeo A. Risk of venous thromboembolism in patients with idiopathic inflammatory myositis: a systematic review and meta-analysis. *Rheumatol Int.* 2014;34(10):1455–1458.

106. Ungprasert P, et al. Risk of venous thromboembolism in patients with rheumatoid arthritis: a systematic review and meta-analysis. *Clin Rheumatol.* 2014;33(3):297–304.

107. Ungprasert P, Srivali N, Kittanamongkolchai W. Risk of venous thromboembolism in patients with Sjogren's syndrome: a systematic review and meta-analysis. *Clin Exp Rheumatol.* 2015;33(5):746–750.

108. Tobin RW, et al. Increased prevalence of gastroesophageal reflux in patients with idiopathic pulmonary fibrosis. *Am J Respir Crit Care Med.* 1998;158(6):1804–1808.

109. Raghu G, et al. High prevalence of abnormal acid gastro-oesophageal reflux in idiopathic pulmonary fibrosis. *Eur Respir J.* 2006;27(1):136–142.

110. Raghu G, et al. Sole treatment of acid gastroesophageal reflux in idiopathic pulmonary fibrosis: a case series. *Chest.* 2006;129(3):794–800.

111. Ghebre YT, Raghu G. Idiopathic pulmonary fibrosis: novel concepts of proton pump inhibitors as antifibrotic drugs. *Am J Respir Crit Care Med.* 2016;193(12):1345–1352.

112. Christmann RB, et al. Gastroesophageal reflux incites interstitial lung disease in systemic sclerosis: clinical, radiologic, histopathologic, and treatment evidence. *Semin Arthritis Rheum.* 2010;40(3):241–249.

113. de Souza RB, et al. Centrilobular fibrosis: an underrecognized pattern in systemic sclerosis. *Respiration.* 2009;77(4):389–397.

114. Miura Y, et al. Gastroesophageal reflux disease in patients with rheumatoid arthritis. *Mod Rheumatol.* 2014;24(2):291–295.

115. Bredenoord AJ, Pandolfino JE, Smout AJ. Gastro-oesophageal reflux disease. *Lancet*. 2013;381(9881):1933–1942.

116. Foocharoen C, et al. Effectiveness of add-on therapy with domperidone vs alginic acid in proton pump inhibitor partial response gastro-oesophageal reflux disease in systemic sclerosis: randomized placebo-controlled trial. *Rheumatology (Oxford)*. 2016;kew216.

117. Patti MG, et al. The intersection of GERD, aspiration, and lung transplantation. *J Laparoendosc Adv Surg Tech A*. 2016;26(7):501–505.

118. Patel NM, et al. Pulmonary hypertension in idiopathic pulmonary fibrosis. *Chest*. 2007;132(3):998–1006.

119. Goldberg A. Pulmonary arterial hypertension in connective tissue diseases. *Cardiol Rev*. 2010;18(2):85–88.

120. Corte TJ, Wort SJ, Wells AU. Pulmonary hypertension in idiopathic pulmonary fibrosis: a review. *Sarcoidosis Vasc Diffuse Lung Dis*. 2009;26(1):7–19.

121. Mittoo S, et al. Treatment of pulmonary hypertension in patients with connective tissue disease and interstitial lung disease. *Can Respir J*. 2010;17(6):282–286.

122. Hassoun PM. Pulmonary arterial hypertension complicating connective tissue diseases. *Semin Respir Crit Care Med*. 2009;30(4):429–439.

123. Volkmann ER, et al. Improved transplant-free survival in patients with systemic sclerosis-associated pulmonary hypertension and interstitial lung disease. *Arthritis Rheumatol*. 2014;66(7):1900–1908.

124. Saggar R, et al. Systemic sclerosis and bilateral lung transplantation: a single centre experience. *Eur Respir J*. 2010;36(4):893–900.

125. Gasper WJ, et al. Lung transplantation in patients with connective tissue disorders and esophageal dysmotility. *Dis Esophagus*. 2008;21(7):650–655.

126. Shitrit D, et al. Lung transplantation in patients with scleroderma: case series, review of the literature, and criteria for transplantation. *Clin Transplant*. 2009;23(2):178–183.

127. Crespo MM, et al. Lung transplant in patients with scleroderma compared with pulmonary fibrosis. Short- and long-term outcomes. *Ann Am Thorac Soc*. 2016;13(6):784–792.

128. O'Beirne S, Counihan IP, Keane MP. Interstitial lung disease and lung transplantation. *Semin Respir Crit Care Med*. 2010;31(2):139–146.

129. Martinez FJ, et al. The clinical course of patients with idiopathic pulmonary fibrosis. *Ann Intern Med*. 2005;142(12 Pt 1):963–967.

130. Mogulkoc N, et al. Pulmonary function in idiopathic pulmonary fibrosis and referral for lung transplantation. *Am J Respir Crit Care Med*. 2001;164(1):103–108.

131. Merlo CA, Orens JB. Candidate selection, overall results, and choosing the right operation. *Semin Respir Crit Care Med*. 2010;31(2):99–107.

132. Aletaha D, et al. 2010 Rheumatoid arthritis classification criteria: an American College of Rheumatology/European League Against Rheumatism collaborative initiative. *Arthritis Rheum*. 2010;62(9):2569–2581.

133. Klareskog L, Catrina AI, Paget S. Rheumatoid arthritis. *Lancet*. 2009;373(9664):659–672.

134. Gabriel SE, Michakud K. Epidemiological studies in incidence, prevalence, mortality, and comorbidity of the rheumatic diseases. *Arthritis Res Ther*. 2009;11(3):229.

135. Spector TD. Rheumatoid arthritis. *Rheum Dis Clin North Am*. 1990;16(3):513–537.

136. Mori S, et al. A simultaneous onset of organizing pneumonia and rheumatoid arthritis, along with a review of the literature. *Mod Rheumatol*. 2008;18(1):60–66.

137. Gochuico BR, et al. Progressive preclinical interstitial lung disease in rheumatoid arthritis. *Arch Intern Med*. 2008;168(2):159–166.

138. Suzuki A, et al. Cause of death in 81 autopsied patients with rheumatoid arthritis. *J Rheumatol*. 1994;21(1):33–36.

139. Hakala M. Poor prognosis in patients with rheumatoid arthritis hospitalized for interstitial lung fibrosis. *Chest*. 1988;93(1):114–118.

140. King TE, et al. Connective tissue diseases. In: Schwarz MI, King TE, eds. *Interstitial Lung Disease*. London: BC Decker Inc; 2003:535–598.

141. Kelly CA, et al. Rheumatoid arthritis-related interstitial lung disease: associations, prognostic factors and physiological and radiological characteristics–a large multicentre UK study. *Rheumatology (Oxford)*. 2014;53(9):1676–1682.

142. Christie GS. Pulmonary lesions in rheumatoid arthritis. *Australas Ann Med*. 1954;3(1):49–58.

143. Dixon AS, Ball J. Honeycomb lung and chronic rheumatoid arthritis; a case report. *Ann Rheum Dis*. 1957;16(2):241–245.

144. Ellman P, Ball RE. Rheumatoid disease with joint and pulmonary manifestations. *Br Med J*. 1948;2(4583):816–820.

145. Catterall M, Rowell NR. Respiratory function studies in patients with certain connective tissue diseases. *Br J Dermatol*. 1965;77:221–225.

146. Dawson JK, et al. Fibrosing alveolitis in patients with rheumatoid arthritis as assessed by high resolution computed tomography, chest radiography, and pulmonary function tests. *Thorax*. 2001;56(8):622–627.

147. Gabbay E, et al. Interstitial lung disease in recent onset rheumatoid arthritis. *Am J Respir Crit Care Med*. 1997;156(2 Pt 1):528–535.

148. Bilgici A, et al. Pulmonary involvement in rheumatoid arthritis. *Rheumatol Int*. 2005;25(6):429–435.

149. Turesson C, et al. Occurrence of extraarticular disease manifestations is associated with excess mortality in a community based cohort of patients with rheumatoid arthritis. *J Rheumatol*. 2002;29(1):62–67.

150. Cimmino MA, et al. Extra-articular manifestations in 587 Italian patients with rheumatoid arthritis. *Rheumatol Int*. 2000;19(6):213–217.

151. Brannan HM, et al. Pulmonary disease associated with rheumatoid arthritis. *JAMA*. 1964;189:914–918.

152. Gizinski AM, et al. Rheumatoid arthritis (RA)-specific autoantibodies in patients with interstitial lung disease and absence of clinically apparent articular RA. *Clin Rheumatol*. 2009;28(5):611–613.

153. Akira M, Sakatani M, Hara H. Thin-section CT findings in rheumatoid arthritis-associated lung disease: CT patterns and their courses. *J Comput Assist Tomogr.* 1999;23(6):941–948.

154. Sumikawa H, et al. Nonspecific interstitial pneumonia: histologic correlation with high-resolution CT in 29 patients. *Eur J Radiol.* 2009;70(1):35–40.

155. Hubbard R, Venn A. The impact of coexisting connective tissue disease on survival in patients with fibrosing alveolitis. *Rheumatology (Oxford).* 2002;41(6):676–679.

156. Cannon GW. Methotrexate pulmonary toxicity. *Rheum Dis Clin North Am.* 1997;23(4):917–937.

157. Ito S, Sumida T. Interstitial lung disease associated with leflunomide. *Intern Med.* 2004;43(12):1103–1104.

158. Kamata Y, et al. Rheumatoid arthritis complicated with acute interstitial pneumonia induced by leflunomide as an adverse reaction. *Intern Med.* 2004;43(12):1201–1204.

159. Suissa S, Hudson M, Ernst P. Leflunomide use and the risk of interstitial lung disease in rheumatoid arthritis. *Arthritis Rheum.* 2006;54(5):1435–1439.

160. Huggett MT, Armstrong R. Adalimumab-associated pulmonary fibrosis. *Rheumatology (Oxford).* 2006;45(10):1312–1313.

161. Tournadre A, et al. Exacerbation of interstitial lung disease during etanercept therapy: two cases. *Joint Bone Spine.* 2008;75(2):215–218.

162. Villeneuve E, St-Pierre A, Haraoui B. Interstitial pneumonitis associated with infliximab therapy. *J Rheumatol.* 2006;33(6):1189–1193.

163. Saag KG, et al. Rheumatoid arthritis lung disease. Determinants of radiographic and physiologic abnormalities. *Arthritis Rheum.* 1996;39(10):1711–1719.

164. Kinder AJ, et al. The treatment of inflammatory arthritis with methotrexate in clinical practice: treatment duration and incidence of adverse drug reactions. *Rheumatology (Oxford).* 2005;44(1):61–66.

165. Imokawa S, et al. Methotrexate pneumonitis: review of the literature and histopathological findings in nine patients. *Eur Respir J.* 2000;15(2):373–381.

166. Chang HK, Park W, Ryu DS. Successful treatment of progressive rheumatoid interstitial lung disease with cyclosporine: a case report. *J Korean Med Sci.* 2002;17(2):270–273.

167. Kelly C, Saravanan V. Treatment strategies for a rheumatoid arthritis patient with interstitial lung disease. *Expert Opin Pharmacother.* 2008;9(18):3221–3230.

168. Saketkoo LA, Espinoza LR. Experience of mycophenolate mofetil in 10 patients with autoimmune-related interstitial lung disease demonstrates promising effects. *Am J Med Sci.* 2009;337(5):329–335.

169. Saketkoo LA, Espinoza LR. Rheumatoid arthritis interstitial lung disease: mycophenolate mofetil as an antifibrotic and disease-modifying antirheumatic drug. *Arch Intern Med.* 2008;168(15):1718–1719.

170. Hartung W, et al. Effective treatment of rheumatoid arthritis-associated interstitial lung disease by B-cell targeted therapy with rituximab. *Case Rep Immunol.* 2012;2012:272–303.

171. Franzen D, et al. Effect of rituximab on pulmonary function in patients with rheumatoid arthritis. *Pulm Pharmacol Ther.* 2016;37:24–29.

172. Chartrand S, et al. Rituximab for the treatment of connective tissue disease-associated interstitial lung disease. *Sarcoidosis Vasc Diffuse Lung Dis.* 2015;32(4):296–304.

173. Vassallo R, Matteson E, Thomas Jr CF. Clinical response of rheumatoid arthritis-associated pulmonary fibrosis to tumor necrosis factor-alpha inhibition. *Chest.* 2002;122(3):1093–1096.

174. Iqbal K, Kelly C. Treatment of rheumatoid arthritis-associated interstitial lung disease: a perspective review. *Ther Adv Musculoskelet Dis.* 2015;7(6):247–267.

175. Yazdani A, et al. Survival and quality of life in rheumatoid arthritis-associated interstitial lung disease after lung transplantation. *J Heart Lung Transplant.* 2014;33(5):514–520.

176. Hassoun P. Lung involvement in systemic sclerosis. *Presse Med.* 2011;40(1 Pt 2):e3–e17.

177. Castelino FV, Varga J. Interstitial lung disease in connective tissue diseases: evolving concepts of pathogenesis and management. *Arthritis Res Ther.* 2010;12(4):213.

178. Steen VD, Medsger TA. Changes in causes of death in systemic sclerosis, 1972-2002. *Ann Rheum Dis.* 2007;66(7):940–944.

179. Wells AU, Steen V, Valentini G. Pulmonary complications: one of the most challenging complications of systemic sclerosis. *Rheumatology (Oxford).* 2009;48(suppl 3):iii40–iii44.

180. De Santis M, et al. Functional, radiological and biological markers of alveolitis and infections of the lower respiratory tract in patients with systemic sclerosis. *Respir Res.* 2005;6:96.

181. Highland KB, Garin MC, Brown KK. The spectrum of scleroderma lung disease. *Semin Respir Crit Care Med.* 2007;28(4):418–429.

182. D'Angelo WA, et al. Pathologic observations in systemic sclerosis (scleroderma). A study of fifty-eight autopsy cases and fifty-eight matched controls. *Am J Med.* 1969;46(3):428–440.

183. Ostojic P, Damjanov N. Different clinical features in patients with limited and diffuse cutaneous systemic sclerosis. *Clin Rheumatol.* 2006;25(4):453–457.

184. Toya SP, Tzelepis GE. The many faces of scleroderma sine scleroderma: a literature review focusing on cardiopulmonary complications. *Rheumatol Int.* 2009;29(8):861–868.

185. Walker UA, et al. Clinical risk assessment of organ manifestations in systemic sclerosis: a report from the EULAR Scleroderma Trials and Research group database. *Ann Rheum Dis.* 2007;66(6):754–763.

186. Briggs DC, et al. Immunogenetic prediction of pulmonary fibrosis in systemic sclerosis. *Lancet.* 1991;338(8768):661–662.

187. Wells AU, et al. Interstitial lung disease in systemic sclerosis. *Semin Respir Crit Care Med.* 2014;35(2):213–221.

188. Wells AU, et al. Fibrosing alveolitis in systemic sclerosis: indices of lung function in relation to extent of disease on computed tomography. *Arthritis Rheum.* 1997;40(7):1229–1236.

189. Steen V, Medsger Jr TA. Predictors of isolated pulmonary hypertension in patients with systemic sclerosis and limited cutaneous involvement. *Arthritis Rheum.* 2003;48(2):516–522.

190. Bouros D, et al. Histopathologic subsets of fibrosing alveolitis in patients with systemic sclerosis and their relationship to outcome. *Am J Respir Crit Care Med.* 2002;165(12):1581–1586.

191. Plastiras SC, et al. Scleroderma lung: initial forced vital capacity as predictor of pulmonary function decline. *Arthritis Rheum.* 2006;55(4):598–602.

192. Assassi S, et al. Clinical and genetic factors predictive of mortality in early systemic sclerosis. *Arthritis Rheum.* 2009;61(10):1403–1411.

193. Steen VD, et al. Severe restrictive lung disease in systemic sclerosis. *Arthritis Rheum.* 1994;37(9):1283–1289.

194. Assassi S, et al. Predictors of interstitial lung disease in early systemic sclerosis: a prospective longitudinal study of the GENISOS cohort. *Arthritis Res Ther.* 2010;12(5):R166.

195. Garin MC, et al. Limitations to the 6-minute walk test in interstitial lung disease and pulmonary hypertension in scleroderma. *J Rheumatol.* 2009;36(2):330–336.

196. Pignone A, et al. High resolution computed tomography in systemic sclerosis. Real diagnostic utilities in the assessment of pulmonary involvement and comparison with other modalities of lung investigation. *Clin Rheumatol.* 1992;11(4):465–472.

197. Desai SR, et al. CT features of lung disease in patients with systemic sclerosis: comparison with idiopathic pulmonary fibrosis and nonspecific interstitial pneumonia. *Radiology.* 2004;232(2):560–567.

198. Launay D, et al. High resolution computed tomography in fibrosing alveolitis associated with systemic sclerosis. *J Rheumatol.* 2006;33(9):1789–1801.

199. Shah RM, Jimenez S, Wechsler R. Significance of ground-glass opacity on HRCT in long-term follow-up of patients with systemic sclerosis. *J Thorac Imaging.* 2007;22(2):120–124.

200. Kim HG, et al. A computer-aided diagnosis system for quantitative scoring of extent of lung fibrosis in scleroderma patients. *Clin Exp Rheumatol.* 2010;28(5 suppl 62): S26–S35.

201. Camiciottoli G, et al. Lung CT densitometry in systemic sclerosis: correlation with lung function, exercise testing, and quality of life. *Chest.* 2007;131(3):672–681.

202. Goh NS, et al. Interstitial lung disease in systemic sclerosis: a simple staging system. *Am J Respir Crit Care Med.* 2008;177(11):1248–1254.

203. Strollo D, Goldin J. Imaging lung disease in systemic sclerosis. *Curr Rheumatol Rep.* 2010;12(2):156–161.

204. Ebert EC. Esophageal disease in progressive systemic sclerosis. *Curr Treat Options Gastroenterol.* 2008;11(1):64–69.

205. Johnson DA, et al. Pulmonary disease in progressive systemic sclerosis. A complication of gastroesophageal reflux and occult aspiration? *Arch Intern Med.* 1989;149(3):589–593.

206. Denis P, et al. Esophageal motility and pulmonary function in progressive systemic sclerosis. *Respiration.* 1981;42(1):21–24.

207. Lock G, et al. Association of esophageal dysfunction and pulmonary function impairment in systemic sclerosis. *Am J Gastroenterol.* 1998;93(3):341–345.

208. Marie I, et al. Esophageal involvement and pulmonary manifestations in systemic sclerosis. *Arthritis Rheum.* 2001;45(4):346–354.

209. Steen VD, Medsger Jr TA. Case-control study of corticosteroids and other drugs that either precipitate or protect from the development of scleroderma renal crisis. *Arthritis Rheum.* 1998;41(9):1613–1619.

210. Steen VD, et al. Therapy for severe interstitial lung disease in systemic sclerosis. A retrospective study. *Arthritis Rheum.* 1994;37(9):1290–1296.

211. Akesson A, et al. Improved pulmonary function in systemic sclerosis after treatment with cyclophosphamide. *Arthritis Rheum.* 1994;37(5):729–735.

212. White B, et al. Cyclophosphamide is associated with pulmonary function and survival benefit in patients with scleroderma and alveolitis. *Ann Intern Med.* 2000;132(12):947–954.

213. Tashkin DP, et al. Cyclophosphamide versus placebo in scleroderma lung disease. *N Engl J Med.* 2006;354(25):2655–2666.

214. Martinez FJ, McCune WJ. Cyclophosphamide for scleroderma lung disease. *N Engl J Med.* 2006;354(25):2707–2709.

215. Tashkin DP, et al. Effects of 1-year treatment with cyclophosphamide on outcomes at 2 years in scleroderma lung disease. *Am J Respir Crit Care Med.* 2007;176(10):1026–1034.

216. Wells AU, Latsi P, McCune WJ. Daily cyclophosphamide for scleroderma: are patients with the most to gain underrepresented in this trial? *Am J Respir Crit Care Med.* 2007;176(10):952–953.

217. Hoyles RK, et al. A multicenter, prospective, randomized, double-blind, placebo-controlled trial of corticosteroids and intravenous cyclophosphamide followed by oral azathioprine for the treatment of pulmonary fibrosis in scleroderma. *Arthritis Rheum.* 2006;54(12):3962–3970.

218. Yiannopoulos G, et al. Combination of intravenous pulses of cyclophosphamide and methylprednisolone in patients with systemic sclerosis and interstitial lung disease. *Rheumatol Int.* 2007;27(4):357–361.

219. Zamora AC, et al. Use of mycophenolate mofetil to treat scleroderma-associated interstitial lung disease. *Respir Med.* 2008;102(1):150–155.

220. Gerbino AJ, Goss CH, Molitor JA. Effect of mycophenolate mofetil on pulmonary function in scleroderma-associated interstitial lung disease. *Chest.* 2008;133(2):455–460.

221. Owen C, et al. Mycophenolate mofetil is an effective and safe option for the management of systemic sclerosis-associated interstitial lung disease: results from the Australian Scleroderma Cohort Study. *Clin Exp Rheumatol.* 2016;34 Suppl 100(5):170–176.

222. Clements P, Tashkin D, et al. The scleroderma lung study II (SLS II) shows that both oral cyclophosphamide (CYC) and mycophenolate mofitil (MMF) are efficacious in treating progressive interstitial lung disease (ILD) in patients with systemic sclerosis (SSc). In: *ACR/ARHP Annual Meeting.* 2015;4(9):708–719.

223. Dheda K, et al. Experience with azathioprine in systemic sclerosis associated with interstitial lung disease. *Clin Rheumatol.* 2004;23(4):306–309.

224. Berezne A, et al. Therapeutic strategy combining intravenous cyclophosphamide followed by oral azathioprine to treat worsening interstitial lung disease associated with systemic sclerosis: a retrospective multicenter open-label study. *J Rheumatol.* 2008;35(6):1064–1072.

225. Seibold JR, et al. Randomized, prospective, placebo-controlled trial of bosentan in interstitial lung disease secondary to systemic sclerosis. *Arthritis Rheum.* 2010;62(7):2101–2108.

226. Spiera RF, et al. Imatinib mesylate (Gleevec) in the treatment of diffuse cutaneous systemic sclerosis: results of a 1-year, phase IIa, single-arm, open-label clinical trial. *Ann Rheum Dis.* 2010;70(6):1003–1009.

227. Daniels CE, et al. Imatinib treatment for idiopathic pulmonary fibrosis: randomized placebo-controlled trial results. *Am J Respir Crit Care Med.* 2009;181(6):604–610.

228. Daoussis D, et al. Experience with rituximab in scleroderma: results from a 1-year, proof-of-principle study. *Rheumatology (Oxford).* 2010;49(2):271–280.

229. Sharp C, et al. Rituximab in autoimmune connective tissue disease-associated interstitial lung disease. *Rheumatology (Oxford).* 2016;55(7):1318–1324.

230. Jordan S, et al. Effects and safety of rituximab in systemic sclerosis: an analysis from the European Scleroderma Trial and Research (EUSTAR) group. *Ann Rheum Dis.* 2015;74(6):1188–1194.

231. Nakamura K, et al. The first case report of fatal acute pulmonary dysfunction in a systemic sclerosis patient treated with rituximab. *Scand J Rheumatol.* 2016;45(3):249–250.

232. Udwadia ZF, et al. Improved pulmonary function following pirfenidone treatment in a patient with progressive interstitial lung disease associated with systemic sclerosis. *Lung India.* 2015;32(1):50–52.

233. Miura Y, et al. Clinical experience with pirfenidone in five patients with scleroderma-related interstitial lung disease. *Sarcoidosis Vasc Diffuse Lung Dis.* 2014;31(3):235–238.

234. Tsukamoto H, et al. A phase I-II trial of autologous peripheral blood stem cell transplantation in the treatment of refractory autoimmune disease. *Ann Rheum Dis.* 2006;65(4):508–514.

235. Farge D, Nash R, Laar JM. Autologous stem cell transplantation for systemic sclerosis. *Autoimmunity.* 2008;41(8):616–624.

236. Rosas V, et al. Lung transplantation and systemic sclerosis. *Ann Transplant.* 2000;5(3):38–43.

237. Miele CH, et al. Lung transplant outcomes in systemic sclerosis with significant esophageal dysfunction. A comprehensive single-center experience. *Ann Am Thorac Soc.* 2016;13(6):793–802.

238. Spiera R, Kagen L. Extramuscular manifestations in idiopathic inflammatory myopathies. *Curr Opin Rheumatol.* 1998;10(6):556–561.

239. Frazier AR, Miller RD. Interstitial pneumonitis in association with polymyositis and dermatomyositis. *Chest.* 1974;65(4):403–407.

240. Schwarz MI, et al. Interstitial lung disease in polymyositis and dermatomyositis: analysis of six cases and review of the literature. *Medicine (Baltimore).* 1976;55(1):89–104.

241. Cottin V, et al. Interstitial lung disease in amyopathic dermatomyositis, dermatomyositis and polymyositis. *Eur Respir J.* 2003;22(2):245–250.

242. Dalakas MC, Hohlfeld R. Polymyositis and dermatomyositis. *Lancet.* 2003;362(9388):971–982.

243. Targoff IN, et al. Classification criteria for the idiopathic inflammatory myopathies. *Curr Opin Rheumatol.* 1997;9(6):527–535.

244. Hall VC, Keeling JH, Davis MD. Periorbital edema as the presenting sign of dermatomyositis. *Int J Dermatol.* 2003;42(6):466–467.

245. Mii S, et al. A histopathologic study of mechanic's hands associated with dermatomyositis: a report of five cases. *Int J Dermatol.* 2009;48(11):1177–1182.

246. Marie I, et al. Interstitial lung disease in polymyositis and dermatomyositis. *Arthritis Rheum.* 2002;47(6):614–622.

247. Danko K, et al. Long-term survival of patients with idiopathic inflammatory myopathies according to clinical features: a longitudinal study of 162 cases. *Medicine (Baltimore).* 2004;83(1):35–42.

248. Hepper NG, Ferguson RH, Howard Jr FM. Three types of pulmonary involvement in polymyositis. *Med Clin North Am.* 1964;48:1031–1042.

249. Dickey BF, Myers AR. Pulmonary disease in polymyositis/dermatomyositis. *Semin Arthritis Rheum.* 1984;14(1):60–76.

250. Braun NM, Arora NS, Rochester DF. Respiratory muscle and pulmonary function in polymyositis and other proximal myopathies. *Thorax.* 1983;38(8):616–623.

251. Johnson C, et al. Assessment of mortality in autoimmune myositis with and without associated interstitial lung disease. *Lung.* 2016;194(5):733–737.

252. Fathi M, et al. Interstitial lung disease in polymyositis and dermatomyositis: longitudinal evaluation by pulmonary function and radiology. *Arthritis Rheum.* 2008;59(5):677–685.

253. Richards TJ, et al. Characterization and peripheral blood biomarker assessment of anti-Jo-1 antibody-positive interstitial lung disease. *Arthritis Rheum.* 2009;60(7):2183–2192.

254. Friedman AW, Targoff IN, Arnett FC. Interstitial lung disease with autoantibodies against aminoacyl-tRNA synthetases in the absence of clinically apparent myositis. *Semin Arthritis Rheum.* 1996;26(1):459–467.

255. Ideura G, et al. Interstitial lung disease associated with amyopathic dermatomyositis: review of 18 cases. *Respir Med.* 2007;101(7):1406–1411.

256. Fathi M, et al. Interstitial lung disease, a common manifestation of newly diagnosed polymyositis and dermatomyositis. *Ann Rheum Dis.* 2004;63(3):297–301.

257. Mukae H, et al. Clinical differences between interstitial lung disease associated with clinically amyopathic dermatomyositis and classic dermatomyositis. *Chest.* 2009;136(5):1341–1347.

258. Love LA, et al. A new approach to the classification of idiopathic inflammatory myopathy: myositis-specific autoantibodies define useful homogeneous patient groups. *Medicine (Baltimore).* 1991;70(6):360–374.

259. Marguerie C, et al. Polymyositis, pulmonary fibrosis and autoantibodies to aminoacyl-tRNA synthetase enzymes. *Q J Med.* 1990;77(282):1019–1038.

260. Labirua A, Lundberg IE. Interstitial lung disease and idiopathic inflammatory myopathies: progress and pitfalls. *Curr Opin Rheumatol.* 2010;22(6):633–638.

261. Sato S, Kuwana M, Hirakata M. Clinical characteristics of Japanese patients with anti-OJ (anti-isoleucyl-tRNA synthetase) autoantibodies. *Rheumatology (Oxford).* 2007;46(5):842–845.

262. Kalluri M, et al. Clinical profile of anti-PL-12 autoantibody. Cohort study and review of the literature. *Chest.* 2009;135(6):1550–1556.

263. La Corte R, et al. In patients with antisynthetase syndrome the occurrence of anti-Ro/SSA antibodies causes a more severe interstitial lung disease. *Autoimmunity.* 2006;39(3):249–253.

264. Connors GR, et al. Interstitial lung disease associated with the idiopathic inflammatory myopathies: what progress has been made in the past 35 years? *Chest.* 2010;138(6):1464–1474.

265. Ikezoe J, et al. High-resolution CT findings of lung disease in patients with polymyositis and dermatomyositis. *J Thorac Imaging.* 1996;11(4):250–259.

266. Mino M, et al. Pulmonary involvement in polymyositis and dermatomyositis: sequential evaluation with CT. *AJR Am J Roentgenol.* 1997;169(1):83–87.

267. Hayashi S, et al. High-resolution computed tomography characterization of interstitial lung diseases in polymyositis/dermatomyositis. *J Rheumatol.* 2008;35(2):260–269.

268. Tazelaar HD, et al. Interstitial lung disease in polymyositis and dermatomyositis. Clinical features and prognosis as correlated with histologic findings. *Am Rev Respir Dis.* 1990;141(3):727–733.

269. Webb DR, Currie GD. Pulmonary fibrosis masking polymyositis. Remission with corticosteroid therapy. *JAMA.* 1972;222(9):1146–1149.

270. Marie I, Mouthon L. Therapy of polymyositis and dermatomyositis. *Autoimmun Rev.* November 2011;11(1):6–13.

271. Nawata Y, et al. Corticosteroid resistant interstitial pneumonitis in dermatomyositis/polymyositis: prediction and treatment with cyclosporine. *J Rheumatol.* 1999;26(7):1527–1533.

272. Rowen AJ, Reichel J. Dermatomyositis with lung involvement, successfully treated with azathioprine. *Respiration.* 1983;44(2):143–146.

273. Tanaka F, et al. Successful combined therapy of cyclophosphamide and cyclosporine for acute exacerbated interstitial pneumonia associated with dermatomyositis. *Intern Med.* 2000;39(5):428–430.

274. Yamasaki Y, et al. Intravenous cyclophosphamide therapy for progressive interstitial pneumonia in patients with polymyositis/dermatomyositis. *Rheumatology (Oxford).* 2007;46(1):124–130.

275. Lateef O, Shakoor N, Balk RA. Methotrexate pulmonary toxicity. *Expert Opin Drug Saf.* 2005;4(4):723–730.

276. Gruhn WB, Diaz-Buxo JA. Cyclosporine treatment of steroid resistant interstitial pneumonitis associated with dermatomyositis/polymyositis. *J Rheumatol.* 1987;14(5):1045–1047.

277. Wilkes MR, et al. Treatment of antisynthetase-associated interstitial lung disease with tacrolimus. *Arthritis Rheum.* 2005;52(8):2439–2446.

278. Hervier B, et al. Long-term efficacy of mycophenolate mofetil in a case of refractory antisynthetase syndrome. *Joint Bone Spine.* 2009;76(5):575–576.

279. Suzuki Y, et al. Intravenous immunoglobulin therapy for refractory interstitial lung disease associated with polymyositis/dermatomyositis. *Lung.* 2009;187(3):201–206.

280. Sem M, et al. Rituximab treatment of the anti-synthetase syndrome: a retrospective case series. *Rheumatology (Oxford).* 2009;48(8):968–971.

281. Rios Fernandez R, et al. Rituximab in the treatment of dermatomyositis and other inflammatory myopathies. A report of 4 cases and review of the literature. *Clin Exp Rheumatol.* 2009;27(6):1009–1016.

282. Marie I, et al. Rituximab therapy for refractory interstitial lung disease related to antisynthetase syndrome. *Respir Med.* 2012;106(4):581–587.

283. Unger L, et al. Rituximab therapy in patients with refractory dermatomyositis or polymyositis: differential effects in a real-life population. *Rheumatology (Oxford).* 2014;53(9):1630–1638.

284. Andersson H, et al. Long-term experience with rituximab in anti-synthetase syndrome-related interstitial lung disease. *Rheumatology (Oxford).* 2015;54(8):1420–1428.

285. Papiris SA, Tsonis IA, Moutsopoulos HM. Sjogren's Syndrome. *Semin Respir Crit Care Med.* 2007;28(4):459–471.

286. Kokosi M, Riemer EC, Highland KB. Pulmonary involvement in Sjogren syndrome. *Clin Chest Med.* 2010;31(3):489–500.

287. Hatron PY, et al. Pulmonary manifestations of Sjogren's syndrome. *Presse Med.* 2011;40(1 Pt 2):e49–64.

288. Amarasena R, Bowman S. Sjogren's syndrome. *Clin Med.* 2007;7(1):53–56.

289. Garcia-Carrasco M, et al. Primary Sjogren syndrome: clinical and immunologic disease patterns in a cohort of 400 patients. *Medicine (Baltimore)*. 2002;81(4):270–280.

290. Vitali C, et al. Classification criteria for Sjogren's syndrome: a revised version of the European criteria proposed by the American-European Consensus Group. *Ann Rheum Dis*. 2002;61(6):554–558.

291. Davidson BK, Kelly CA, Griffiths ID. Ten year follow up of pulmonary function in patients with primary Sjogren's syndrome. *Ann Rheum Dis*. 2000;59(9):709–712.

292. Ramos-Casals M, et al. Primary Sjogren syndrome in Spain: clinical and immunologic expression in 1010 patients. *Medicine (Baltimore)*. 2008;87(4):210–219.

293. Segal I, et al. Pulmonary function abnormalities in Sjogren's syndrome and the sicca complex. *Thorax*. 1981;36(4):286–289.

294. Papathanasiou MP, et al. Reappraisal of respiratory abnormalities in primary and secondary Sjogren's syndrome. A controlled study. *Chest*. 1986;90(3):370–374.

295. Constantopoulos SH, et al. Xerotrachea and interstitial lung disease in primary Sjogren's syndrome. *Respiration*. 1984;46(3):310–314.

296. Parambil JG, et al. Interstitial lung disease in primary Sjogren syndrome. *Chest*. 2006;130(5):1489–1495.

297. Papiris SA, et al. Lung involvement in primary Sjogren's syndrome is mainly related to the small airway disease. *Ann Rheum Dis*. 1999;58(1):61–64.

298. Kelly C, et al. Lung function in primary Sjogren's syndrome: a cross sectional and longitudinal study. *Thorax*. 1991;46(3):180–183.

299. Franquet T, et al. Primary Sjogren's syndrome and associated lung disease: CT findings in 50 patients. *AJR Am J Roentgenol*. 1997;169(3):655–658.

300. Koyama M, et al. Pulmonary involvement in primary Sjogren's syndrome: spectrum of pulmonary abnormalities and computed tomography findings in 60 patients. *J Thorac Imaging*. 2001;16(4):290–296.

301. Meyer CA, et al. Inspiratory and expiratory high-resolution CT findings in a patient with Sjogren's syndrome and cystic lung disease. *AJR Am J Roentgenol*. 1997;168(1):101–103.

302. Voulgarelis M, Skopouli FN. Clinical, immunologic, and molecular factors predicting lymphoma development in Sjogren's syndrome patients. *Clin Rev Allergy Immunol*. 2007;32(3):265–274.

303. Honda O, et al. Differential diagnosis of lymphocytic interstitial pneumonia and malignant lymphoma on high-resolution CT. *AJR Am J Roentgenol*. 1999;173(1):71–74.

304. Franquet T, et al. Air trapping in primary Sjogren syndrome: correlation of expiratory CT with pulmonary function tests. *J Comput Assist Tomogr*. 1999;23(2):169–173.

305. Ito I, et al. Pulmonary manifestations of primary Sjogren's syndrome: a clinical, radiologic, and pathologic study. *Am J Respir Crit Care Med*. 2005;171(6):632–638.

306. Deheinzelin D, et al. Interstitial lung disease in primary Sjogren's syndrome. Clinical-pathological evaluation and response to treatment. *Am J Respir Crit Care Med*. 1996;154(3 Pt 1):794–799.

307. Isaksen K, Jonsson R, Omdal R. Anti-CD20 treatment in primary Sjogren's syndrome. *Scand J Immunol*. 2008;68(6):554–564.

308. Seror R, et al. Tolerance and efficacy of rituximab and changes in serum B cell biomarkers in patients with systemic complications of primary Sjogren's syndrome. *Ann Rheum Dis*. 2007;66(3):351–357.

309. Gottenberg JE, et al. Efficacy of rituximab in systemic manifestations of primary Sjogren's syndrome: results in 78 patients of the AutoImmune and Rituximab registry. *Ann Rheum Dis*. 2013;72(6):1026–1031.

310. Kamen DL, Strange C. Pulmonary manifestations of systemic lupus erythematosus. *Clin Chest Med*. 2010;31(3):479–488.

311. Tan EM, et al. The 1982 revised criteria for the classification of systemic lupus erythematosus. *Arthritis Rheum*. 1982;25(11):1271–1277.

312. Matthay RA, et al. Pulmonary manifestations of systemic lupus erythematosus: review of twelve cases of acute lupus pneumonitis. *Medicine (Baltimore)*. 1975;54(5):397–409.

313. Torre O, Harari S. Pleural and pulmonary involvement in systemic lupus erythematosus. *Presse Med*. 2011;40(1 Pt 2):e19–e29.

314. Inoue T, et al. Immunopathologic studies of pneumonitis in systemic lupus erythematosus. *Ann Intern Med*. 1979;91(1):30–34.

315. Matthay RA, Hudson LD, Petty TL. Acute lupus pneumonitis: response to azathioprine therapy. *Chest*. 1973;63(1):117–120.

316. Schnabel A, Reuter M, Gross WL. Intravenous pulse cyclophosphamide in the treatment of interstitial lung disease due to collagen vascular diseases. *Arthritis Rheum*. 1998;41(7):1215–1220.

317. Zamora MR, et al. Diffuse alveolar hemorrhage and systemic lupus erythematosus. Clinical presentation, histology, survival, and outcome. *Medicine (Baltimore)*. 1997;76(3):192–202.

318. Schwab EP, et al. Pulmonary alveolar hemorrhage in systemic lupus erythematosus. *Semin Arthritis Rheum*. 1993;23(1):8–15.

319. Santos-Ocampo AS, Mandell BF, Fessler BJ. Alveolar hemorrhage in systemic lupus erythematosus: presentation and management. *Chest*. 2000;118(4):1083–1090.

320. Myers JL, Katzenstein AA. Microangiitis in lupus-induced pulmonary hemorrhage. *Am J Clin Pathol*. 1986;85(5):552–556.

321. Erickson RW, Franklin WA, Emlen W. Treatment of hemorrhagic lupus pneumonitis with plasmapheresis. *Semin Arthritis Rheum*. 1994;24(2):114–123.

322. Verzegnassi F, et al. Prompt efficacy of plasmapheresis in a patient with systemic lupus erythematosus and diffuse alveolar haemorrhage. *Clin Exp Rheumatol*. 2010;28(3):445–446.

323. Canas C, et al. Diffuse alveolar hemorrhage in Colombian patients with systemic lupus erythematosus. *Clin Rheumatol.* 2007;26(11):1947–1949.

324. Al Rashidi A, Alajmi M, Hegazi MO. Mycophenolate mofetil as a maintenance therapy for lupus-related diffuse alveolar hemorrhage. *Lupus.* 2011;20(14):1551–1553.

325. Na JO, et al. Successful early rituximab treatment in a case of systemic lupus erythematosus with potentially fatal diffuse alveolar hemorrhage. *Respiration.* 2015;89(1):62–65.

326. Tse JR, et al. Rituximab: an emerging treatment for recurrent diffuse alveolar hemorrhage in systemic lupus erythematosus. *Lupus.* 2015;24(7):756–759.

327. Haupt HM, Moore GW, Hutchins GM. The lung in systemic lupus erythematosus. Analysis of the pathologic changes in 120 patients. *Am J Med.* 1981;71(5):791–798.

328. Bankier AA, et al. Discrete lung involvement in systemic lupus erythematosus: CT assessment. *Radiology.* 1995;196(3):835–840.

329. Boulware DW, Hedgpeth MT. Lupus pneumonitis and anti-SSA(Ro) antibodies. *J Rheumatol.* 1989;16(4):479–481.

330. Mochizuki T, Aotsuka S, Satoh T. Clinical and laboratory features of lupus patients with complicating pulmonary disease. *Respir Med.* 1999;93(2):95–101.

331. Jacobsen S, et al. A multicentre study of 513 Danish patients with systemic lupus erythematosus. I. Disease manifestations and analyses of clinical subsets. *Clin Rheumatol.* 1998;17(6):468–477.

332. de Lauretis A, Veeraraghavan S, Renzoni E. Review series: aspects of interstitial lung disease: connective tissue disease-associated interstitial lung disease: how does it differ from IPF? How should the clinical approach differ? *Chron Respir Dis.* 2011;8(1):53–82.

333. Swigris JJ, et al. Mycophenolate mofetil is safe, well tolerated, and preserves lung function in patients with connective tissue disease-related interstitial lung disease. *Chest.* 2006;130(1):30–36.

334. Lim SW, et al. Rituximab use in systemic lupus erythematosus pneumonitis and a review of current reports. *Intern Med J.* 2006;36(4):260–262.

335. Duskin A, Eisenberg RA. The role of antibodies in inflammatory arthritis. *Immunol Rev.* 2010;233(1):112–125.

336. Self SE. Autoantibody testing for autoimmune disease. *Clin Chest Med.* 2010;31(3):415–422.

337. Peng S, Craft J. In: Firestein GS, ed. *Anti-nuclear Antibodies, in Kelley's Textbook of Rheumatology.* 8th ed. Philadelphia: Saunders Elsevier; 2008:741–754.

# Index

Note: Page numbers followed by "f" indicate figures, "t" indicate tables, and "b" indicates boxes.

Printed and bound by CPI Group (UK) Ltd, Croydon, CR0 4YY

03/10/2024

01040383-0001